A Caregiver's
Bible to Excellence!

A Caregiver's
Bible to Excellence!

VOLUME 2

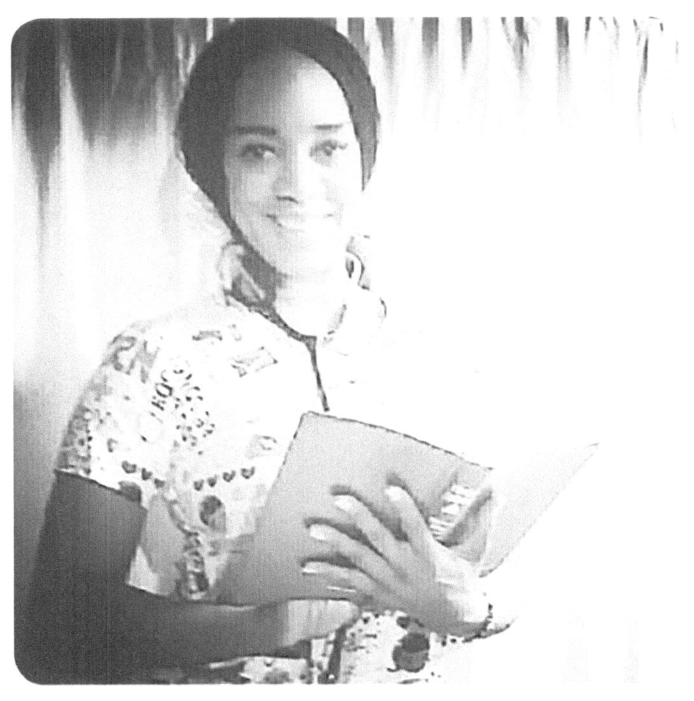

Miss Asondra StarN'air

Ordering Information:

For orders and inquiries, please contact:
1-888-404-1388
www.goldtouchpress.com
book.orders@goldtouchpress.com

Printed in the United States of America

CONTENTS

A Caregiver's Bible To Excellence

Welcome back, and welcome to volume 2

But before we get started I want to take this time out to thank all healthcare workers around the world and abroad. Did you know that you play a vital part to the physical and economic health of every person in the United States? Well you do and right now we want to thank you.

SECTION XIV

Qualities of an Excellent Caregiver

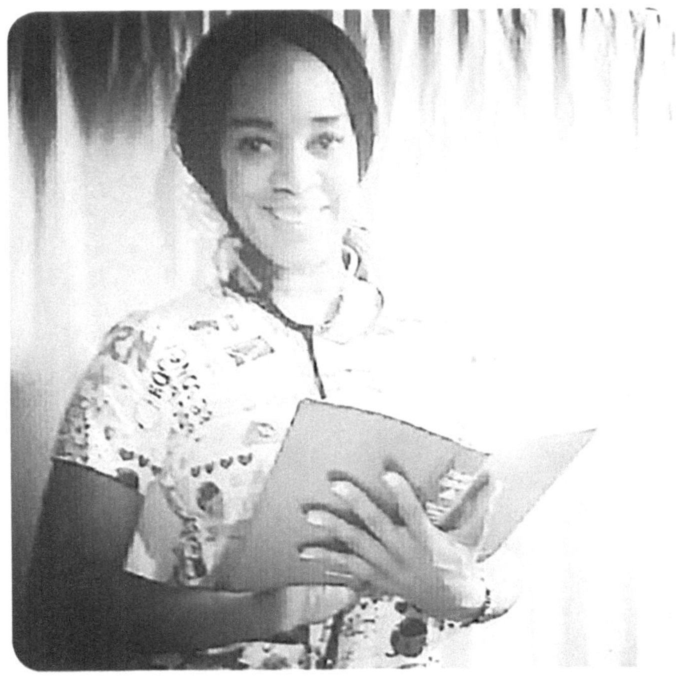

"I Say", it Starts with Jesus and ends with a "Smile!"

"I Say"

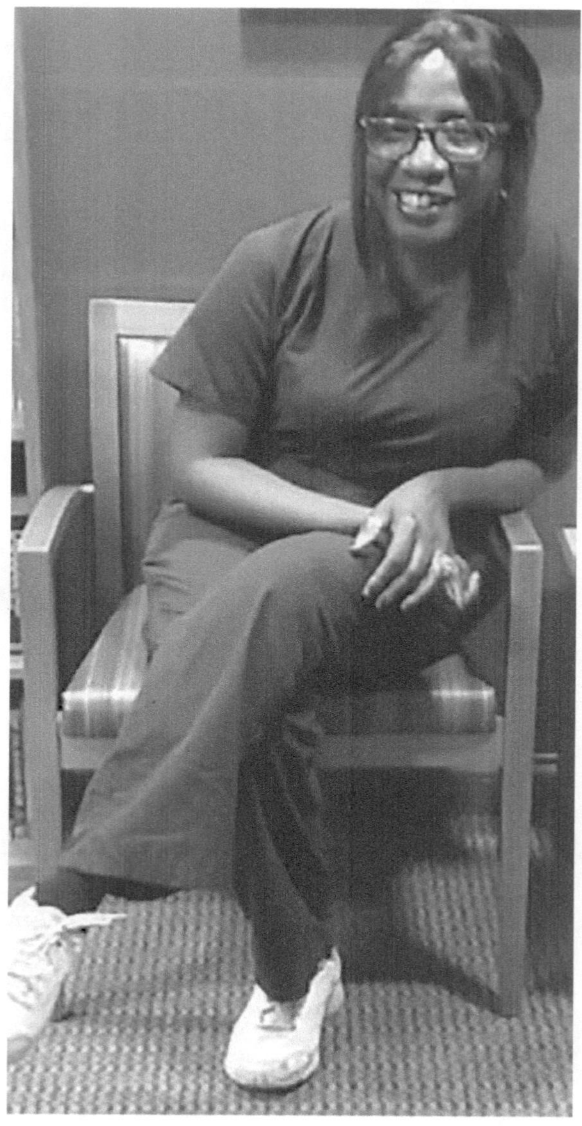

Empathy, Love and Compassion!

"I Say"

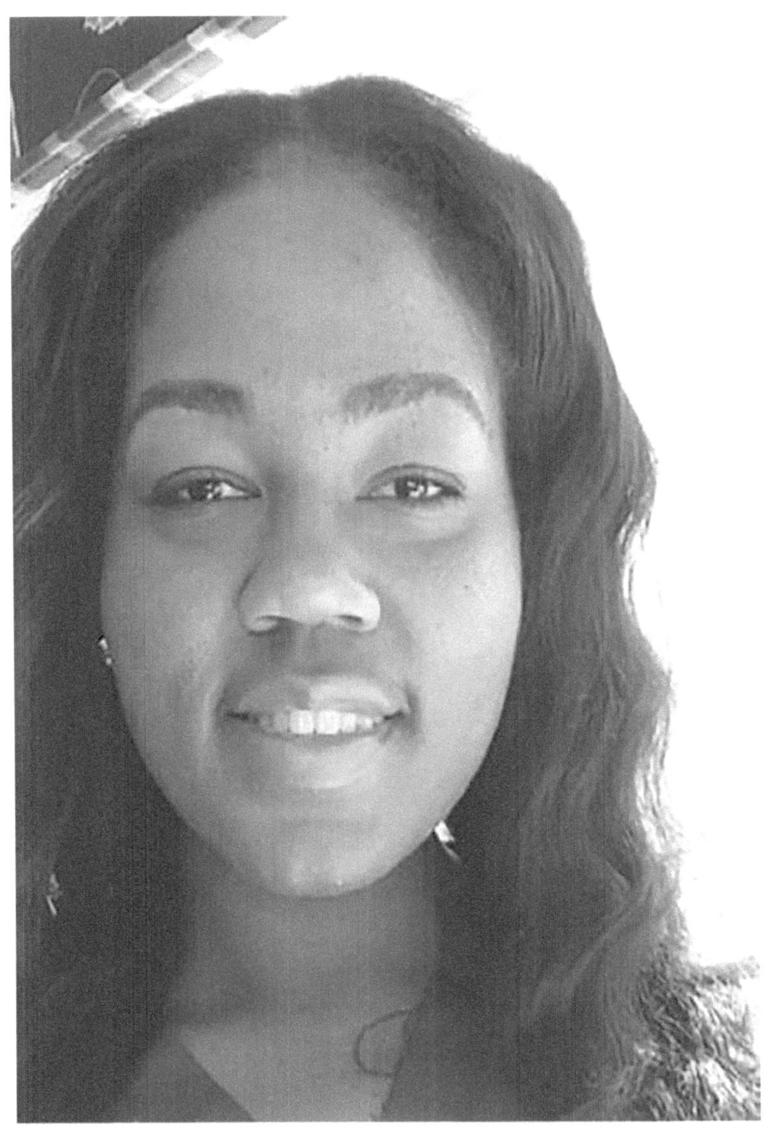

A Good Heart!

"I Say"

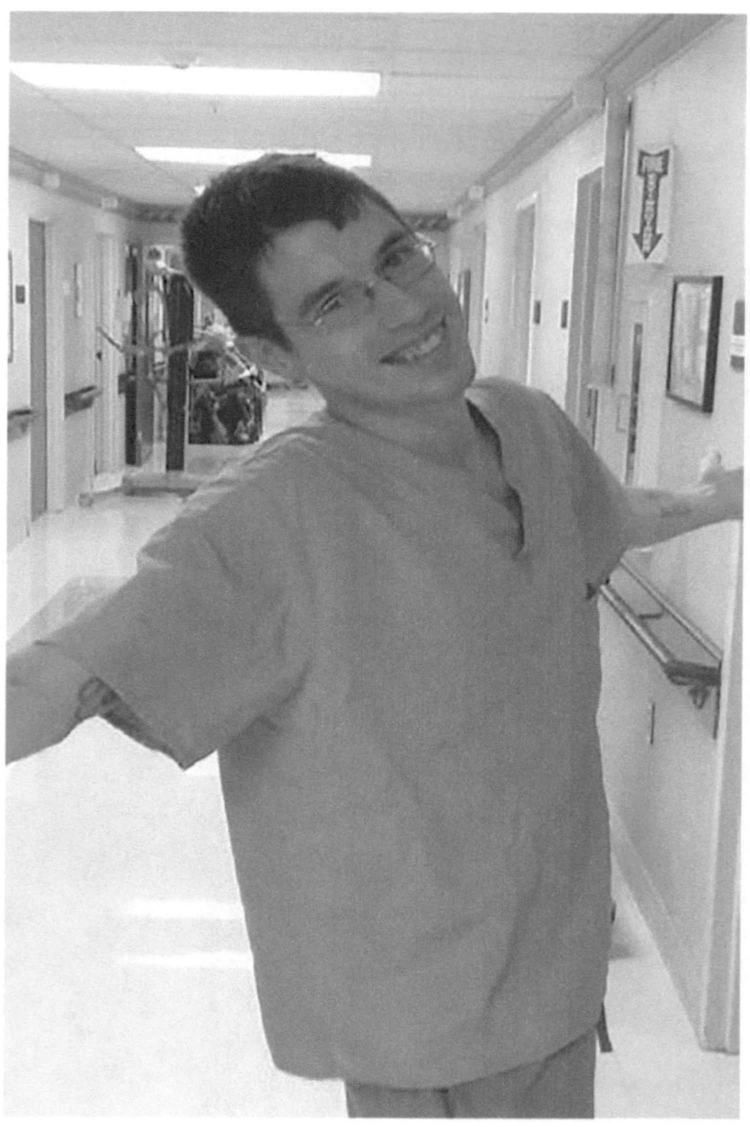

Enthusiasm, and Loving What You Do!

"I Say"

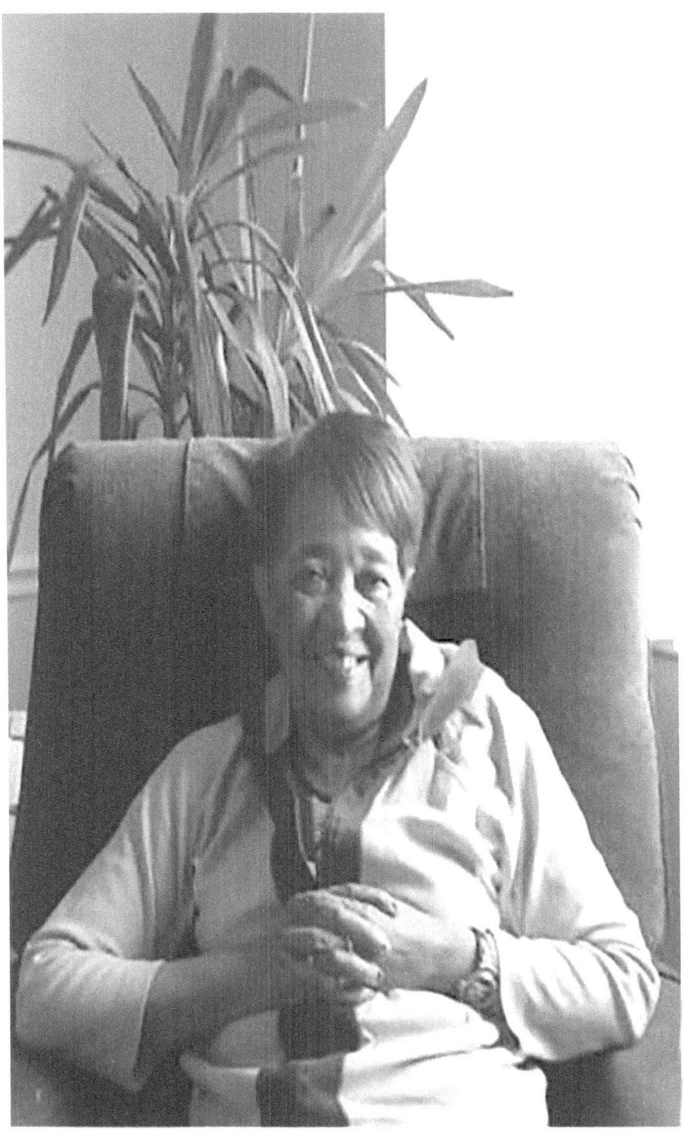

Wisdom, Experience, and Know How!

"I Say"

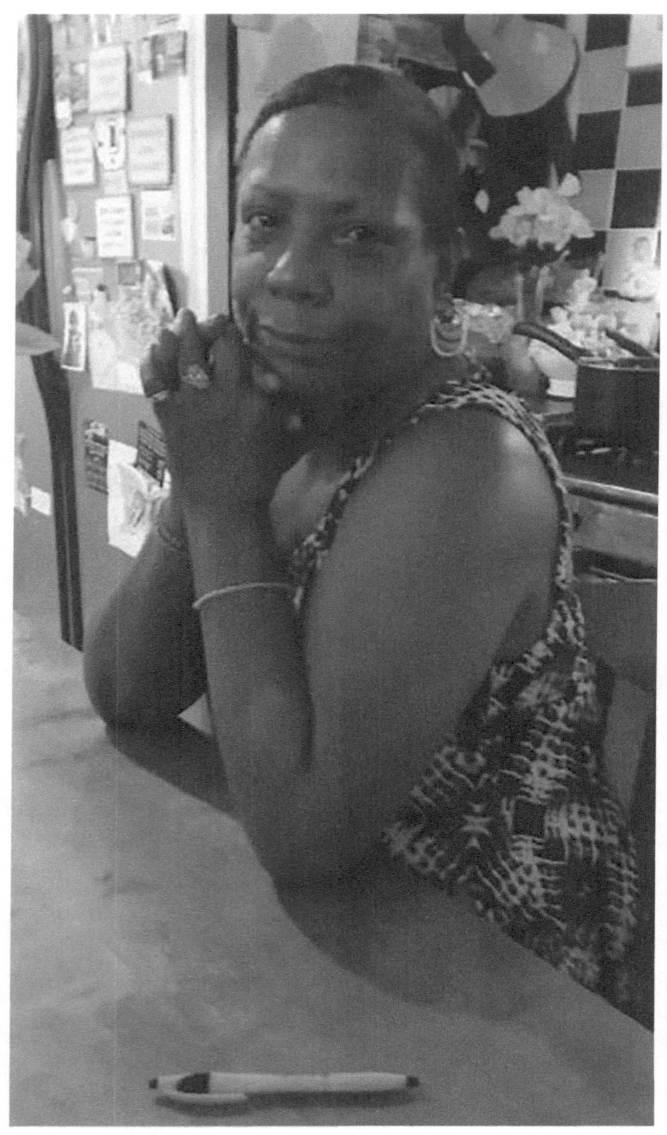

It's Simple, Really Care About People, Want to Serve!

"I Say"

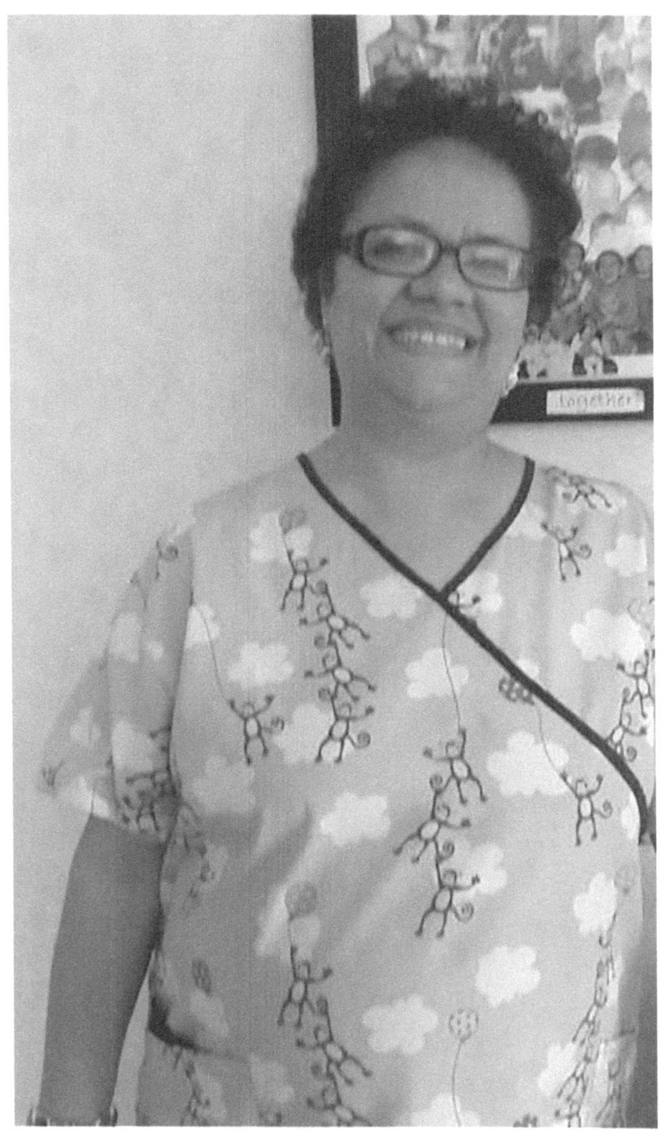

Patience and Understanding!

"I Say"

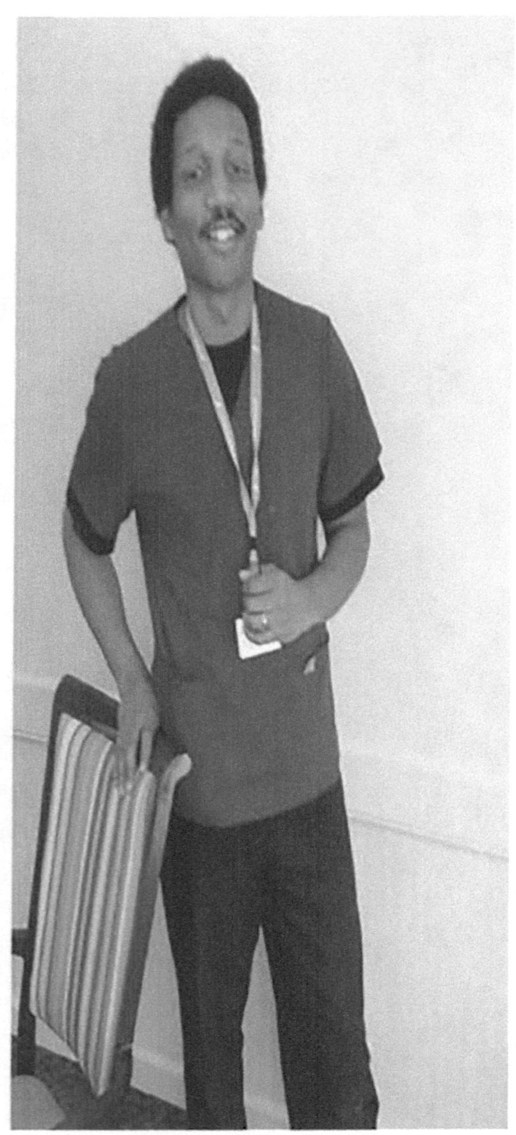

Strength and Endurance!

 Miss Asondra StarN'air

"I Say"

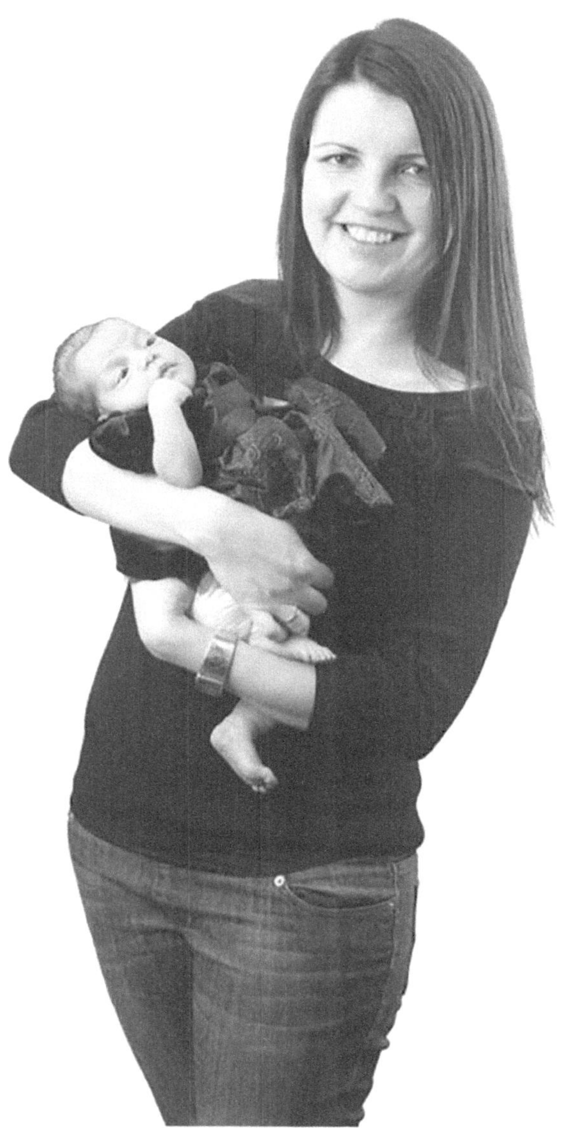

**Being Responsible And Ready to Give of Oneself Always!
Ready to Perform a Task or duty Right Away!**

"I Say"

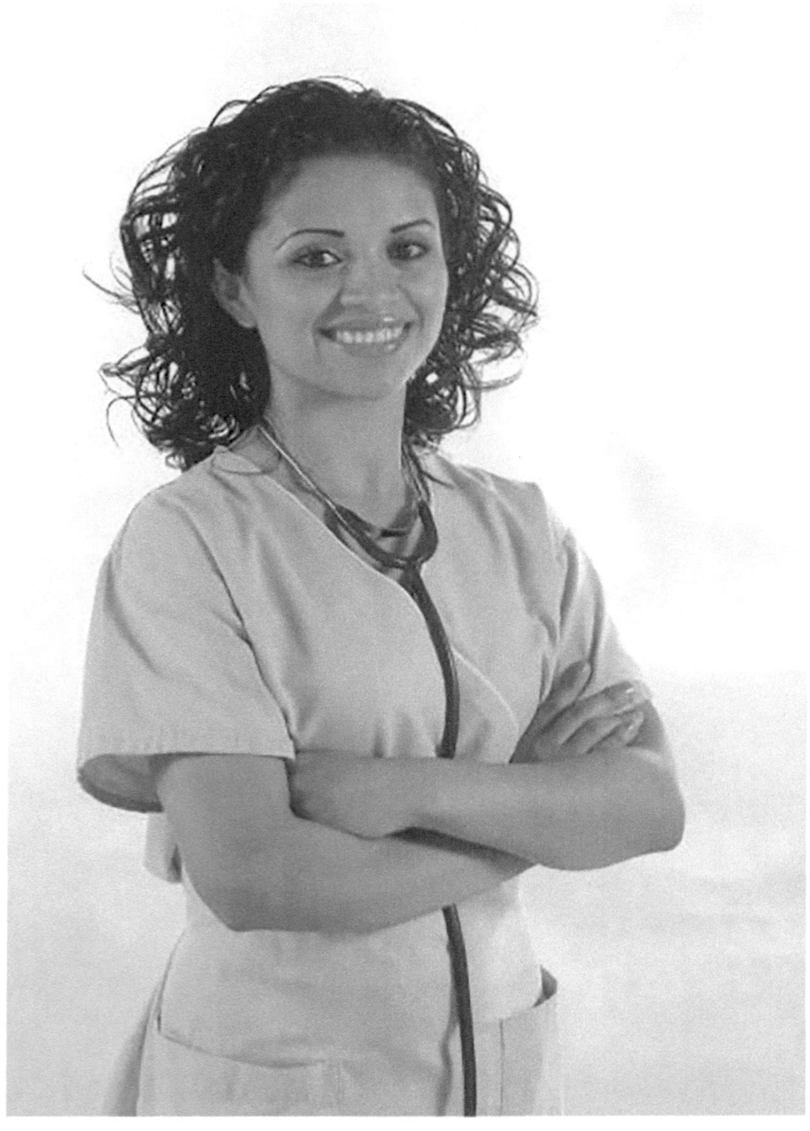

Education, Self-Development, and Commitment is Key!

 Miss Asondra StarN'air

"We're All Right!"

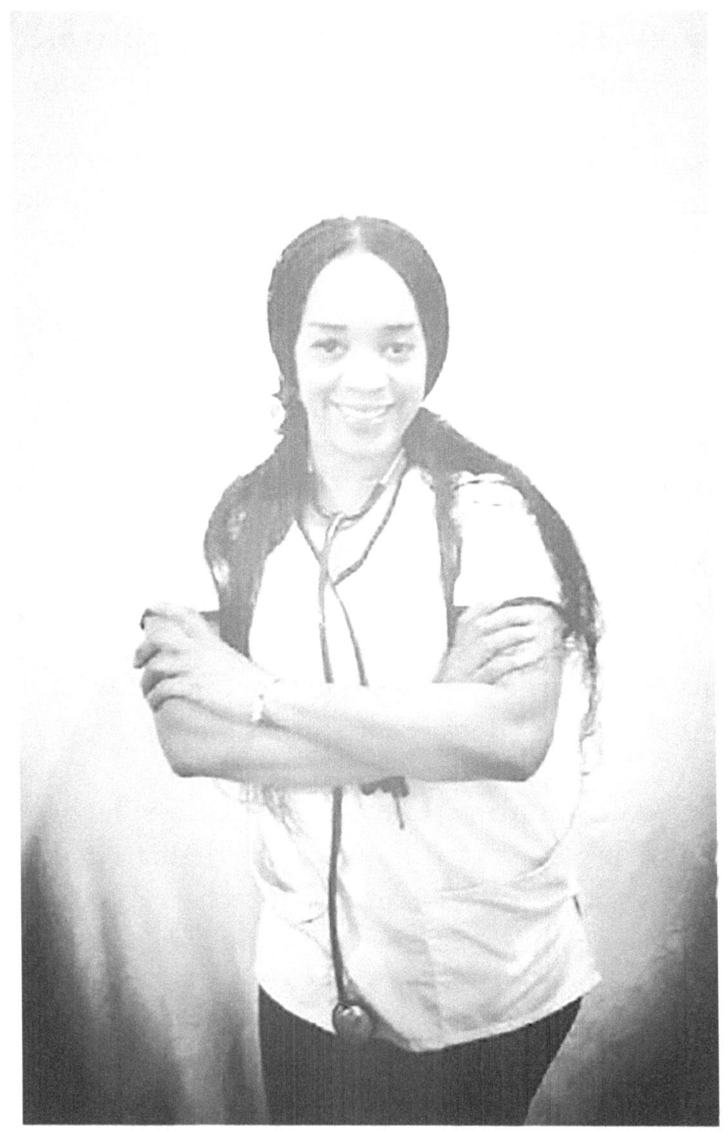

'Care Giving Has No Bounds!'
Just Look At All These "Incredible Caregivers" I Found!

Qualities of an Excellent Caregiver!

*__Patience__—They don't expect things to happen overnight; they have learned to wait on the Lord for everything.

*__Compassion__—A heart like Jesus. Loves everyone, truly cares about that person, and wants to do everything they can to ease the pain of any kind of suffering.

*__Attentive__—See what the need is and take action; they don't ignore their responsibility.

*__Trustworthy__—Keeps promises, tells the truth, and is dependable.

*__Flexible__—Understands there is more than one way to skin a cat; looks for more options to bring about positive results.

*__Listens__—Pays attention to what is going on, what's being communicated, and does it without judgment.

*__Excellent Communication Skills__—Knows how to talk with common sense and without all the drama. Understands caregiving is a profession for many and must be communicated in a professional manner at all times, no matter what the situation.

*__Drama-Free__—Very important. An excellent caregiver knows not to ever, ever, ever, ever bring their problems to the workplace and discuss it with those in their care or with gossiping co-workers for that matter. Because __drama -free__ caregivers are wise; they learn the ways of Christ. They are told to cast __ALL__ their cares on to him, and they do! (1Peter 5:7)

***Respect Administration/Management**—Does not talk about the boss in a negative way with coworkers—respect authority whether they agree or disagree. They want to be the best employee they can be even when the boss is not around. **(Romans 13:13)**

***Will Not Leave Work for Others to do**—These caregivers take full responsibility for their own shift and does everything that needs to be done. They don't believe in saving work for others, especially if they have more than enough time with time to spare to get it done.

Their goal is excellence, not only for the client but also for the entire team.

***Team Oriented**—Through action, believes that: Team -Work Makes The Dream Work!

***Lives A Balanced Life**—Understands the importance of rest and spending quality time with **GOD** and reading his word.

***Skilled**—Having a good personality and kind heart is not enough when you are going to be working as a professional caregiver. I wish it was, but it is not enough. Therefore, one must also be *competent*. Having the necessary experience, ability, knowledge, or skills to do something successfully.

***Appearance**—Professional caregivers understands that looking the part is smart! They are always well groomed and in work gear/scrubs that say I am a professional person the loves what I do! You won't see them in spandex or out of dress code. That's a no, no!

Excellent Caregivers!

Love What They do, and It Shows! They are full of joy, they smile a lot, and are very warm and kind to everyone. They are always willing to help anyone in need.

These caregivers emulate **Jesus** in so many ways that they stand out from the rest of the world. They are the kind of caregivers that deserve all the blessings and prosperity that comes their way. They will succeed in all they do because **Jesus** has become their role model of success.

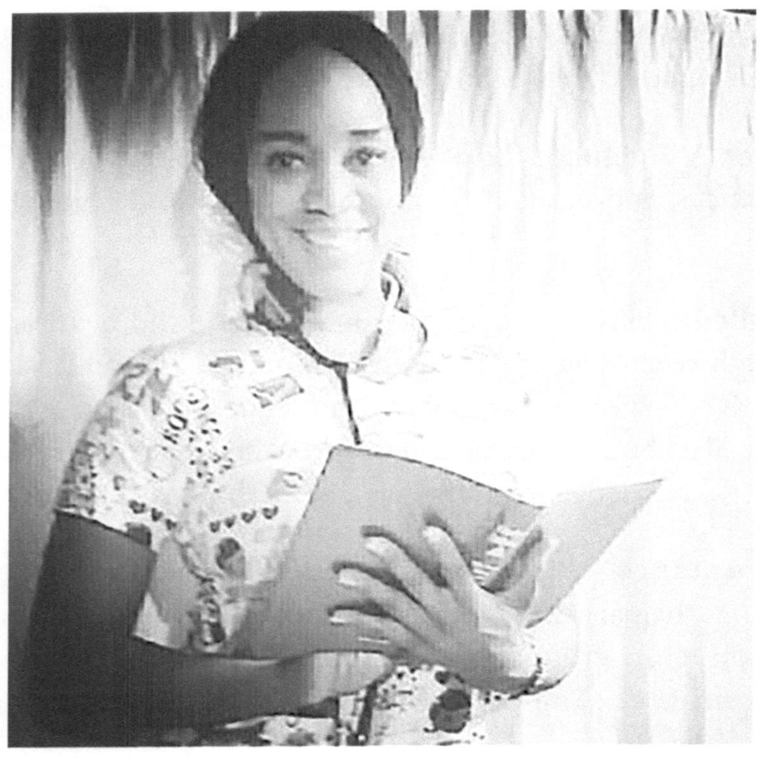

Without Further Ado

Let's Meet The Caregivers!

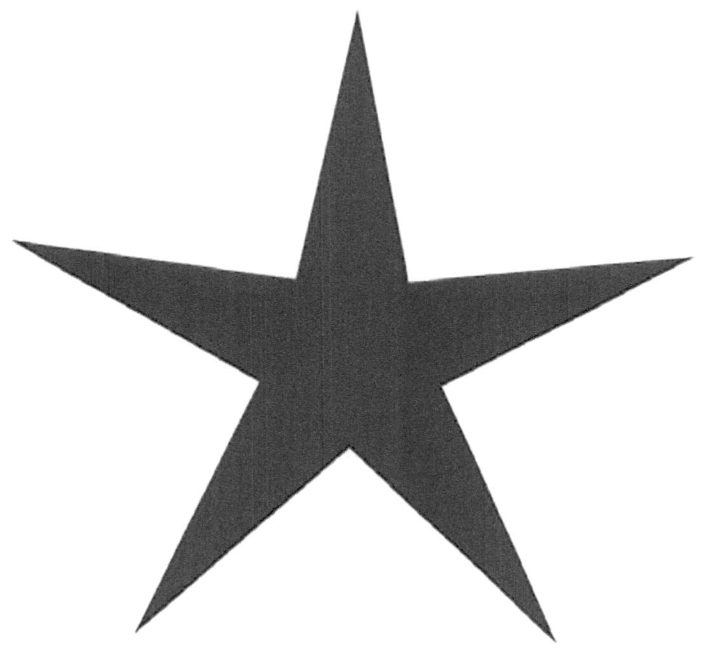

Hello, I'm Amy Fortson

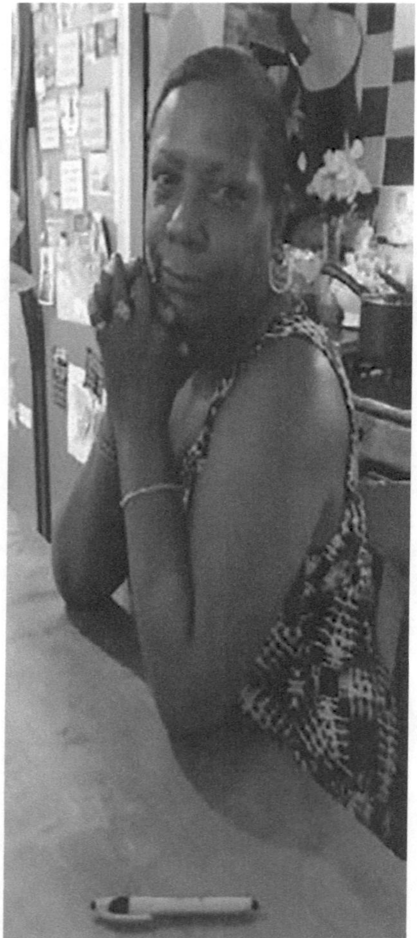

I've been a caregiver now for ten years, foster caring for three years. I am a Christian. I love serving and caring for people. I like to share—lending a helping hand is what I do.

For those thinking about becoming a foster care provider, fostering requires a heart that is willing to help nurture, uplift, and comfort those in need of a good, loving home.

Foster care also requires skills and there are plenty of classes free of charge for those individuals that are serious about being professional, loving providers. I am one of them!

I recommend you take advantage of every opportunity that's presented to you. This will help both you and the person in your care.

They're your family now! To all the foster care caregivers out there, I just want to say thank you!

And to my dear, dear friend Asondra, we've had a very long friendship. You are my sister. I am so proud of you.

You are such a loving person whose love I will forever cherish. May God continue to pour down his blessing upon you!

Hello, I'm Dana and this is my son Jaylon

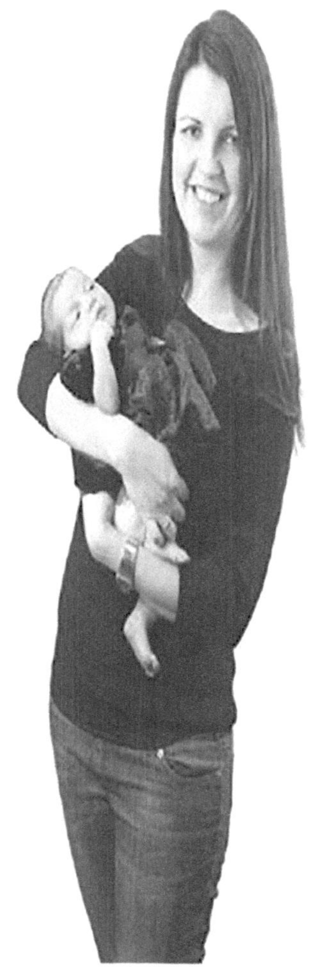

I love being a mother, what an incredible feeling it is, yet a huge responsibility. So I guess you can call me a caregiver too! I love this book Asondra created for all of us, it is dynamite, incredible, it's is truly a Caregiver's Bible, a must have.

What I want say to other new moms out there, love your child. Give them the world, they are truly a gift from God.

Utilizes The Baby Journal in "First Time Mom" section of the book, it's there for us too. I am so overwhelmed by all the thoughtfulness and details she added to making things a whole lot easier for first time moms like me. My family and I will treasure this book for a lifetime. It's a book to be passed on from generation to generation. Timeless!

Thank you so much "Star"

You are an inspiration to the world.

So nice to have met you
God Bless You!!!

Dana Clark

Hello, I'm Erica Long

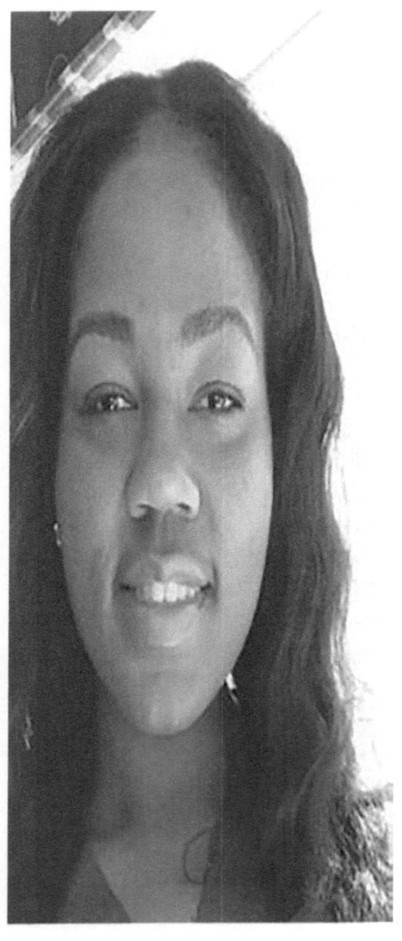

I've been a caregiver now for six years and love it. I like working with the elderly and young children.

I love my residence but what I dislike is the pay, we work so hard and should be paid a respectable wage.

That's the change I'd like to see, higher wages for all caregiver globally.

What I would like to say to new caregivers is this, it is not an easy job but if you have patience and a heart they won't be just residence or someone you get paid to care for, they will be family!

I also want to say to management, appreciate us "we do a lot".

Lastly, Miss StarN'air **(Star)** Is a very lovable and happy bright person, always makes you smile no matter how you're feeling on the job, she's a bright light that keeps us all moving in a positive direction.

Hello my name is Sean Henry

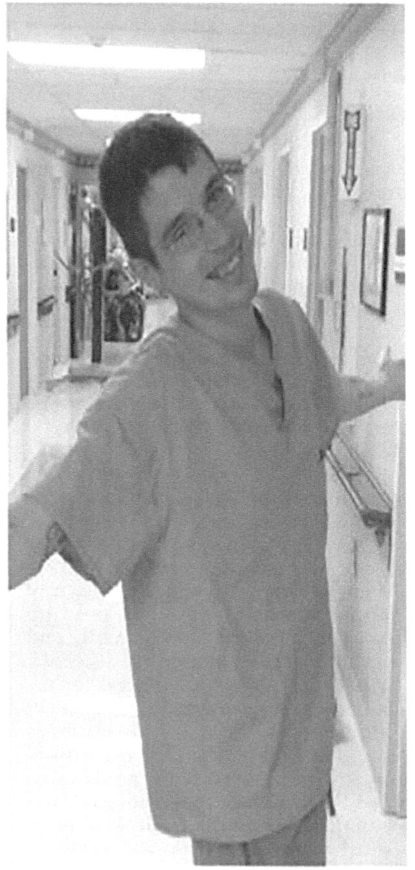

I've been a caregiver for five years. I decided to be a caregiver because I enjoy helping others and I am very Empathetic when it comes to others

What I like the most about being a care- giver, I am able to help the elderly population. Just seeing them smile and the appreciation they give "makes my day"!

To all you new caregivers out there don't just become a caregiver for the money, our residence deserve better than that from you. Come and make a difference in their lives, form relationships with those in your care. We need caregivers who are truly going to be caregivers.

This is what I want to say also to management everywhere, keep up the good work, but acknowledge us and all the hard work we do.

Lastly, Star, I would have to say working with you is an honor, how you got started as a caregiver is inspiring, gives me more reason to strive for excellence. StarN'air you are more than a co-worker but a wonderful inspirational friend.

Hi, I'm Mary, but "You" can call me Grandma!

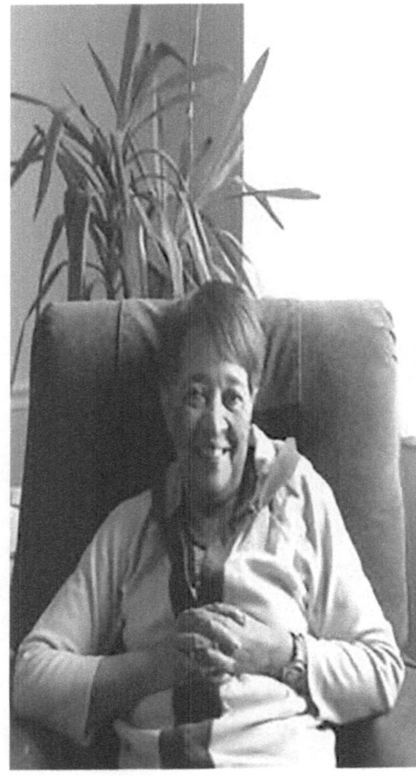

I know all there is to know about being a Caregiver, yes I do! I had eleven children, 10 girls and 1 boy.

Along with that I became a private duty nurse, back then we did not need certification, all we needed was a good kind loving heart and a strong desire to love and care for others.

I have been so blessed and fortunate to have met so many wonderful people, I worked hospitals cases too but mostly private duty care-giving in homes.

Most of my career was with one lady I cared for her and her family for twenty-five years, seven days a week I only took time off for vacation time, which were paid by the family.

With so much time being spent with this person, we became inseparable, when she hurt, I hurt, caregiving for me was the best thing that ever happen, it created a job for me, doing what I always love to do, care for people. I was able to travel, open up a restaurant, provided for my family and more. Plus it worked around my schedule, I was still able to cook a hot meal for my children when they came home from school.

I'm told a lot of things have changed since way back then, now everyone needs to be certified, but just remember, all you caregiver out there, no one can certify your heart if you are who you say you are it will be reviled by your work and attitude.

Here's another thing to always remember, I tell this to my children, and grandchildren all the time, Love does not require two, it only requires one of you.

So do the right thing, be good to those you care for and blessing will surely come your way. I lived a good life and so can you.

Caregiver StarN'air!

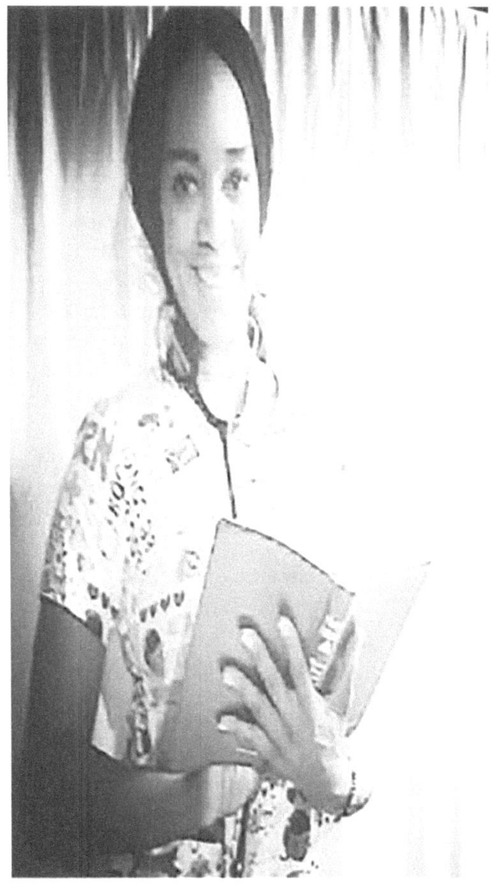

The Holy Bible

Basic Instructions **B**efore Leaving Earth
A Caregivers Bible to Excellence
wants to be a part of your life too
Don't leave home without it!

Caregivers In Christ Sounds Nice!

I'm a Caregiver for the Lord, it is my belief without a good leader we will become mediocre, not very good.

Everyone needs a role model why not Jesus? Because He's *"The Greatest Caregiver of All"!*

Pick up the bible read it daily, everything we need to know about excellence is right inside this incredible book the one I'm holding in my hands right now. Love, kindness, patients, endurance, forgiveness, Jesus Sermon on the Mount "The Beatitudes" along with all that. Thousands of tools caregivers can use.

My advice to new caregivers let Jesus lead. Step aside and let him make you into the kind of caregiver He wants you to be.

What I am hoping for is a change, a global movement toward **"Excellence!"** Yes I want to see the day when Caregivers all over the world get the recognition and respect they deserve. Professional pay rates and more.

The Holy Spirit Opens Doors!

Maria Chapel, Caregiver / Nursing Student

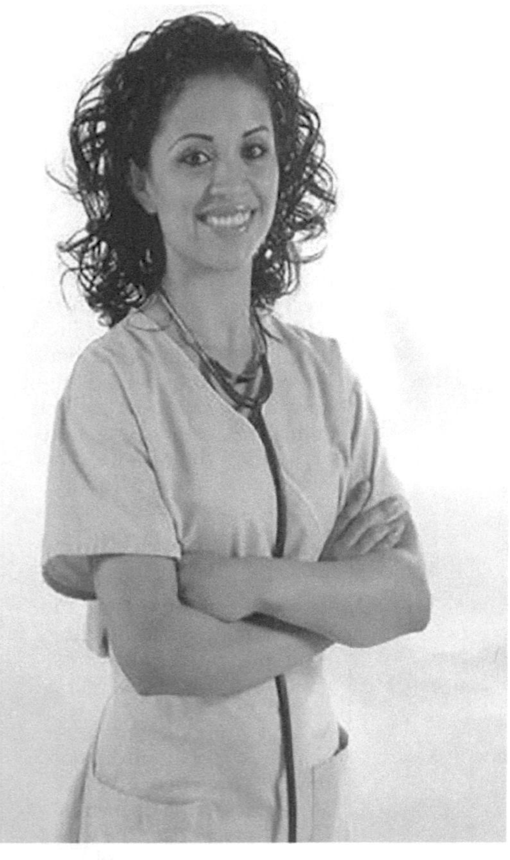

Caregivers, For Us, The Sky Is The Limit!

Today Is A Great Time To Be

"A Caregiver"!

It takes a lot of guts to stand up for what is NOT right, **Miss Asondra StarN'air** is truly a pioneer. Never before in history has there been anyone to fight for caregivers this way, and under such constant pressure, losing one job after the other, while still fighting for equality. Most people would have given up a long time ago or change professions, but not Star, I agree with Asondra once a caregiver always one, especially if you know it's your calling and it certainly is hers. My advice to caregivers is **"UNITE"** become one body because that's what it's going to take for real change. I love being a Caregiver, it is such a rewarding career. It offer so much flexibility and opportunities for those perusing nursing degrees like me. What an incredible book! Never seen anything like it or met anyone like Miss Asondra StarN'air This is truly *"A Caregiver's Bible To Excellence"* book.

"All I can say is Wow!"

What Ah Book!

Maria Chapel

Greeting, I'm Richard Douglas Crawford

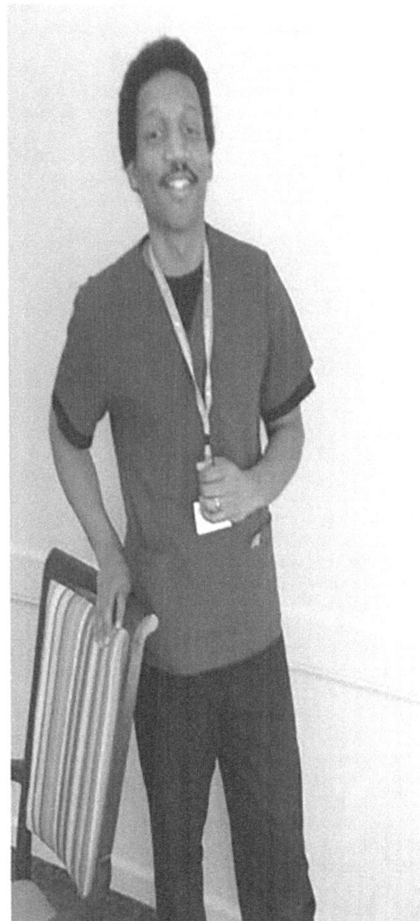

I been a male caregiver for two years, and have gain a great respect for this field. I even notice some positive changes in me since I've become a Caregiver, I'm more patient and loving, my wife notices it too.

My hope is more men come on board.

Advice I'd give to New Caregivers is to really get to know those in your care especially when working in memory care, dementia /Alzheimer's units in particular, where you may run into behavior problems, I have found, if you make a mistake, or upset them, **"Apologize"**, they will forgive you, just change your approach and start over, that's all.

Let me say this too, caregivers come to work to make a difference or stay home. These people really need our help.

And to my male caregivers out there, man, it's **"OK"** to smile dude.

Being A Male Caregiver Is Cool!

And to Star, let me say, it has been an honor working with you. Wish you all the success. You are truly a blessing to us all.

I'm Sharron Cummings, "A Caregiver!"

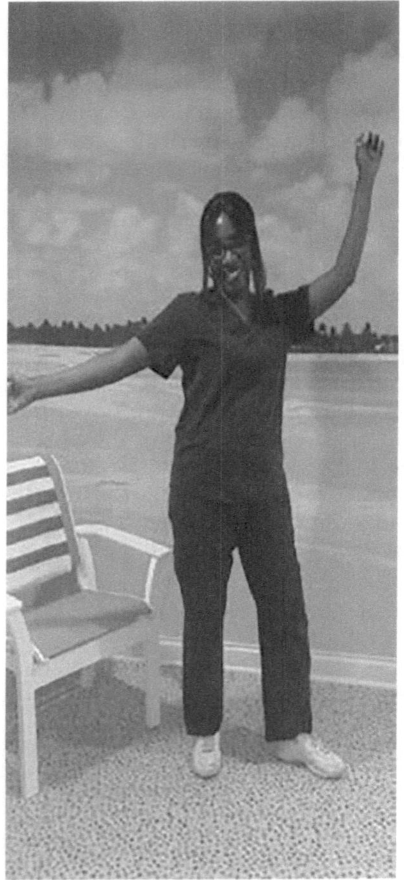

I've been a caregiver now for 10 years and I love it!

I will never forget the moment I felt in my heart that taking care of seniors is what I wanted to do. One day my daughter and I was out shopping and we came upon a very sweet fragile elderly lady but something was wrong we both noticed she seemed disorientated as if she was dizzy, lost or something to that effect.

My daughter and I went over to see if we could help her, are you okay we asked? Why are you out here by yourself? and her response was" I came to be with my companion, my friend, but they did not come today.

Next we asked where is your family? And this is what she said. "I don't have one".

My daughter and I looked at each other with heart break, love and compassion for this little old lady and knew in our hearts we had to take care of her.

So I said to her, from now on we will be your family. We put her in our car and gave her a ride home. After that we became her family, we did all her grocery shopping. We prepared her meals and whatever else she needed.

Soon after that experience, I was too moved in my heart to stop, so I contacted the department of aging to find out the process of becoming a fulltime caregiver.

My first call was very disappointing and heartbreaking, I was told I was too young to be working with the aging community. But then God somehow intervened and the next thing I knew I was hired as a caregiving fulltime at a very respectable agency full time and the rest is history.

This is what I want other caregivers to know, you must have love and compassion in your heart when working with the elderly. Our clients deserve our empathy, compassion and understanding and a staff with a warm heart and that would be me that's what I bring.

For a long time before I had that encounter with that lady, I did not know what I was going to do, had no clue, but God knew. God had a plan for me and it was perfect, he made me a CareGiver.

Jeremiah 29:11

Hi, I'm Susan Morgan

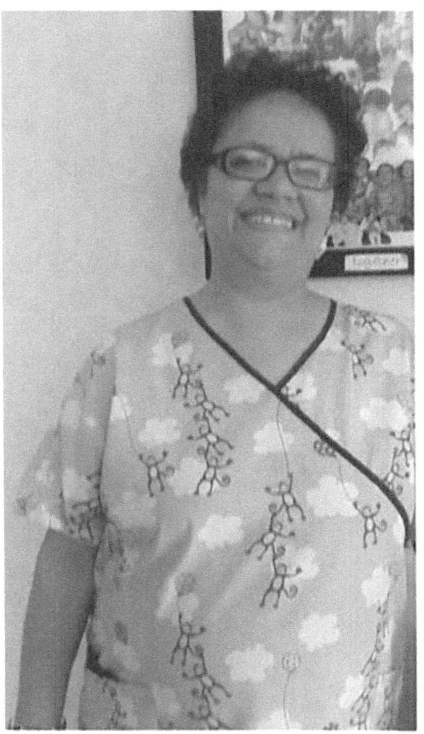

I have been a caregiver for 3 years.

It was a bold switch from customer service rep to the caregiving field. However when my mom and dad passed away I saw a great need for homecare and nursing home providers.

So I made the switch I became a healthcare worker. I see the need and the satisfaction it brings to me and the client.

What I like the most is when a resident responds positive to my assistance, such as a smile, and the desire to select me as their caregiver. Physical and mental progress is definitely a plus also however, what I dislike is being abruptly taken off a case without notifying the family and when my client passes away. It sadden me, I feel the loss too.

What I would like to say to new caregivers, be patient and avoid being bored with a resident find out about their past activities or accomplishments, likes and dislikes. Get to know the family if possible, to discuss their private needs and how you can help enhance their lives.

A word to management, don't observe care- givers just for an evaluation listen also to what caregivers suggest , because we are the ones doing the work and know what would help make the team successful. And another thing, make resources readily available, establish a rapport at least once a month with us, we matter.

Final remarks, it is wonderful when you meet a co-workers who really loves what she does, working with Star, she has a genuine sincere personality, I admire her outspokenness to get the attention of management to solve an issue, she displays a very professional and caring attitude toward the residents and employees around her. She's a great leader for us all. Hardworker too.

"She's Wonderful"!

Hello My Name Is

Add your photo

SECTION XV

Boot Camp For Caregivers

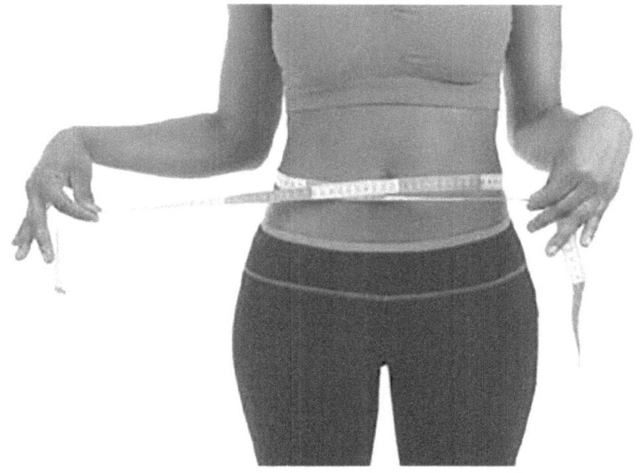

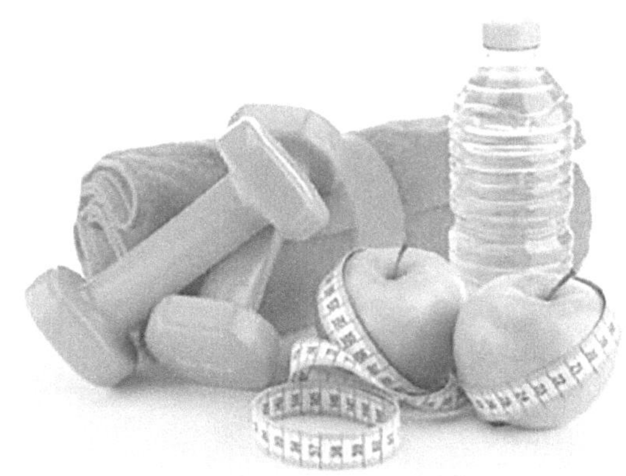

Don't Forget Your Bibles

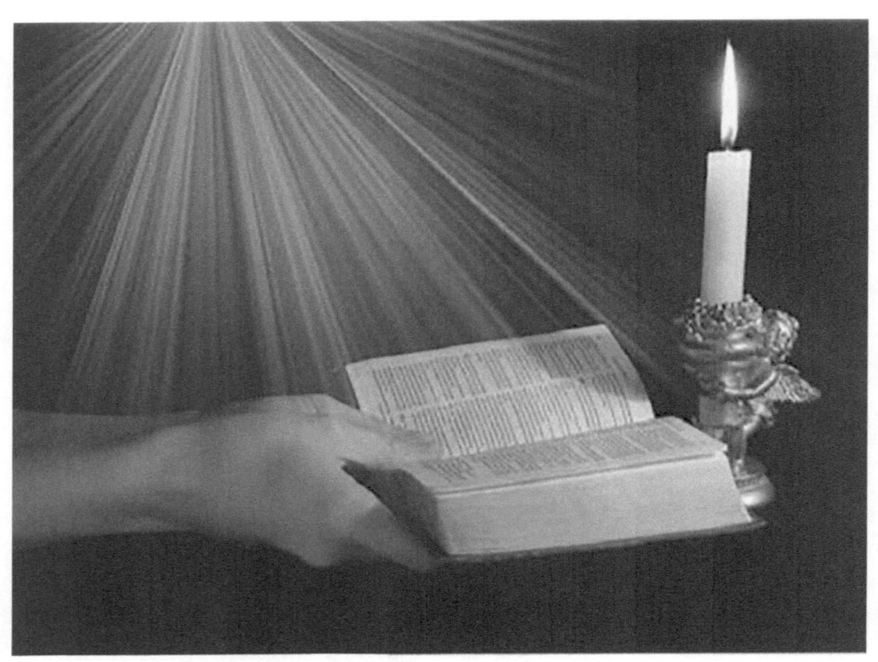

1 Corinthians 10:31
"Therefore, whether you eat or drink or whatever
you do, do all to the glory of God."

"Welcome To Boot Camp!"

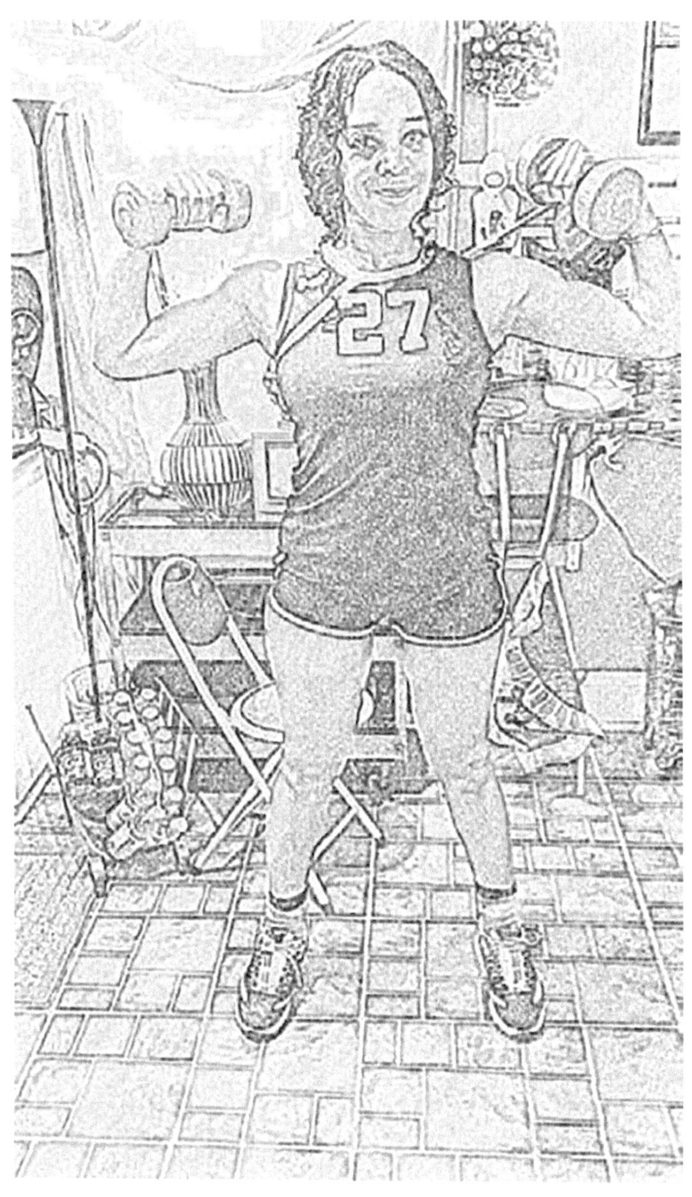

Introduction

Hello to all you caregivers out there are you ready to get fit and fabulous? Well, you've come to the right place.

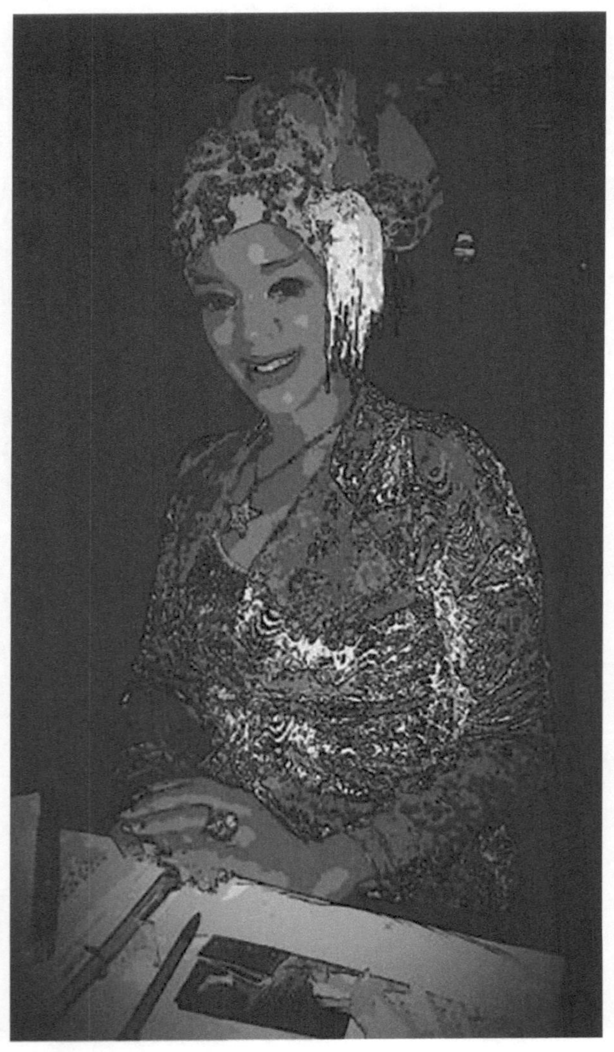

 Miss Asondra StarN'air

Caregiver's Boot Camp!

When it comes to health and fitness, it is very important to be dedicated and consistent. There is no other way to take control of your body; you must get up and fight the good fight of healthy living.

I have been the same size since high school, give or take a few pounds. How I maintain my lean body is simple and easy. And if you follow my formula—the one I have been using for more than twenty years—then you are sure to see amazing and lasting results too.

But first let me say this, this is not a diet plan; **"They don't Work"** no this is a life plan!

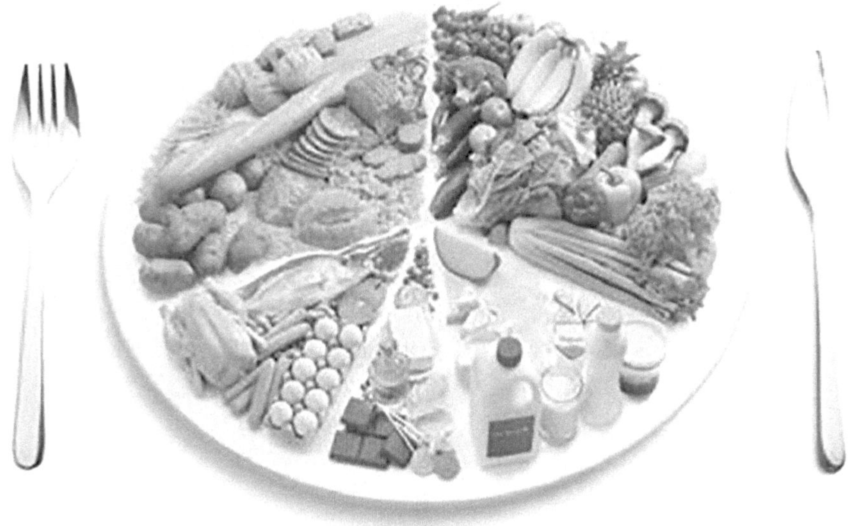

Let's Get Started!

Five-day Boot Camp for Caregivers

Five-day boot camp is designed to help caregivers develop a Christian foundation in care-giving and fitness, So, if we are not fit we are not able to perform as well as we could. Being in 'Good Shape' is important and necessary.

Today we are going get fit God's way, and I will share with you what I do to get in shape and stay in shape. So come on, let's get ready, let's get fit.

Here is a list of items you will need:

- ✓ Bible
- ✓ *A Caregiver's Bible To Excellence*
- ✓ Journal
- ✓ writing utensils and a note pad
- ✓ Water bottle
- ✓ Open heart to receive God's messages
- ✓ Time to pray and meditate
- ✓ A quiet place/room

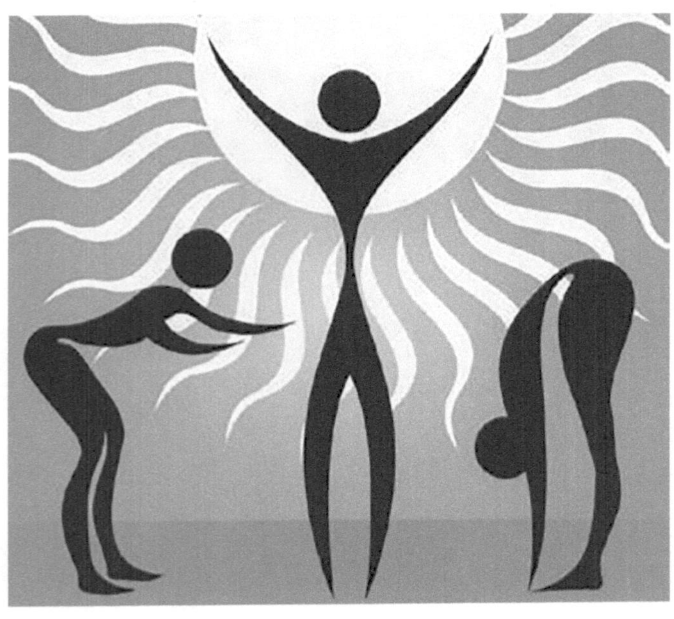

You'll Need These Too!

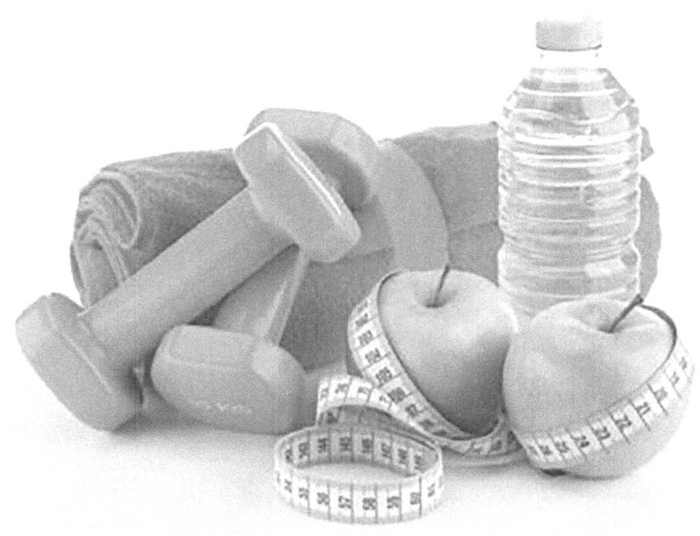

Fitness Begins with God, Get Right With God!

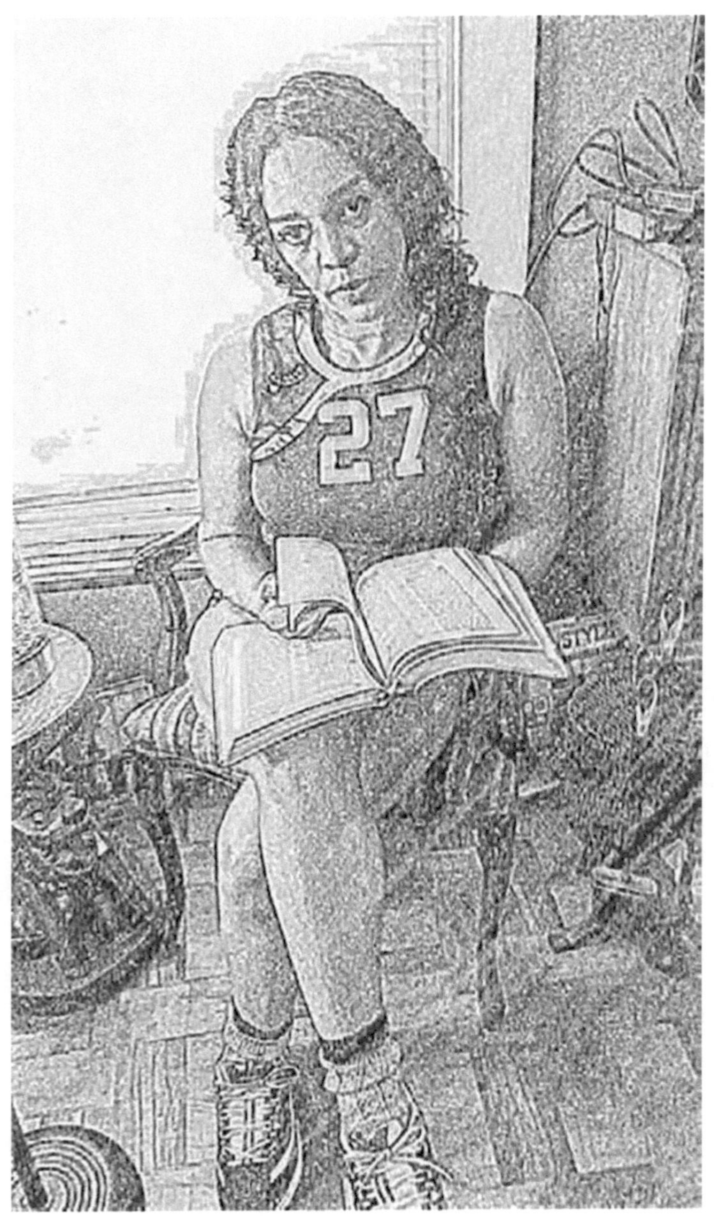

Day One: Monday

We will start with a warm-up. Take your bibles out and go to 1st Corinthians 6:19-20. Ready! read, *"Or do you not know that your body is the temple of the Holy Spirit who is in you, whom you have from God, and you are not your own? For you were brought with a price; therefore glorify God in your body and in your spirit which are God's."*

All day long and all this week meditate on that scripture, ask God to help you treat and respect your body better.

Fitness starts in the mind, not in the body.

Today you will reduce your food intake by 10 percent.

And replace it with God's word, you will start (eating) devouring Scriptures. By this, I mean you will find five scriptures regarding HEALTH in the Bible. Write them out and, every Monday, study and meditate on them; share them with coworkers, family, and friends too if you like. Each time you read those scripture, meditate on them, then apply them during meal time, think before you eat. Ask yourself this question, is this God for my body? That's right I said is this God for my body? Meaning would God keep eating these kinds of foods and stay healthy and physically fit? If not, **"dump it"!** Don't eat it, choose something else.

Next, today you are to reduce your sugar intake by 50 percent until you are at 90 percent, drinking only living water from now on. The kind that Jesus offers, guaranteeing you'll never thirst again. Regular water will be your supplemental drink. No more soda or sugary sweet drinks; get rid of that junk!

Class do one hour of physical exercise today—no excuses!

Be creative; find unique ways to do it, if you have full schedules, **"So What"**, **"Me Too"**, get up an hour early each day. **"Just do It!"**

Cool down: Tonight, before you go to bed, say this weight loss prayer: Lord thank you for taking over my body, thank you for finally making me understand that I have no choice but to get in shape and stay in shape because my body doesn't belong to me Lord, it belongs to you. Father thank you for this incredible vessel you have entrusted me with. In Jesus name, help me change the way I eat. **Amen**

Back On Your Feet!

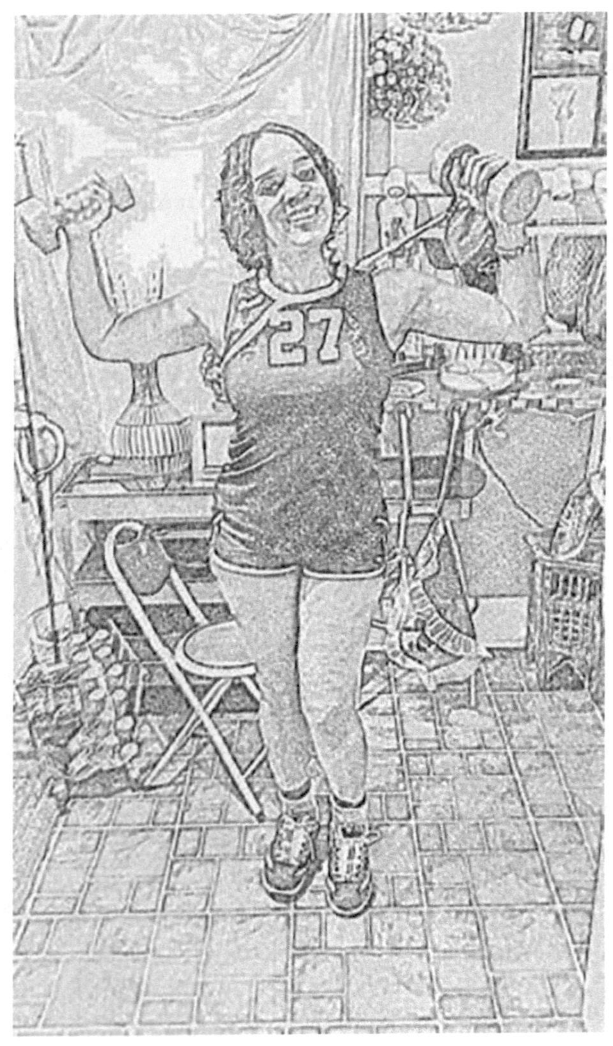

Take back control, don't let the devil tempt you anymore
Tell him to take his junk food and shove it!
Eat smart, and drop those pounds!

 Miss Asondra StarN'air

Day Two: Tuesday

I see you made it back, **"Welcome!"**

Let's warm up, go to **Proverbs 23:2**. Ready, read: *"And put a knife to thy throat, if thou (be) a man given to appetite."*

If you don't take back control of your life and body, it is going to destroy you in the end—kill you too. When we give into our desires over and over and over and over again, we can't win. Eventually our appetites and lifestyle catches up with us.

Today we are going to reduce our food intake by 20 percent and increasing your bible study time too, by that same amount, 20 percent.

You are now starting to eat less and less, now the scale will do the rest. What I am doing is shrinking your stomach, so that you can get the weight off, without dieting and keep the weight off. But remember, choose what God would choose, I guarantee you will lose!

Now what I want you to do today is find five scriptures in the Bible on food. Oh, it's in there. Google it if you can't find it. Ask Google to pull up scriptures on food, drinking and overeating. Pick out your favorite ones. Write them down and meditate on those five scriptures every Tuesday. Take your scriptures to work with you, and read them every chance you get. Share it with everyone you know.

Next, you are going to increase your water intake four to six cups a day, and you are now going to drink one full cup of that water right before you take your first bite of food at "Each Meal" from this day forward.

Today, get those workout clothes back on and do one hour of cardiovascular exercise. Go do a fast one hour walk, step -aerobic or cycling whatever, I don't care, you choose. Just move that body! If you are in poor shape, you'll get there, but you have to start somewhere, so just walk as long as you can. Hey class, make sure you have your water bottles with you, slowdown and drink some water, don't overdo it. After each work out slowly cool down and stretch OK? OK! Today you will start a journal—yes a journal. You are going to start talking to God, journaling your thoughts, situations, pain, broken heartedness if that's you, and anything else you have inside of you that needs to get out. So go purchase your journal; make sure you record dates and your weight too. Oh yes. You can share everything about you with God. God will get you in tip-top shape, watch and see. He helped me; now he's has me helping all of you. And let me tell you, I used Jesus and every scripture I could find to help lose weight and keep it off. And of course I worked out too. Look, caregivers if you want the pounds off you have some sweating to do, this is boot-camp and it's for champs!

Just do what I tell you, look I dropped 50 lbs. a long time ago, doing exactly what I'm telling you. I still wear some of my high school clothes; I kid you not. Just stay with me and this book for one year, and I promise you, you will never be the same; **"Never"**! You are going to start to do things in Jesus's name when I'm done with you.

Cool down: Tell God how thankful you are before you go to bed tonight and when you wake up. Good night, caregivers. See you tomorrow.

Hump day, Well On Your Way!

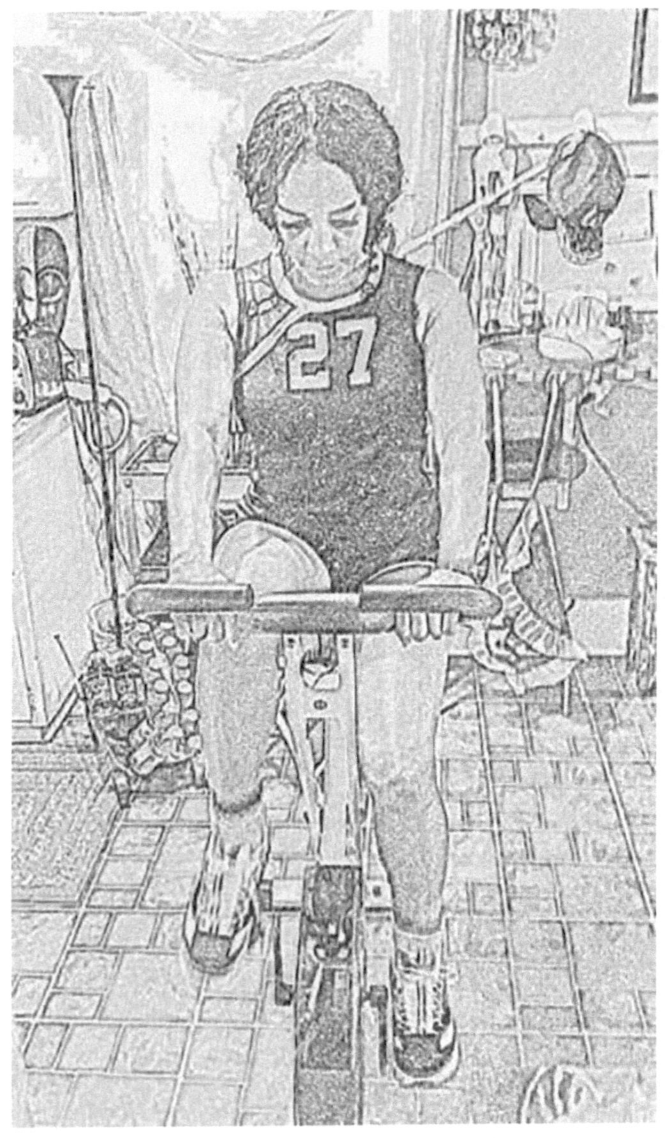

Press Through, don't Give up Now!

Day 3: Wednesday

It's hump day! Let's warm up. Caregivers, get your bibles out and go to the book of **Philippians 4:13**. Ready, read: *"I can do all things through Christ which strengtheneth me."*

If you are a caregiver, I know how busy your day is. We are often overwhelmed by the needs of others. We are only one person and just can't do it all, right? Plus, we have our own life to contend with. Where do we find the time and strength to do it all? Caregiver, we find it in Christ and only in Christ. He will give us the strength to do all he has called us to do including losing weight. Right now cast all your cares on him and get on the bike and ride for an hour or so, if you don't have one, save money and get one, we are trying to get you fit for life, not for a wedding dress or your favorite outfit.

Get Fit, Invest, Always Be Able to Wear "That dress"!

Today we are reducing our food intake by 30 percent and replacing it with God's word by the same amount 30 percent. Now we are spending more and more time in God's word as well. You should be up to thirty minutes a day studying your Bible now. If you don't have one, don't come back to this class until you get one. This is boot-camp and we're on the third day already. By now, everyone should own a bible, are you kidding me? Don't come back in here without it!

We are not playing games if you want to receive all that God has for you, then you have to invest time and effort in learning God's word. And in order to do that, you need a Bible. *The CareGiver's Bible to Excellence* is designed to give caregivers tools they need to become excellent at what they do, but it is not the Bible. It is, however, a friend of the Bible, because it's going to help lead souls to Christ.

Therefore, I don't have time to play games, this is boot-camp yawl. I'm out to help win as many souls as I can for Christ, "Many are called, but few are chosen"! That's right it is written in **Matthews 22:14** that many are called but few are chosen, and suspect it's because people just aren't willing to put in the time or work to get where God is trying to take them. Hope this is not you. if it's not, do what the word is calling you to do! Respect your body and temple, this boot-camp isn't hard, it's simple!

And another thing, while we're on the subject of the bible, mightiest well sit down and consider this day lecture hall. **"Sit down!"**

Listen up Everybody, Everywhere, I have an announcement to make, 'I'm not ashamed of the gospel, Jesus is what I do" and he called me an oracle, which means a **'Speaker of the LORD!'** He has asked me, **Miss Asondra StarN'air** to speak for him through these pages and address fitness, especially concerning his caregivers; Don't roll your eyes, listen! Obesity is still on the rise, the average caregiver in America is fat, some obese. Lets get serious, and stop playing around, too many caregivers have let themselves go, you've become "Fat not Fit" I heard you in the back row, ("oh, how dare she') yes, you're fat; know some of you are not trying to hear that! Stop crying "suck it up", this is boot-camp, my goal is to make you a champ! Stop your whinnying, get off your "hiney" and get in shape, stop trying to use food as an escape. Time to get physical, caregivers it's time to get fit. But here the secret to it all, are you ready? Here's the secret, **"Get Fit for Christ First"**, "not for you". To do this all you have to do is **"Watch What You Say and Do!"** Here it is in a nutshell, the lack of respect for God's body is hurting all of **"YOU"**! But the good news is today is a new day, and I've been called to show you a new way. That new way is Jesus!

He can get those pounds off and keep them off. You won't need diet pills or pay for plans that still don't work. I am a living testimony of what God can do for those who are willing to do the work his way. Don't leave this class. "Stay"!

Get a Bible today! Your assignment today is to explore the Bible; just take a look around. Write down all the names of the sixty-six books, dividing the Old and New Testament.

Make 'Wednesdays', bible study days and a day to spend more time with God. Find out what He wants you to start doing, then do it. That's how I keep my weight off, I talk to God about everything and so should you.

Cool down: Ooh- wee, we covered a lot and now I'm hottt with a triple t! I don't want worldly water, no, I'll have what Jesus is having! Scriptures that keeps him faithful , fit, so he don't quit, and focused on his father's business. didn't you know that? Yeah that's how Christ kept his body in such good shape and he was physical too, he walked a lot and he also watched what he ate, what's on your plate? Tonight pray this simple prayer: **Jesus Show Me Your Ways!**

Good night caregivers see you on Thursday and don't forget your bibles.

Good Job Today!

 MISS ASONDRA STARN'AIR

Hello World, Look Out!

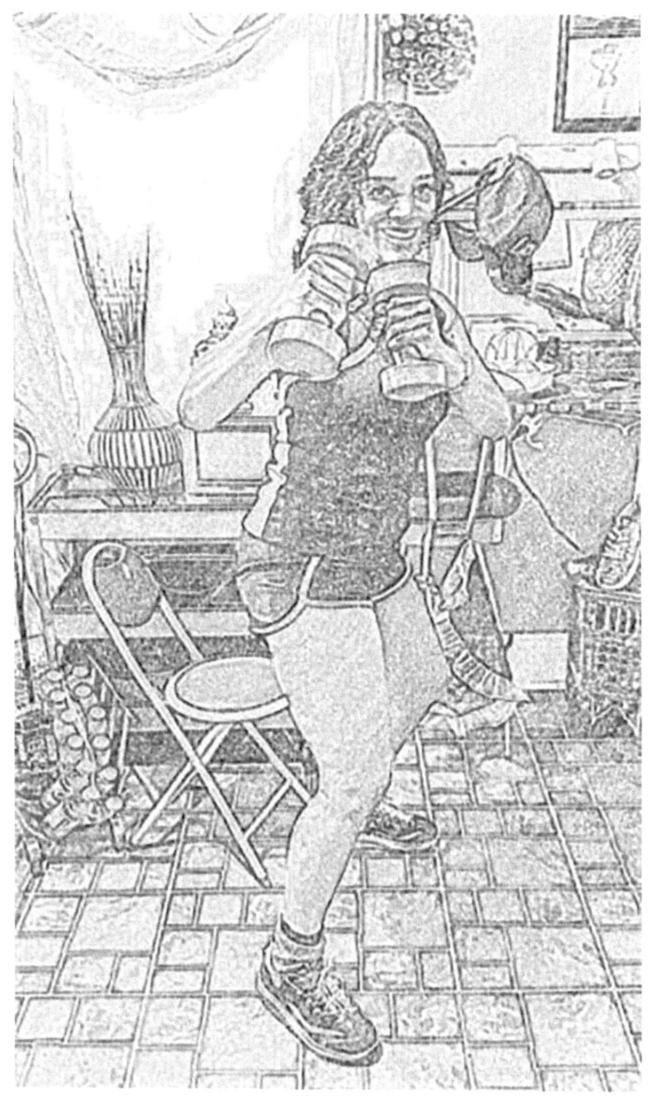

**Fit or Fat "Take That"!
A Healthy Body's Where's It's At!**

Day 4: Thursday

Hello, I see some of you weren't afraid to come back, glad to see ya, come in grab your water bottles and let's get ready to warm up. Hopefully, by now, everyone has their own Bibles. ("we do") great!

Open them up and let's go back to **1 Corinthians 6:19–20** Ready, read, "Do you not know that your bodies are temples of the Holy Spirit, who is in you, whom you have received from God? You are not your own; you were bought with a price. Therefore, honor God with your bodies."

Need I say more? I think I do, Stop shacking up with your lovers or baby's daddy! This is not honoring God. This is honoring fornication; **Sex outside of marriage is wrong**. Those who live this way are living a lie, and disrespecting God and will suffer behind it, perhaps this is where some of the heavy weight gain and depression is all coming from, I'm just sayin' if you are not living right, you probably aren't eating right either, think about that one tonight. Stop living and eating like the world.

Give "All" Your Life to Christ, That's My "Real Fitness Advice!"

Sorry, but I had to go there. Too many women are caught up in sexual bondage by men who pretend to love them—but instead, using you ladies for their own purpose. Many of you call that kind of relationship love; I call it loss.

Look, I'm not holding back the punches, this is boot -camp, hence the name. You cannot pick and choose how you are going to serve God. Your body, sisters and brothers is not your own. I had to learn this too, over and over again, until I got tired of the fortification life, robbing me and leaving me devastated, brokenhearted, and depressed.

And when I was depressed I ate, and gained weight too, so I've been there, **"Me Too"**! But, enough is enough, I got tired and grew, I started sticking with God and his will for my life **"Like Glue"**. Now all I'm trying to do here is help you. Once I gave all my life to Christ and started reading my bible daily, I quickly woke up, I saw the sin, I saw what sex outside of marriage was out to do to me. Use me, like it's using some of you right now. Those who have ears, please listen, 'charming snakes' are just that, charming and are real good looking too and some come with jobs, houses, nice cars, even fame and degrees; oh. but listen, don't let all that fool you, because if they are not living for God, you will get hurt in the end. If you belong to this world. you belong to a fornicating world too, but the choice is all up to you. This oracle telling you something, you won't get in school. And why do you supposed that is? Because this world is corrupt, and the bible tells us so, in fact it says clearly, that men have become lovers of themselves. God is not a God that he would lie, to females, We mean the world to him, he love us like he loves the church. However, the men of this world, the one you call your boyfriend don't, if he's getting you to lay with him outside the will of God. He's a fraud! A liar and a player too, what you do with all this wisdom is up to you. Not only is this guy taking you to hell with him, he's making sure there's no more purity! Come on, you know locker room talk, why buy the milk when you can get it for free? Ladies I have been where some of you are. Looking for love in all the wrong places, yes, I was blind but now I can see, I will not let sex destroy me, my advice is for you to get out as soon as you can, whether it be a woman or man. we do not belong to ourselves, we belong to God.

Ooh wee, that was a hard but I had to go there, because getting into shape God's way require ***Holiness, Self-Discipline and Righteous Living.*** We can't be fit and live like the world does. for the wages of sin is still death. And besides what good is it to be fit, **"But Not It"**! God Can't use you, because you belong to the world. Okay, I think I made my point and have said enough, read your bible daily God will pick up where I left off, I'm tired, now it's time to cool down! Somebody please grab me a towel!

Today we are reducing our food intake by 40 percent and increasing our Bible study time by the same amount, 40 percent. If you have been working this boot camp faithfully, everyone should start to notice changes—not only are you starting to lose weight, but your mind and soul is getting a makeover too, you are growing stronger and stronger in the Lord, and that the goal here as well. I love you and I want to see caregivers set free! Yes I can see you, all of you. 👁 I'm watching over you with my spiritual eye; you are indeed changing getting fit too, all of you. You're transitioning, you're getting a lot more than you signed up for. You're becoming a new creature in Christ and that's nice! It's wonderful and it's a joy to be a part of all that! Wow! look what God can do! Caregivers, God can use you too, He can use **"Everybody, Everywhere"**, a bum, prostitutes, carpenters, animals in a cage, blacks, whites, those who got it made, he don't care! With that being said, stay focus, those pounds are coming off, never give up!

From this day forward, you will no longer eat on a regular plate. Your new plate will be saucers, or snack-size plates. For simplicity, let's just eat on medium-size saucers. To avoid confusion. Notice I never asked you to give up your favorite foods, did I? No, because what I learned twenty years ago through experiment is simply this: if you want to lose half the weight, eat half the food. It's just that simple!

It takes 3,500 calories to gain one pound. If you keep reducing your food intake by half that number everyday then you are guaranteed to lose unwanted pounds without giving up any of your favorite foods.

Today we are going to work out one for hour doing sculpting and toning, we will also be using weights and doing a few sets of planks. Go online and YouTube a plank session video for those who do not know what planks are or how to do them.

Next, I want you to find a workout buddy, someone who will do this boot camp with you from now on. Both of you can become bible study partners as well. God said in **Matthew 18:20** and I quote "For where two or three gather in my name, (and we getting in shape for him, not us) there I am with them". Trust me, once your others start seeing all these incredible changes in you and your appearance, they'll want to do what you are doing too! And of course God and **'A Caregivers Bible To Excellence'** is very, very happy about all this, who can ask for anything more.

Now, before we end this session, you have another homework assignment tonight I want all of you to get on your knees and ask God to forgive you for your sins and for taking so long to come to him. Tonight is a night of repentance. It is time we come clean with God although he already know everything about us and what we have been doing and how we have been living. Nevertheless repentance is due. People if you want it all, great mind, nice fit body plus success and abundance too, then live true, that's whatcha' do. Otherwise the wages of sinful living with sneak back up on you. You think you have problems now you haven't seen nothing yet. Don't love this world, don't be a fool, Get fit for God, and stay fit in every way for God! Repent and tell God you are sorry for everything you have ever done and want to start living for him, not yourself anymore. Be quiet and listen to what God has to say to you.

Cool down: Spend this evening confessing and accepting God back into your life. Before you go to bed, ask God to help you come out of the world. Tell him you can't do it without him. Tell him you are lost and in need of a savior and that you are beginning to see the light, and that want to start living right. Next, thank him and go to sleep, he will take it from there. He will slowly get you where you need to be, because you asked him to. And that's all God has been waiting for anyway for you to come to him on your own. Yes, I tell you there truth, he's been waiting and waiting patiently for all of you to come back to your first love, **"HIM"**!

  MISS ASONDRA STARN'AIR

What an incredible way to end the day. This is fitness at its highest level don't you think? It's working for me, today I am still fit, stable and able to do all things in Christ who strengthens me! I will see all of you tomorrow, grab a towel and some water, this was a tough but great workout class today. See you on Friday, bye for now! **"Body By Christ!"**

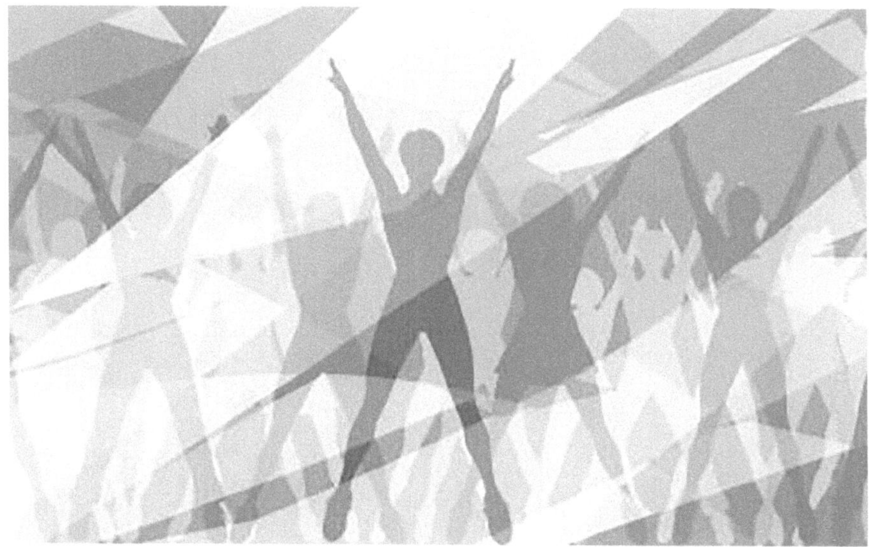

Get Fit For The Lord!

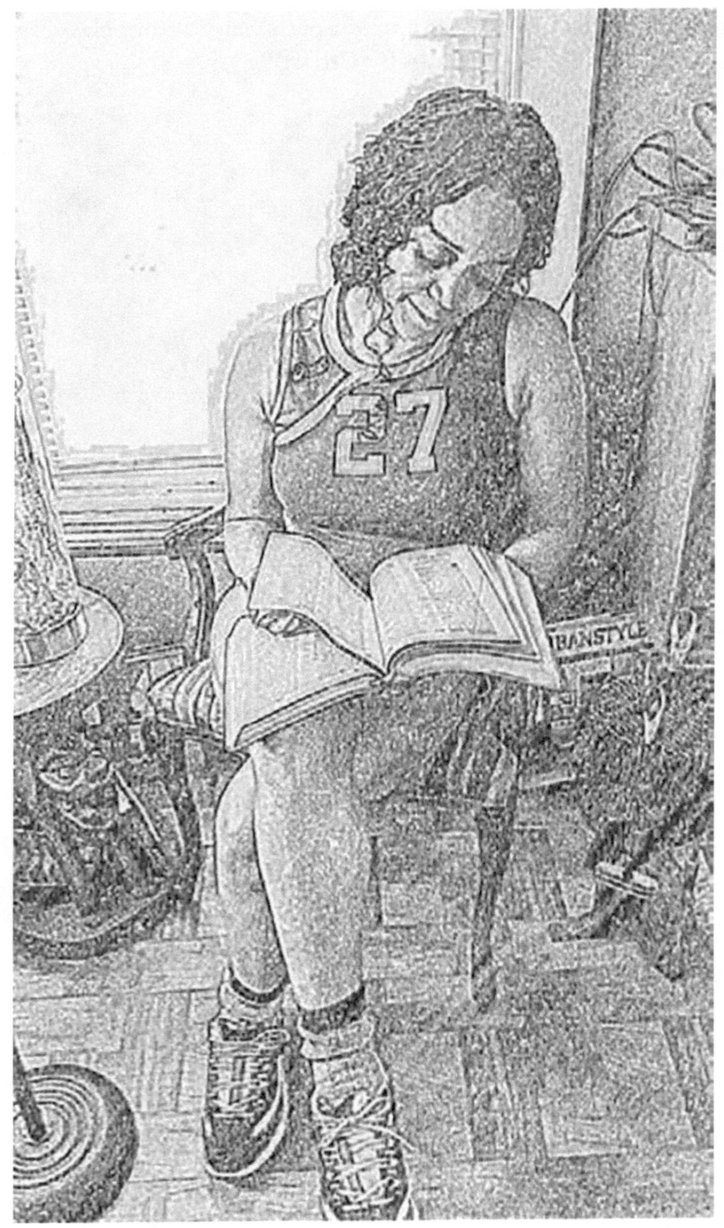

It's almost time to celebrate, laugh!

Day 5: Friday

You made it all the way to day 5, time to take total control of your Christian life. Let's warm up! Go to **Jeremiah 29:11** Ready, read, *"'For I know the plans I have for you,' says the **LORD**, 'plans to prosper you and not to harm you, plans to give you hope and a future.'"*

It is my suspicion that many of you are very overweight, fat not fit because of personal problems. Sometimes when we can't cope with stuff **"We Eat"** or do other things like sin against God instead of trusting God to help us with our troubles. We look for other ways to cope! Some use dope, some sex, and I think it is safe to say if you are in this class, many of you have used food to cope with your problems but today that's all about to end. God knows what's best for you, re-read that scripture every Friday for a year until it syncs in. Wake up to that scripture and at night before you fall asleep think about that scripture. No matter what's going on in your life, God is still going to use you if you let him. For heaven sakes class for once in your life why don't everybody just trust him? I trust in the Lord for everything. If anyone out there is lost, experiencing hopelessness, brokenhearted, unemployed, or struggling financially or dealing with health issues or just can't seem to find peace and happiness nowhere—that used to be me. Yes me, but not anymore, of course life stuff still happen. According to our bibles there's always going to be trials and tribulations. However, I learned over the years to cast it all on Christ and class suggest everybody do the same. That's right, cast your cares on him and keep it movin'. **"Today I'm Movin"**, God has placed a call on my life, He spoken to me, *"Write my book and call it **A Caregiver's Bible to Excellence!"** "And In it, I want a fitness boot-camp!"* Yes Lord, done! So you see just like Jesus was about his father's business we have to be also. Caregivers if you want to live the best life possible, we can't get caught up in fake comforts, fake love or the world, We must be about our father's business, which means constantly in his word, meditating on it day and night, and we must live right. The core message of this boot- camp is this: Get Fit for God, Not You! No matter what you do in life, if God is not the builder, it won't last. Be wise now, learn from your past. Class the bible puts it this way in **Psalms 127:1** In fact, turn to that page with me, ready, read: *"Unless the **LORD** builds the house, the builders labor in vain."* Caregivers not only let him rebuild your body and get you back in shape but let him rebuild your entire life. Don't allow this world to corrupt you any longer. Today you are stronger! Say no to over-eating, no to sex outside of marriage, no to unclean living of any kind. And say yes to the best, Jesus Christ Our Lord and Savior! Tell everybody else, don't do no favor! Moving forward, on Fridays for one years and on your own time take the time out to start educating yourself on the dangers of being overweight in food, sex, sin, then do something about it! I did! I gave this world up and let Jesus in. I Sincerely hope, class you've enjoyed this boot-camp, it's about to end. For the record, this boot camp has never been about making you super model thin, it's about teaching you how to win! "YOU" Win over your flesh, when **"YOU"** let Christ in! We All Win!

Oops, almost forgot, today is the day you are going to give up half your food intake for good. You will now reduce your food intake by 50 percent. Wow! That's what I said 50 percent, but just wait and see what starts to happen now, you won't believe your eyes or your thighs! Everyone around you too is going to be amazed and ask you what you are doing? Tell them, you are doing **'A Caregivers Bible to Excellence',** that you are doing Jesus now! Let them all know you are becoming everything God has called you to be. Yes, that's what you are to tell them, tell them you got saved in so many ways, not only in the body, but in the mind and spirit too, say God loves you!

Today is Friday and you made it all the way through the boot-camp. Congratulations to all of you, **"Well done!"** The Lord is so proud of you, **"Me Too"!**

"Great Job!" Do my boot-camp for life and you will never have to worry about being overweight again. Nor be overweight in sin, **"Keep God In!"** That's how we do it, that's how we win!

Cool down: You did it! **Celebrate!!!!** Go do something special to reward yourself. Go and buy yourself some flowers or do something fun but be don't sin, stay on this righteous path you are on now.

Come to boot-camp on Saturday for more tips on how to keep it all off! You will not need your workout clothes, you're done for the week, however, keep doing the boot-camp, repetitions is the key to a fabulous body! See ya on Saturday, bring your bibles, **"Class dismissed"!**

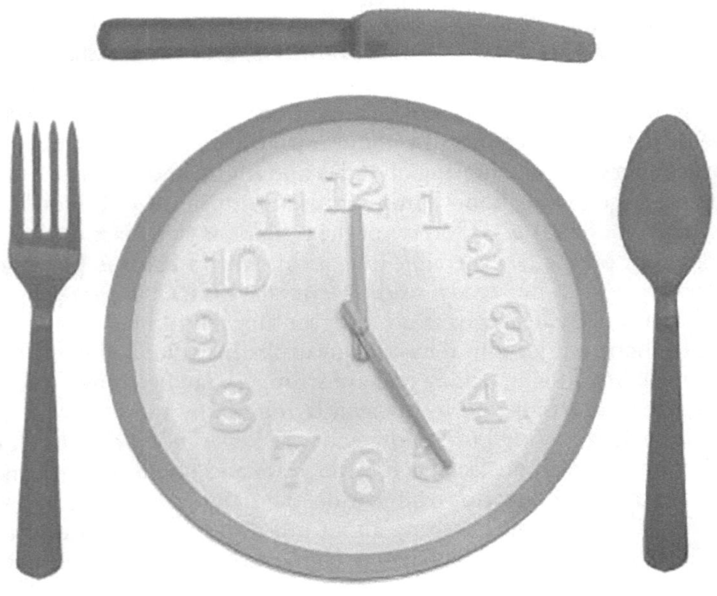

 Miss Asondra StarN'air

Well done Class! Well done!

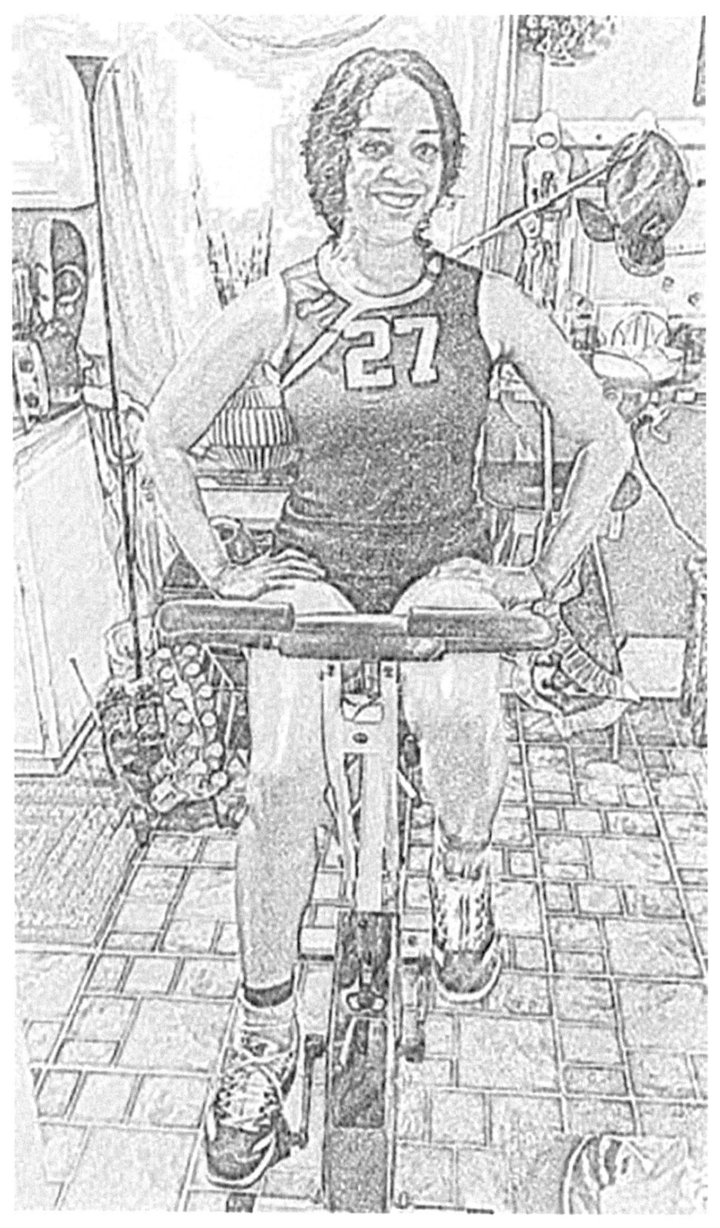

Yawl did It, We did It, Now Stay Committed!

Saturday

Hello everybody, hello! Today is Saturday, and just like I promised, I want to give you some tips on how to keep your weight off and also I'd like to share with you today some other things I do to maintain my healthy body. Class, what I am about to share with you **"Works"** it's a proven formula that's worked for me for over twenty years now and can work for you too. But before we get into foods, fats and workouts, Check this out, *I Eats Scriptures To Stay in Shape!* Class that's right, Food has become secondary to me, God and Scriptures comes first. Some of you in this class may think, this is radical, but for me it's not! No conceit intended, but keep turning the pages, look at me, that picture's recent, I'm fit and beautiful, at least I feel that way. So try it , eat some scriptures today, like milk, it does the body good!

But let me clarify, please allow me explain myself, people when I say, "I eat scripture," what I'm really saying is I study God's word first, and I pray too. Yes I do, I ask God to help me eat right and give me the disciple to get up and work out each day. And those prayers worked, because that's exactly what he did. Everybody open up your bibles to **John 14:13** Ready, read: *You may ask me for anything in my name and I will do it.* Many of you have not lost the weight or gotten your life together because you have not asked God to help you. You are trying to do it and the rest of your life on your own and you're failing each and every time. Caregivers listen to me, I've been where some of you are, grinding trying to make a dollar out of fifteen cents. Want stay in shape, yet can't escape all the pressure and other responsibilities life throws at us. Well I'm here to tell you today, you can escape, we were never meant to do it all on our own, that's where we're going wrong. As long as we have Christ, we have help. Better start believing that, because it's true. He says he will not abandon us, Hebrews 13: 5 and he said he will help us. Isaiah 41:13 But the real problem here is **"You"** and your pride, yes pride, **"YOU"** have not, because **"YOU"** ask not! **James 4:2**

So like many, you went astray, like burger king, have it your way! That's right, some of you have made food your idol, that's why your weight has gotten out of control **"You Live to Eat"** instead of **"Eat to Live"**. But something got to give, and that's why God sent me to help you.

Today is Saturday, and this is what we're going to do. We're going to do what I've learned to do and that is *Trust GOD!* Yes, trust that he is going

 Miss Asondra StarN'air

to fix your life plus get the weight off you and keep it off too! With God all things are possible, too, we don't need diet pills or diet food either, in this plan you can eat what you want.

Enough lecture, now let me introduce all of you to my weekly food regimen:
Monday: hot or cold unsweetened cereal, oatmeal in cold months / cold cereal in warm months. Tea or water.
Morning Snack: yogurt, fruit, water, tea, sometimes coffee, avoid lots of caffeine.
Lunch: half of a homemade sandwich, no fast food or restaurants sandwiches. You can add a side order of fruit and tall glass of water.
Midday Snack: granola, fruit, water, peppermint hard candy throughout the day to help curb cravings.
Dinner: saucer-size portions of food (menu can be anything, no second helping), water, fruit, no after-dinner desserts during the week.
Before-Bedtime Snack: cheese and crackers with tea or 4 cups of popcorn or 1 cup of granola and yogurt/ice cream.

And here's something else I do class, I pick one special day out of the week—say, Saturday or Sunday—and go out to my favorite restaurants if it's in my budget to eat, and I eat whatever I want, including dessert! But guess what, I don't want it! My body's cravings have changed because of my strict regimen. Not only have i loss weight, but I also lost my desire to "pig out," or eat junk food, and drink foolish drinks such as pops and sweet drinks. I'm now eating for God, not for my own fleshly desires anymore. God first, food second. I don't live to eat. I eat to live the life God has intended for me, and obesity is not in his plans for us! God wants us healthy and fit!

I encourage all of you to do this menu for a year and watch the pounds come off. Now I know this would be hard if you have a husband and children to cook for, "me too". But still, I kept my focus on fitness and good health not only for me but for my family as well, I just found a way to do it and it paid off in the end. That was over twenty years ago. Today I'm still in good shape and healthy too and I have God to thank for it! For he cares for the mind , body and soul of all of us. In God I will always trust.

In closing, let me end with this, I really believe that we ought to show more respect for our bodies lifelong. We should realize that our bodies really don't belong to us like the scriptures says and began to make better choices in life . Food can destroy the body as well as sinning against God in fact, the bible says the wages of sin is death. If you want a fit and healthy body, you must first have a fit and healthy mind.

We should all learn to think and do what Christ would do at all times. And if we all learn to do that holistically, we'd all be fine, walking the same line, Healthy body, healthy soul and healthy mind.

Now Go "Get Fit For Christ", and "Stay Fit" for the rest of your life! It has been a pleasure, write to me, let me know how things are going. Don't lose hope, no matter what size you are, you are still a star. And **"YOU"** can do all things in Christ who is with you and gives you the strength. I do hope you feel your time and money on this book has been well spent! Never put a price on excellent advice!

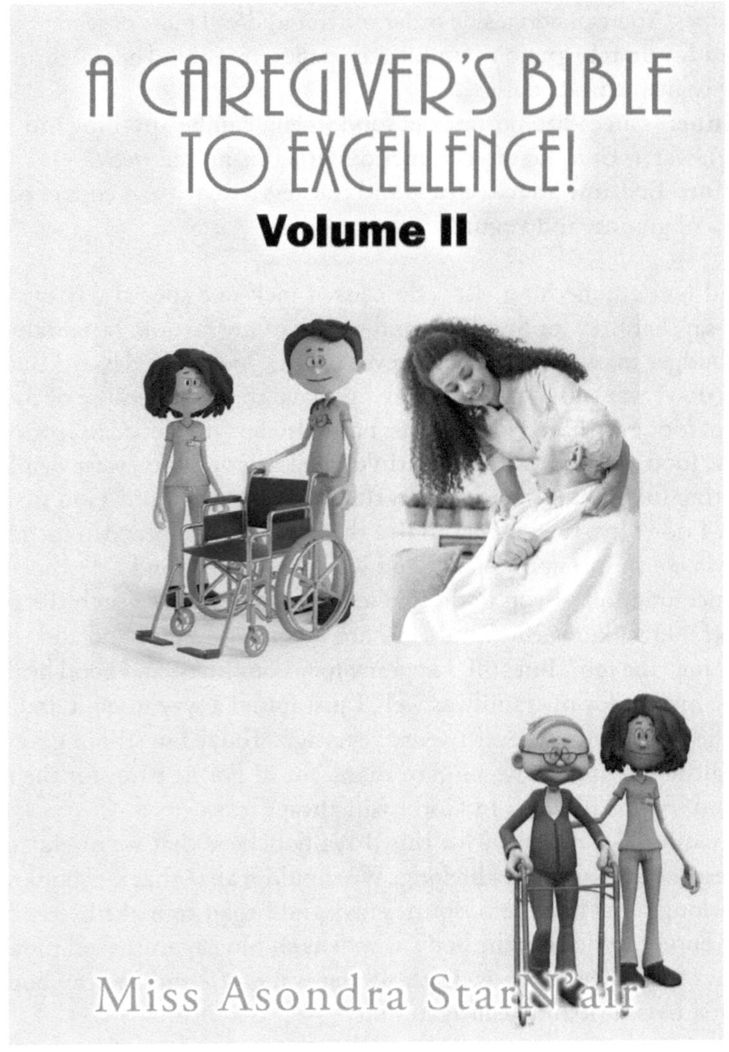

 MISS ASONDRA STARN'AIR

I'm Eating Good In The Neighborhood!

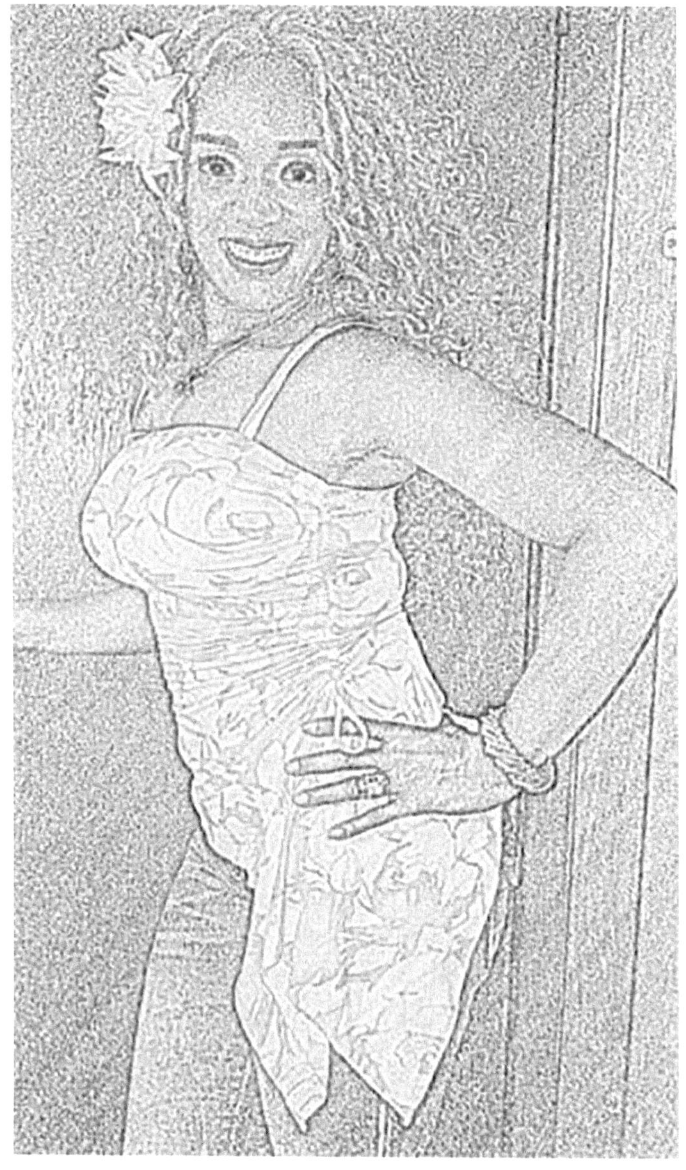

I feel Good, and because of God, I Knew That I Would Yawl!

Sunday

Six days you shall labor,
but on the seventh day you shall rest…
Exodus 34:21

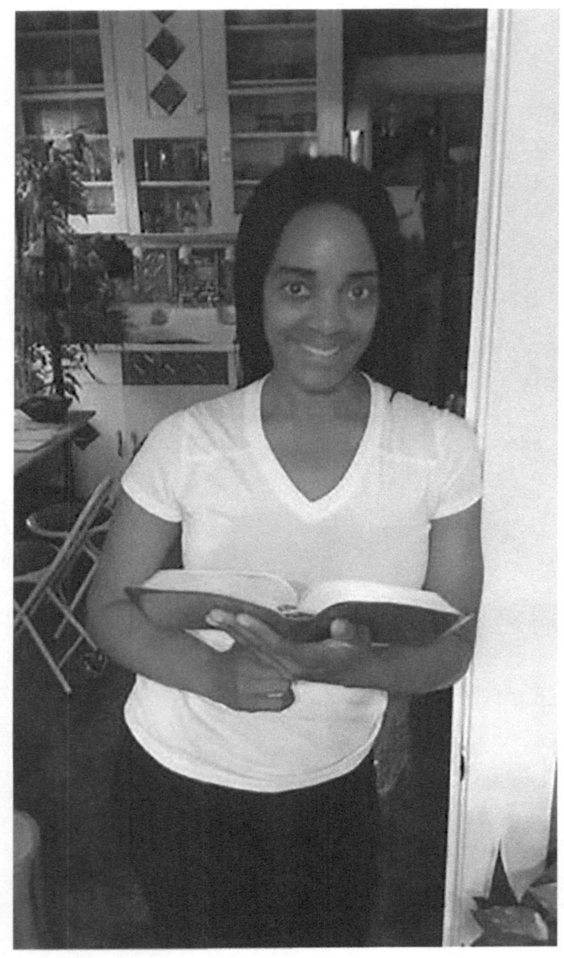

Rest, spend time in the word!

Caregivers Lunch Box

ACT SMART
EAT SMART

- Drink plenty of water.
- Eat half of a Sandwich, your choice.
- Consume more water than food.
- Snack on scripture instead of junk food.
- Eat all the food groups.
- Get off those cakes, cookies and pies, look at your thighs are those sweets really worth it? Instead eat natural sugars like "fresh fruits!"

Say "No" To:

Candy bars
Chips
Cookies
Fried Foods
Large and unhealthy
Sandwiches
Donuts
Pop and Juices
These item should be eliminate from your diet and eaten rarely. If you eliminate these items, you'll see positive results and feel better too!

The Choice Is up To "YOU"

Fit or Fat?

If we want to keep the weight off and achieve good health then we must become very discipline in our eating habits. Follow these simple disciplines:

1. Bring your own lunch!
2. Work out 3 to 5 times a week.
3. Eat the size you want to be. For example if you want to be small, eat small portions, if I want to be medium, eat medium size portions and so on…you get the picture.
4. Give up junk food, because it's just that, Junk!
5. Water only, no juices or sodas.
6. If you over eat, make it up the rest of the week by eating much smaller portions.
7. My 90/10 rule: 90% small portions and smart choices. After that go for it,10% eat whatever you want!
8. Don't eating in front of the television.
9. During lunch time consume more water. and do more fruits and vegetables.
10. Stop sitting around junk food eaters.
11. Purchase clothing in the size you want to be.
12. Reward yourself for looking so fabulous. Looking good takes a lot of work, a brand new outfit couldn't hurt!

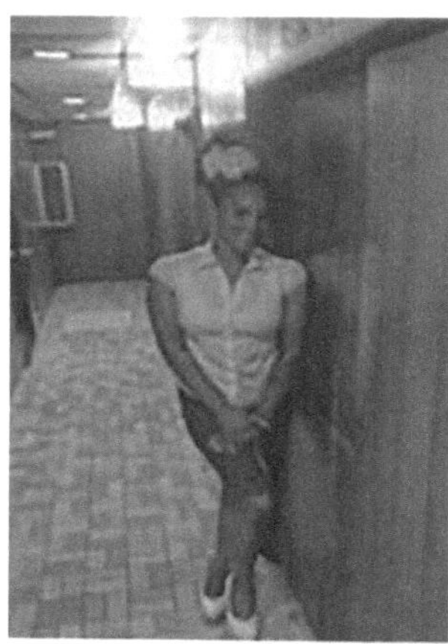

Caregivers Lunch Box Items

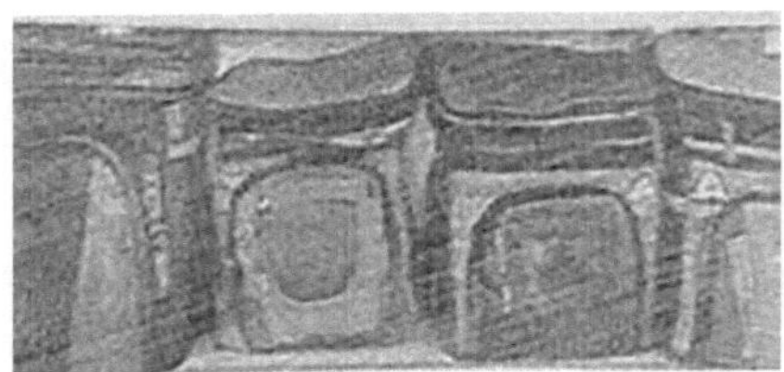

- Make your own lunches, purchase a lunch box.
- An apple a day keeps the doctors away.
- Salad or vegetables
- Half a sandwich
- 8 oz cup of soup/chili
- Favorite crackers to help calm craving.
- Pack a bible too, eat scriptures for lunch, spend time with God!
- Grab some peppermint hard candy, it helps calm junk food craving throughout the day as well.
- You will need a large water bottle, with only water in it, no juice or sodas, WATER! drink it all day.

Lastly, no left over dinners for your lunch box, wait until you get home and watch your portions too, no second helpings.

You Are What You Eat!

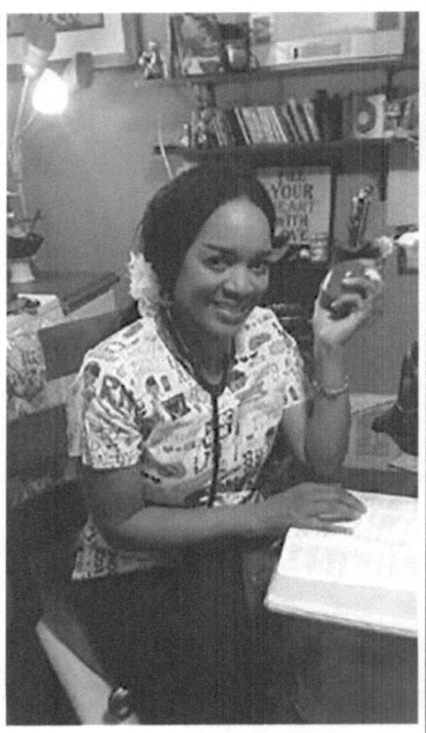

Fit or Fat?

Beauty comes in many sizes, you choose the size you want to be. Remember Jesus and discipline is the key!

Being Overweight is a Trap!

Remember **"YOU"** are what you eat!

Caregiver Café Fit or Fat

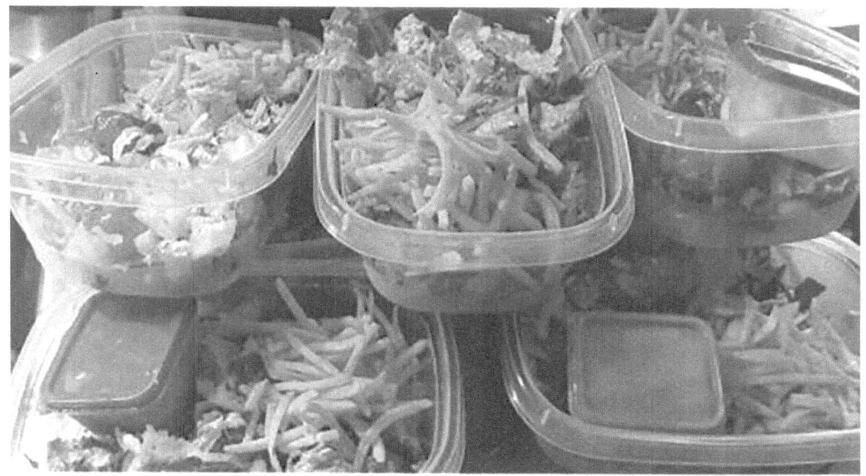

**Prep your lunches for the week.
'Preparation is Key!"**

Fitness Matters!

Today's caregivers are starting to make fitness a priority! After all, come on, we are health care providers, shouldn't we look the part too? Shouldn't we be a role model of good health and fitness to the people we're taking care of, shouldn't we? Yes, I think so. Well then "Go" take action, start taking better care of yourself. **It's Never Too Late To "Make That Change!"**

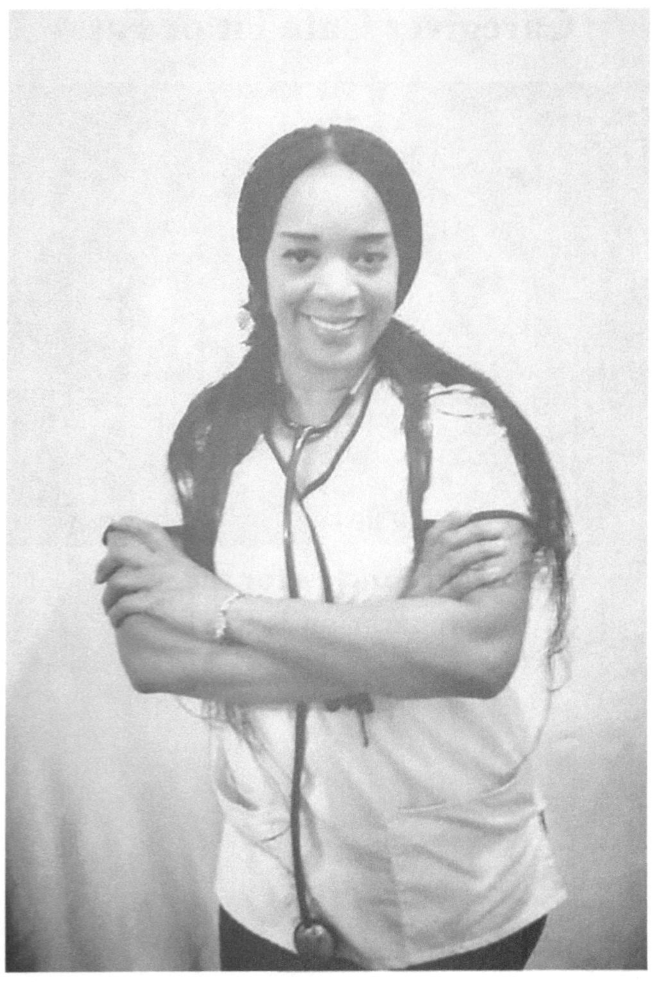

Get Fit, Stay Fit!

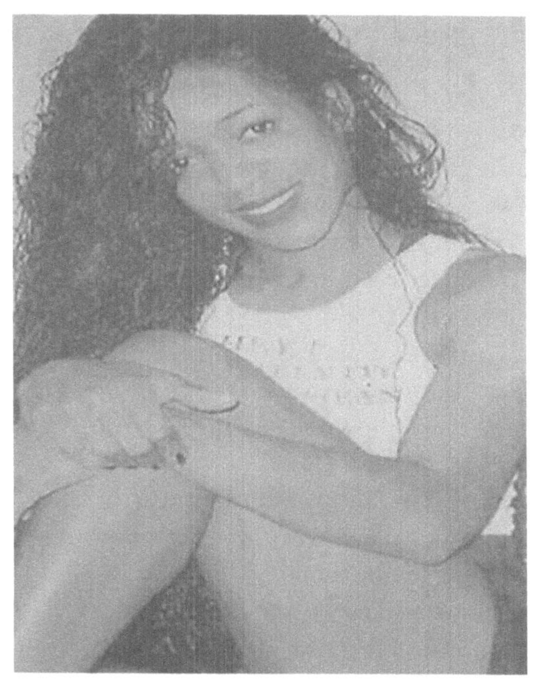

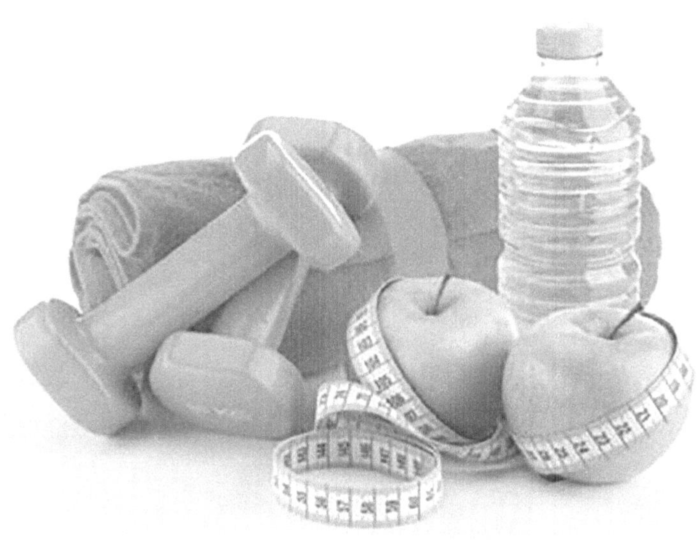

Boot Camps Fitness and Health Affirmations

1. I am eating a lot less and smarter.
2. I am working out four days a week.
3. I enjoy working out now.
4. I am drinking six to eight glasses a water a day.
5. I am starting to feel a lot better.
6. I am determined to lose weight and keep it off this time.
7. I use scriptures to help lose the unwanted pounds.
8. I don't eat junk food because it's just that **"JUNK"**!
9. I am preparing my own smart meals now. Bye -bye- fast-foods!
10. I am reading my bible daily.
11. I do not keep junk foods around me anymore.
12. I believe I can do all things in Christ who strengthens me, I will get my body back in shape.
13. I am patient, I will not rush my weight loss.
14. I'm staying healthy!
15. I am living for Christ now.

 Miss Asondra StarN'air

Obesity

Obesity is a problem, obesity is bad!

There is just no other way to describe it, we must get the weight off and keep it off. Otherwise you are playing a dangerous game with your life.

You're fooling yourself if you think, it's ok to be overweight! It isn't, nor is it healthy.

Being overweight, leads many times to obesity, once that happen you are in real trouble, real big trouble.

Being out of shape or obese is a major health risk. Obesity and overweightness can cause many complications like the following:

- **Hypertension**
- **Type 2 diabetes**
- **Coronary Heart disease**
- **Stroke**
- **Sleep Apnea**
- **Gall Bladder disease**
- **Respiratory problems**
- **Dyslipidemia**
- **Depression /low -self esteem**
- **Negativity, Jealousy and Insecurity**
- **Hatred toward those with a nice physique.**
- **Poor Job Performance**
- **Body aches and pains**
- **Laziness and poor teamwork**
- **Causes accelerating aging**
- **Unusual tiredness, chemical imbalances/sometimes body odor**
- **Gradual physical decline**

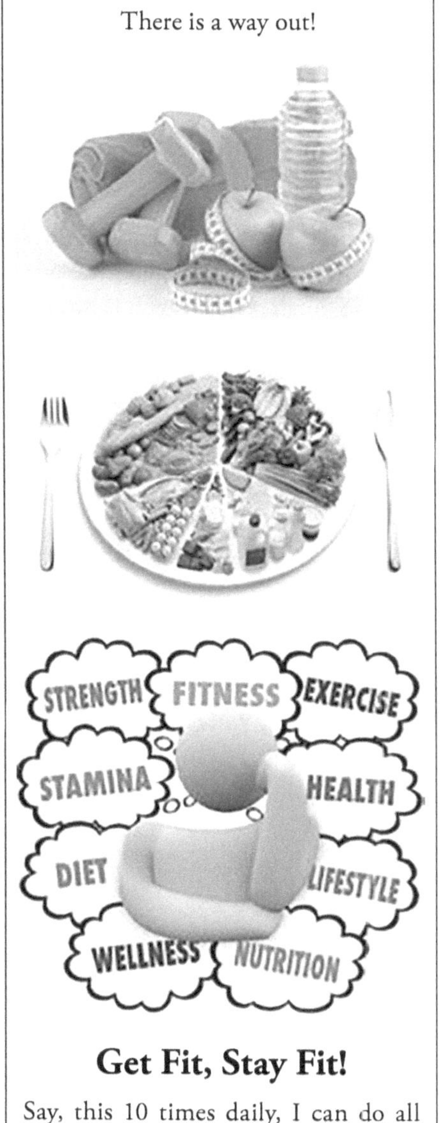

Get Fit, Stay Fit!

Say, this 10 times daily, I can do all things in Christ who Strengthens me!

Philippians 4:13

Say No To Overeating!

Pardon me but, I'm sorry that I could not find anything positive about over-weightiness and obesity. If you finds something positive, post it, let us all know, otherwise see you at boot-camp! You can do it, you MUST do it!

Get The Weight Off And Keep It Off!

Now before I get off the subject of obesity let me make it crystal clear that it is not my intention to offend the overweight population, not at all. I am here to help, you already know it is not healthy to go on this way, your doctor have also told you this. Over eating and not exercising is not good period, it does effect job performance, not only that it effects your entire life and those who will have to care for you later on.

Obesity is NOT good!

It's true obesity or being overweight is not good but today you can change all that, I do believe if you keep doing my boot camp and asking God for help, plus stay in his word, you'll be able to get the weight off and keep it off. It won't be easy, it's going to take at least a year to see major results but it will be well worth it in the end I promise you. Just stay committed and focus you can do it I know you can, look to Jesus he's the man with the real fitness plan!

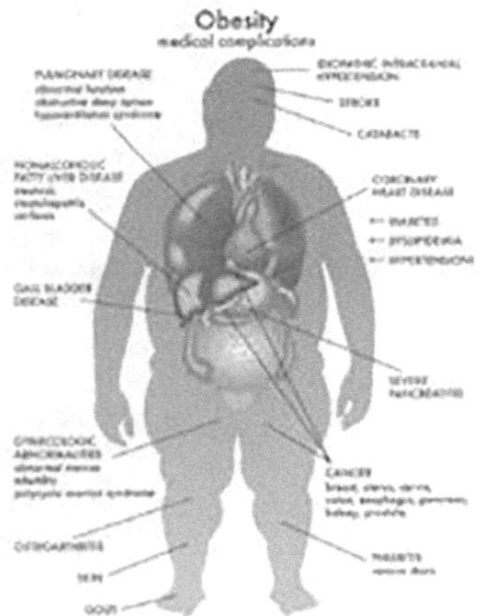

Obviously Yours Is Not Working!

 Miss Asondra StarN'air

Staying Active Matters!

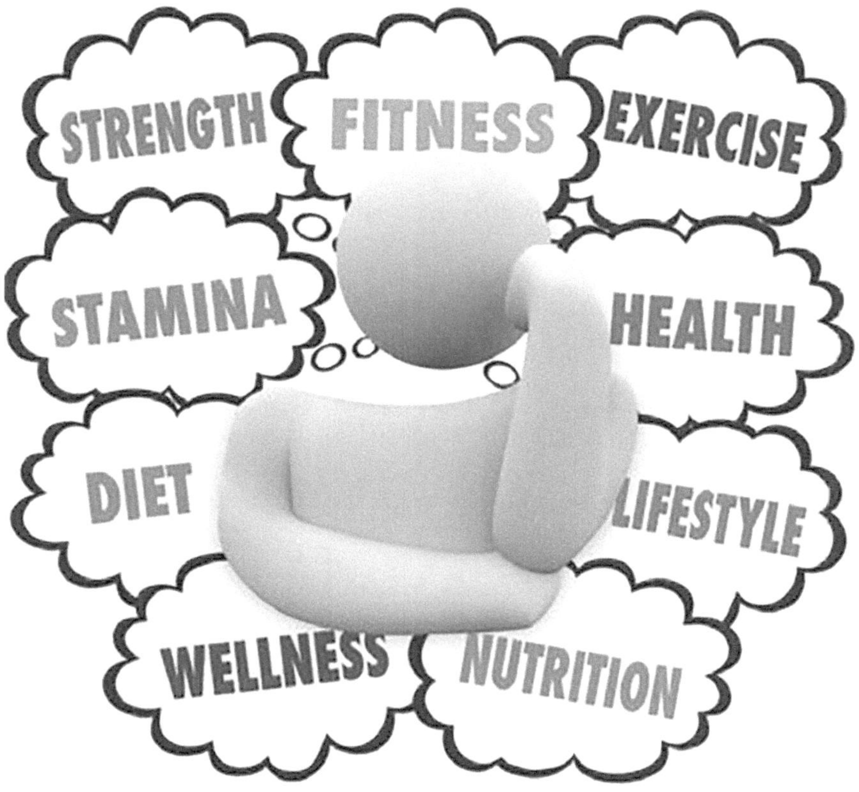

Eating The Right Foods does Too!

Scriptures On Physical Fitness

1 Corinthians 6:19-20 - What? know ye not that your body is the temple of the Holy Ghost [which is] in you, which ye have of God, and ye are not your own? *(Read More...)*

Philippians 4:13 - I can do all things through Christ which strengtheneth me.

1 Corinthians 3:17 - If any man defile the temple of God, him shall God destroy; for the temple of God is holy, which [temple] ye are.

1 Corinthians 9:24-27 - Know ye not that they which run in a race run all, but one receiveth the prize? So run, that ye may obtain.

1 Timothy 4:8 - For bodily exercise profiteth little: but godliness is profitable unto all things, having promise of the life that now is, and of that which is to come.

1 Corinthians 3:16 - Know ye not that ye are the temple of God, and [that] the Spirit of God dwelleth in you?

Corinthians 9:27 - But I keep under my body, and bring [it] into subjection: lest that by any means, when I have preached to others, I myself should be a castaway.

Peter 1:5-6 - And beside this, giving all diligence, add to your faith virtue; and to virtue knowledge;

1 Corinthians 10:31 - Whether therefore ye eat, or drink, or whatsoever ye do, do all to the glory of God.

Romans 12:1 - I beseech you therefore, brethren, by the mercies of God, that ye present your bodies a living sacrifice, holy, acceptable unto God, [which is] your reasonable service.

1 Corinthians 6:19 - What? know ye not that your body is the temple of the Holy Ghost [which is] in you, which ye have of God, and ye are not your own?

Corinthians 9:26 - I therefore so run, not as uncertainly; so fight I, not as one that beateth the air:

Romans 14:20 - For meat destroy not the work of God. All things indeed [are] pure; but [it is] evil for that man who eateth with offence.

   MISS ASONDRA STARN'AIR

<u>**Galatians 5:22-23**</u> - But the fruit of the Spirit is love, joy, peace, longsuffering, gentleness, goodness, faith,

<u>**Daniel 1:10-16**</u> - And the prince of the eunuchs said unto Daniel, I fear my lord the king, who hath appointed your meat and your drink: for why should he see your faces worse liking than the children which [are] of your sort? then shall ye make [me] endanger my head to the king.

<u>**Isaiah 40:31**</u> - But they that wait upon the LORD shall renew [their] strength; they shall mount up with wings as eagles; they shall run, and not be weary; [and] they shall walk, and not faint.

<u>**1 Corinthians 6:12**</u> - All things are lawful unto me, but all things are not expedient: all things are lawful for me, but I will not be brought under the power of any.

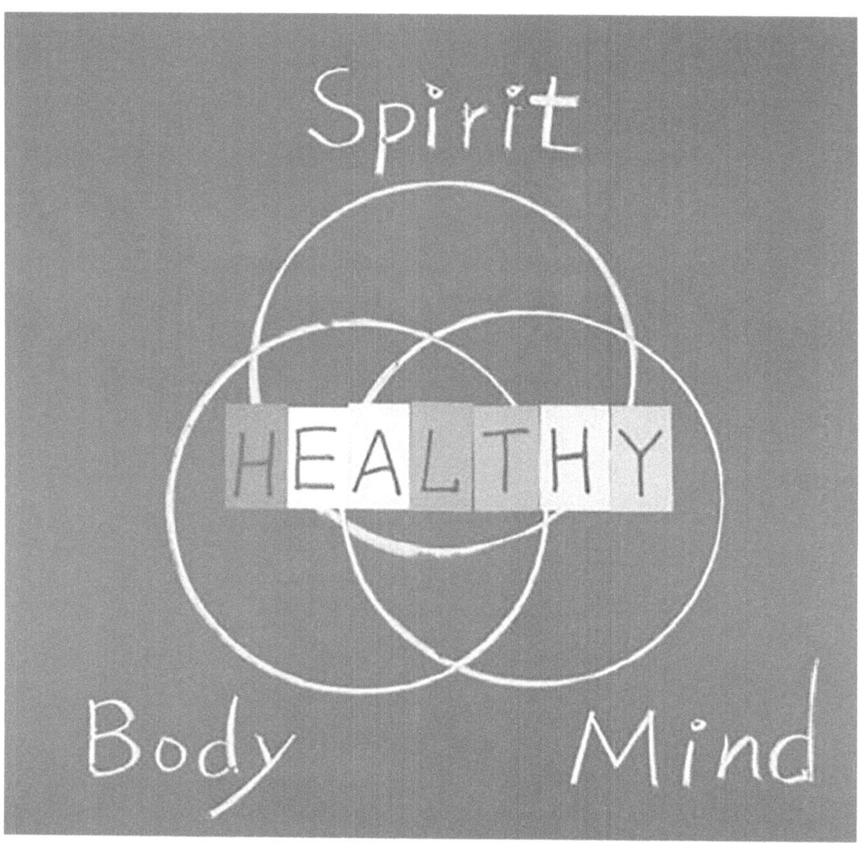

SECTION XVI

Debt Free Caregivers

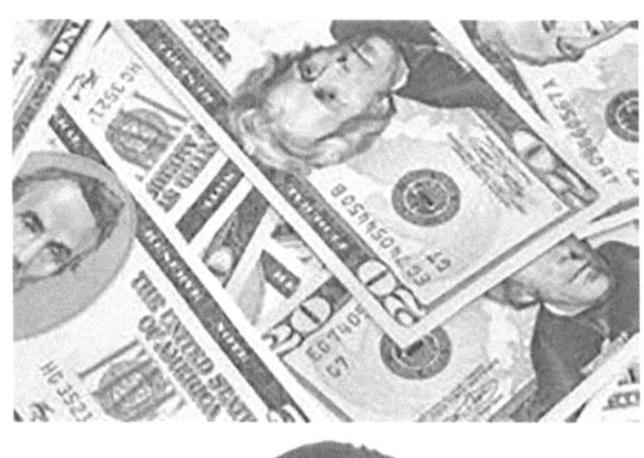

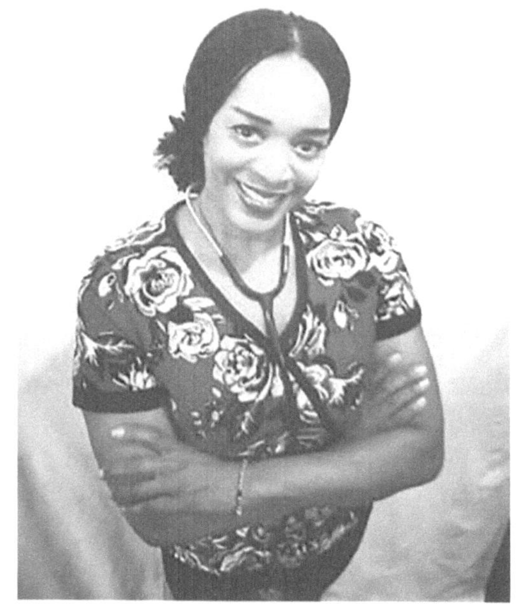

**Being in debt, Keeps us in Bondage
Let's Get Out, and Stay Out!**

Let's Eliminate Reckless Spending Once and For All!

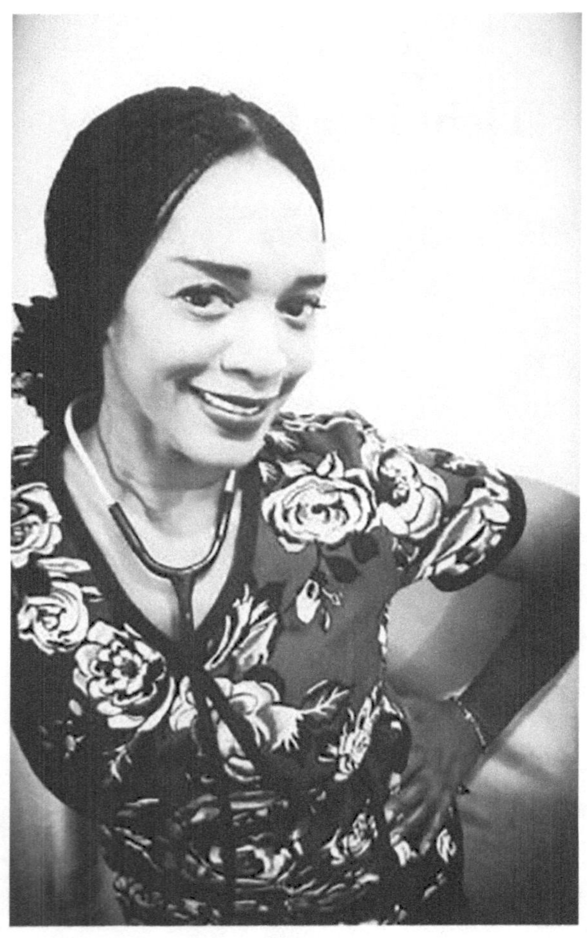

**Follow My debt Free Care Plan
If I Can Get Out Of debt, Anybody Can!**

Debt-Free Caregivers

Today there are so many caregivers working past exhaustion, trying to get out of debt. I used to be one of them, but not anymore. Now I live within my means and have found new ways of doing things.

Caregivers, did you know that when you are in debt, you are also in "slavery"?

Now you have to work, work, work, and keep on working way past retirement or drop dead —whichever comes first. Sorry, but there is no other way to wake some of you up.

Overworking causes stress, and stress is known as **"The Silent Killer."** Why? Because it shows very little symptoms until it's too late. So, caregivers, you cannot continue on this path—you just can't! It is not going to be easy; but like me, you can do it! You have to get started now, not tomorrow—***Right Now*** your life depends on it.

Caregivers, the first thing you need to do is acknowledge you are in financial trouble and you need help. Next, ask God to help you get out of debt. That's what I did and he helped me and he will help you too.

Keep in mind, not all debt is bad. I still owe on a mortgage—many people do. And, of course, big ticket items like, car notes, student loans, and now "mandatory health care." Just those alone can be financial burdens, so we don't want to keep adding to that. No! We cannot afford to keep spending like the "movie stars" we're not. It even catches up with them at some point. I'm sure you've read or heard about celebrities filing for bankruptcy.

Caregivers, listen, I'm looking out for you, and I just want to encourage you to keep fighting for freedom in every way possible especially in your finances. Being in debt allows this world and others to control us, keep us in bondage. And sometimes cause us to do things we ought not be doing; in a "nut shell", we become "The Tail and not The head"! Slaves, overworked, stressed out, sick, and not doing so well. **Deut. 28:13** We don't need that **"GOD Can HELP!"**

Pretty soon, you'll be on your way to debt-free living. It won't be easy, but it'll be worth it in the end. But, let me warn you, it's going to be hard work, it's going to take a lot of discipline over fleshly desires, determination, and patience. Caregivers, you can do it! **"Start Right Now!"**

Tools You Can Use

You Can do it!

Make That Change!

- Make changes inside your home, down grade services. home phone, cell phone and cable.
- Home owners turn down your hot water and save 20 to 30 dollars per month. Want to save even more, put your hot water tank on vacation in the summer time.
- Do all your own personal grooming, learn to do your own eye lashes ladies.
- Cut up all your credit cards except one—for emergencies.
- Contact a debt consolidator.
- Choose free entertainment.
- Have your wine at home, drink ginger ale at social events.
- Reduce grocery bill by 30 percent or more if you can.
- Eat at home more. eat out once a month.
- Purchase a newly used car; never pay sticker price.
- Shop at trendy thrift stores.
- Homeowners, contact your mortgage company see if you can get a modification on your mortgage all you have to do is apply. I did and my house note decrease significantly.
- Stay in prayer and work with God!

Overworking is bad for us in the end the key to getting out of debt is GOD!

Debt Free Prayer For Caregivers

Dear God, I have finally realized, I need help. I can no longer go on this way. Being in debt puts a lot of pressure on me and my family.

Show me how to get and stay out of Debt. I want to be the lender not the borrower, the head and not the tail.

I am ready to make changes right now, just tell me what you want me to do and I'll start to do it. I can't do it without you Lord, please help me!

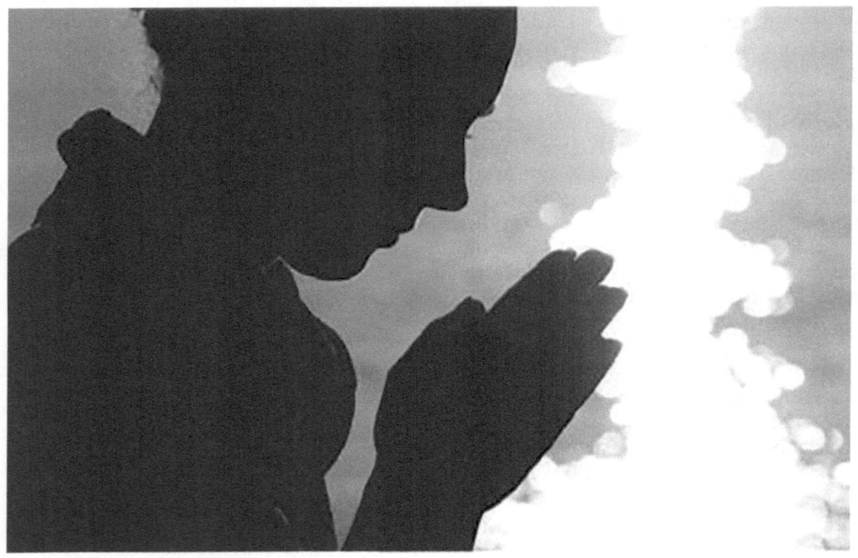

In Jesus name **Amen**

 MISS ASONDRA STARN'AIR

Debt Free Affirmations

1. I am Debt free
2. I am making smarter spend choices
3. I realized I do not need what I think I need.
4. I am cutting up my credit card except one for emergencies
5. I will began to pay debt off one by one, starting now
6. I will ask God to help me be a better steward over my money
7. I will give God his first fruits from now on, 10% of whatever I make now goes to God.
8. I am a giver not a taker
9. I will trust God, to provide all my needs from now on.
10. I will always have more than enough
11. I am prosperous in all I do
12. The less debt, the more blessing I have
13. I will save and save and stay debt free.
14. I have come to realize it is better to give than to receive.
15. I manage my money well, I have taken back control over my spending, I'm a lot happier now.

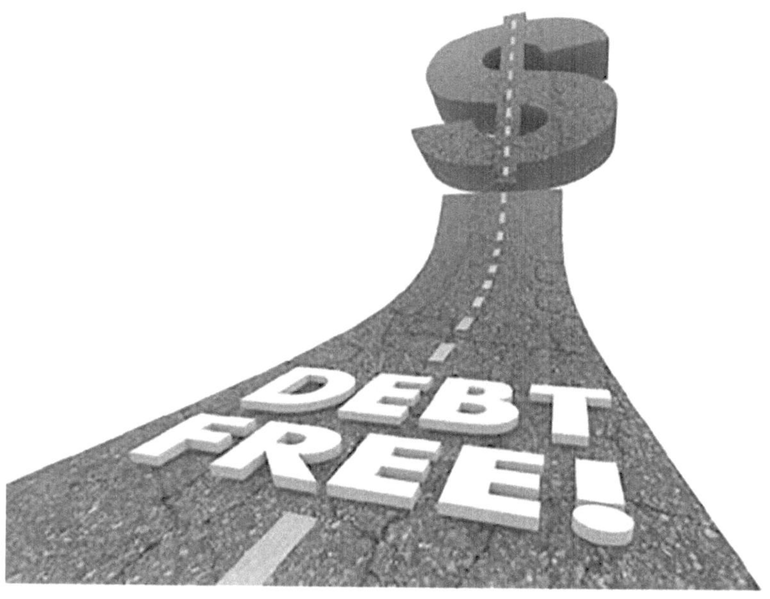

What The Bible Says About debt

Debt, The New Slavery!

Most Relevant Verses

Romans 13:8
Verse Concepts
Owe nothing to anyone except to love one another; for he who loves his neighbor has fulfilled the law.

Proverbs 22:7
Verse Concepts
The rich rules over the poor, And the borrower becomes the lender's slave.

Psalm 37:21
Verse Concepts
The wicked borrows and does not pay back, But the righteous is gracious and gives.

Matthew 6:24
Verse Concepts
"No one can serve two masters; for either he will hate the one and love the other, or he will be devoted to one and despise the other You cannot serve God and wealth.

Ecclesiastes 5:5
Verse Concepts
It is better that you should not vow than that you should vow and not pay.

Proverbs 21:5
Verse Concepts
The plans of the diligent lead surely to advantage, But everyone who is hasty comes surely to poverty.

Proverbs 13:11
Verse Concepts
Wealth obtained by fraud dwindles, But the one who gathers by labor increases it.

Deuteronomy 15:6
Verse Concepts
"For the LORD your God will bless you as He has promised you, and you will lend to many nations, but you will not borrow; and you will rule over many nations, but they will not rule over you.

Proverbs 17:18
Verse Concepts
A man lacking in sense pledges and becomes guarantor in the presence of his neighbor.

  MISS ASONDRA STARN'AIR

Caregiver's Old Monthly Budget Expense Sheet

Tithes and offering Amount _______________________________________

Mortgage /Rent Amount ____

Mortgage insurance Amount ______________________________________

Car loan Amount ____

Car Insurance Amount ____

Health Care insurance Amount ____________________________________

Daycare /co pay Amount ____

Electric bill Amount ____

Gas bill Amount ____

Cable Amount ____

Home phone Amount ____

Internet Amount ____

Cell phone bill Amount ____

Garbage Collection Amount ______________________________________

Union Dues Amount ____

Credit Cards Total combined _____________________________________

1 _______________________ Amount ___________________________

2 _______________________ Amount ___________________________

3 _______________________ Amount ___________________________

4 _______________________ Amount ___________________________

5 _______________________ Amount ___________________________

Hair Salon expense Amount ______________________________________

Household item expense Amount ___________________________________

Groceries Amount ____

Pet insurance Amount ____

Pet care / food Amount ____

College loan bill Amount ____

Other Amount ____

Caregiver's New Monthly Budget Expense Sheet

Total Saving _____________________________________
Tithes and offering Amount _____________________________
Mortgage /Rent Amount _________________________________
Mortgage insurance Amount ______________________________
Car loan Amount _______________________________________
Car Insurance Amount ___________________________________
Health Care insurance Amount ___________________________
Daycare /co pay Amount _________________________________
Electric bill Amount __________________________________
Gas bill Amount _______________________________________
Cable Amount ____
Home phone Amount _____________________________________
Internet Amount _______________________________________
Cell phone bill Amount ________________________________
Garbage Collection Amount _____________________________
Union Dues Amount _____________________________________
Credit Cards Total combined ___________________________
1 _____________________ Amount ________________________
2 _____________________ Amount ________________________
3 _____________________ Amount ________________________
4 _____________________ Amount ________________________
5 _____________________ Amount ________________________
Hair Salon expense Amount _____________________________
Household item expense Amount _________________________
Groceries Amount ______________________________________
Pet insurance Amount __________________________________
Pet care / food Amount________________________________
College loan bill _____________________________________

"Prosperity Comes From God, Not From A Job!"

JER 29:11: "For I know the plans I have for you," declares the LORD, "plans to prosper you and not to harm you, plans to give you hope and a future."

ECC 5:19: "Moreover, when God gives someone wealth and possessions, and the ability to enjoy them, to accept their lot and be happy in their toil—this is a gift of God."

ECC 5:19: "Moreover, when God gives someone wealth and possessions, and the ability to enjoy them, to accept their lot and be happy in their toil—this is a gift of God."

Prov 10:22: "The blessing of the LORD brings wealth, without painful toil for it."

PROV 11:25: "A generous person will prosper; whoever refreshes others will be refreshed."

3 John 1:2: "Beloved, I pray that you may prosper in all things and be in health, just as your soul prospers."

ROM 8:32: "He who did not spare his own Son, but gave him up for us all—how will he not also, along with him, graciously give us all things?"

PROV 28:27: "Those who give to the poor will lack nothing..."

Gen 26:12-13: "Isaac planted crops in that land and the same year reaped a hundredfold, because the LORD blessed him. The man became rich, and his wealth continued to grow until he became very wealthy."

Deut 8:18: "But remember the LORD your God, for it is he who gives you the ability to produce wealth, and so confirms his covenant, which he swore to your ancestors, as it is today."

PHIL 4:19: "And my God will meet all your needs according to the riches of his glory in Christ Jesus.

PS 115:13-14: "he will bless those who fear the LORD— small and great alike. May the LORD cause you to flourish, both you and your children. May you be blessed by the LORD, the Maker of heaven and earth."

Ps 37:3-5,11: "Trust in the LORD and do good; dwell in the land and enjoy safe pasture. Take delight in the LORD, and he will give you the desires of your heart..."

COR 9:6-7: "Remember this: Whoever sows sparingly will also reap sparingly, and whoever sows generously will also reap generously. Each of you should give what you have decided in your heart to give, not reluctantly or under compulsion, for God loves a cheerful giver."

Phil 4:19: "And my God shall supply all your need according to His riches in glory by Christ Jesus.

2 Cor 9:8: "And God is able to bless you abundantly, so that in all things at all times, having all that you need, you will abound in every good work."

Rom 8:32: "He who did not spare his own Son, but gave him up for us all— how will he not also, along with him, graciously give us all things?"

ISA 58:10-11: "And if you spend yourselves in behalf of the hungry and satisfy the needs of the oppressed, then your light will rise in the darkness, and your night will become like the noonday... You will be like a well-watered garden, like a spring whose waters never fail."

2 CHR 31:21: "In everything that he undertook in the service of God's temple and in obedience to the law and the commands, he sought his God and worked wholeheartedly. And so he prospered."

2 CHR 26:5: "He sought God during the days of Zechariah, who instructed him in the fear of God. As long as he sought the LORD, God gave him success."

LEV 26:3-5: "If you follow my decrees and are careful to obey my commands, I will send you rain in its season, and the ground will yield its crops and the trees their fruit. Your threshing will continue until grape harvest and the grape harvest will continue until planting, and you will eat all the food you want and live in safety in your land."

 Miss Asondra StarN'air

Deut 6:3: "Hear, Israel, and be careful to obey so that it may go well with you and that you may increase greatly in a land flowing with milk and honey..."

MAL 3:10: "Bring the whole tithe into the storehouse, that there may be food in my house. Test me in this," says the LORD Almighty, "and see if I will not throw open the floodgates of heaven and pour out so much blessing that there will not be room enough to store it."

PROV 3:9-10: "Honor the LORD with your wealth, with the firstfruits of all your crops; 10 then your barns will be filled to overflowing, and your vats will brim over with new wine."

ACTS 14:17: "Yet he has not left himself without testimony: He has shown kindness by giving you rain from heaven and crops in their seasons; he provides you with plenty of food and fills your hearts with joy."

1 JOHN 5:14-15: "This is the confidence we have in approaching God: that if we ask anything according to his will, he hears us. And if we know that he hears us—whatever we ask—we know that we have what we asked of him."

JER 17:7-8: "But blessed is the one who trusts in the LORD, whose confidence is in him. They will be like a tree planted by the water that sends out its roots by the stream. It does not fear when heat comes; its leaves are always green. It has no worries in a year of drought and never fails to bear fruit."

Matt 6:31-33: "So do not worry, saying, 'What shall we eat?' or 'What shall we drink?' or 'What shall we wear?' For the pagans run after all these things, and your heavenly Father knows that you need them. But seek first his kingdom and his righteousness, and all these things will be given to you as well."

Ps 92:12-14: "The righteous will flourish like a palm tree, they will grow like a cedar of Lebanon; planted in the house of the LORD, they will flourish in the courts of our God. They will still bear fruit in old age, they will stay fresh and green,"

Ps 85:12: "The LORD will indeed give what is good, and our land will yield its harvest."

Ps 84:11-12: "For the LORD God is a sun and shield; the LORD bestows favor and honor; no good thing does he withhold from those whose walk is blameless. LORD Almighty, blessed is the one who trusts in you."

Ps 37:25-26: "I was young and now I am old, yet I have never seen the righteous forsaken or their children begging bread. They are always generous and lend freely; their children will be a blessing."

Tim 6:10: "For the love of money is a root of all kinds of evil, for which some have strayed from the faith in their greediness, and pierced themselves through with many sorrows."

Eph 6:8: "because you know that the Lord will reward each one for whatever good they do, whether they are slave or free."

Gal 6:7: "Do not be deceived: God cannot be mocked. A man reaps what he sows."

Cor 9:10: "Now he who supplies seed to the sower and bread for food will also supply and increase your store of seed and will enlarge the harvest of your righteousness."

2 Cor 9:6: "Remember this: Whoever sows sparingly will also reap sparingly, and whoever sows generously will also reap generously."

2 Cor 8:9: "For you know the grace of our Lord Jesus Christ, that though he was rich, yet for your sake he became poor, so that you through his poverty might become rich."

1 Cor 9:14: "In the same way, the Lord has commanded that those who preach the gospel should receive their living from the gospel.

CHR 29:11-12: "Yours, LORD, is the greatness and the power and the glory and the majesty and the splendor, for everything in heaven and earth is yours. Yours, LORD, is the kingdom; you are exalted as head over all. Wealth and honor come from you..."

Luke 6:38: "Give, and it will be given to you. A good measure, pressed down, shaken together and running over, will be poured into your lap. For with the measure you use, it will be measured to you."

 Miss Asondra StarN'air

Luke 5:4-7: "When he had finished speaking, he said to Simon, "Put out into deep water, and let down the nets for a catch."
Simon answered, "Master, we've worked hard all night and haven't caught anything. But because you say so, I will let down the nets."
When they had done so, they caught such a large number of fish that their nets began to break.
So they signaled their partners in the other boat to come and help them, and they came and filled both boats so full that they began to sink."

Matt 7:11: "If you, then, though you are evil, know how to give good gifts to your children, how much more will your Father in heaven give good gifts to those who ask him!"

Matt 6:19-21: "Do not store up for yourselves treasures on earth, where moths and vermin destroy, and where thieves break in and steal. But store up for yourselves treasures in heaven, where moths and vermin do not destroy, and where thieves do not break in and steal. For where your treasure is, there your heart will be also"

Ecc 2:26: "To the person who pleases him, God gives wisdom, knowledge and happiness, but to the sinner he gives the task of gathering and storing up wealth to hand it over to the one who pleases God..."

Prov 3:9-10: "Honor the LORD with your wealth, with the firstfruits of all your crops; then your barns will be filled to overflowing, and your vats will brim over with new wine"

Ps 113:7: "He raises the poor from the dust and lifts the needy from the ash heap;"

Ps 67:6: "The land yields its harvest; God, our God, blesses us. 7 May God bless us still, so that all the ends of the earth will fear him."

Ps 37:4: "Take delight in the LORD, and he will give you the desires of your heart."

Ps 34:9-10: "Fear the LORD, you his holy people, for those who fear him lack nothing."

Deut 11:13-15: "So if you faithfully obey the commands I am giving you today—to love the LORD your God and to serve him with all your heart and with all your soul— then I will send rain on your land in its season, both autumn and spring rains, so that you may gather in your grain, new wine and olive oil. I will provide grass in the fields for your cattle, and you will eat and be satisfied."

Job 36:11: "If they obey and serve him, they will spend the rest of their days in prosperity and their years in contentment"

Chron 1:12: "therefore wisdom and knowledge will be given you. And I will also give you wealth, possessions and honor, such as no king who was before you ever had and none after you will have."

1 Kings 10:1; 7: "When the queen of Sheba heard about the fame of Solomon and his relationship to the LORD, she came to test Solomon with hard questions.

7: But I did not believe these things until I came and saw with my own eyes. Indeed, not even half was told me; in wisdom and wealth you have far exceeded the report I heard."

Deut 30:9: "Then the LORD your God will make you most prosperous in all the work of your hands and in the fruit of your womb, the young of your livestock and the crops of your land. The LORD will again delight in you and make you prosperous, just as he delighted in your ancestors,"

Gen 39:2-4: "The LORD was with Joseph so that he prospered, and he lived in the house of his Egyptian master."

Gen 24:35: "The LORD has blessed my master abundantly, and he has become wealthy. He has given him sheep and cattle, silver and gold, male and female servants, and camels and donkeys."

SECTION XVII

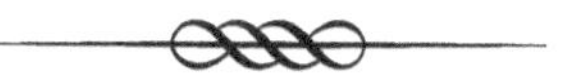

Caregiver's Back Office

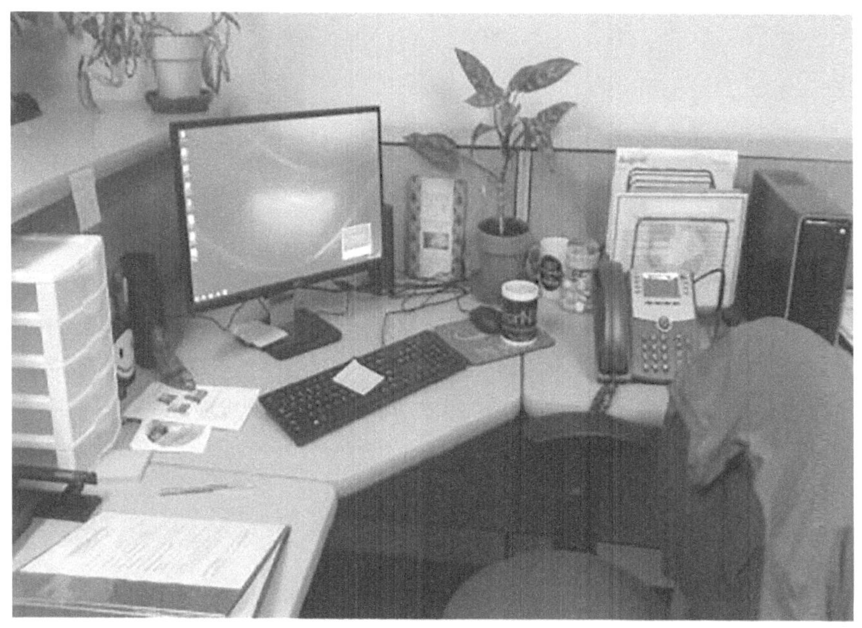

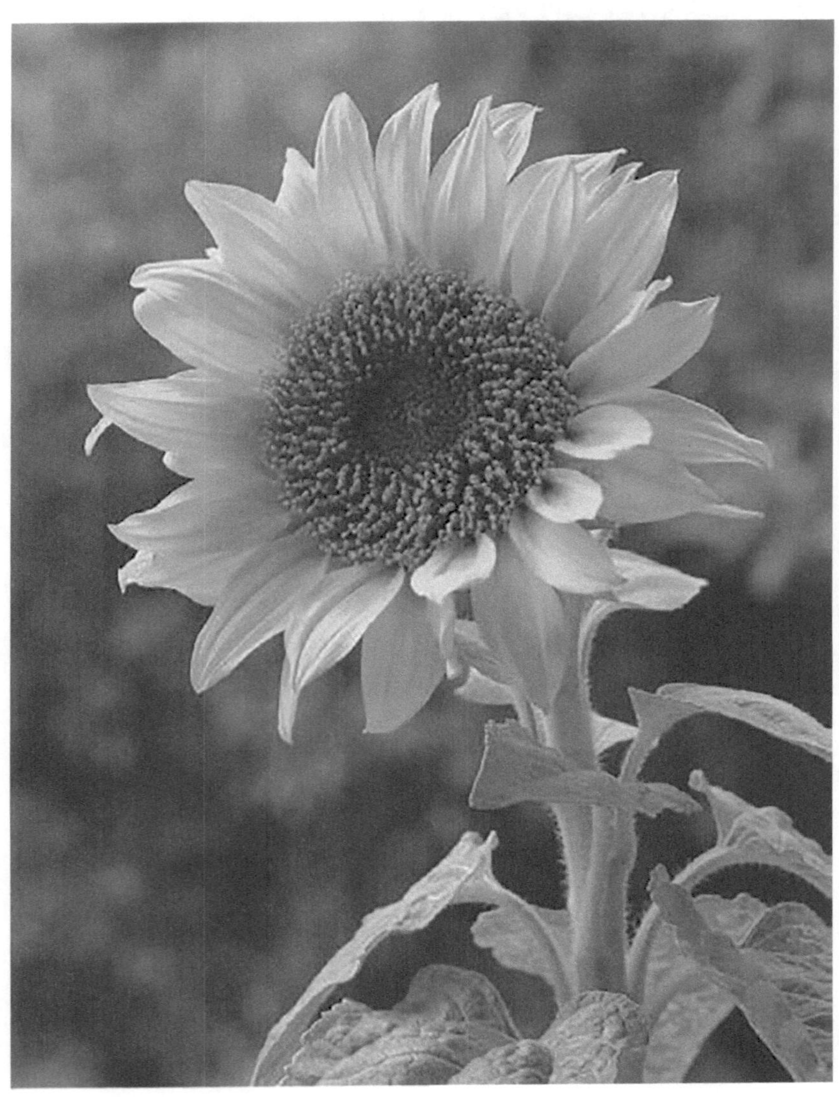

 MISS ASONDRA STARN'AIR

Welcome to your office, your workstation desk is already set up and ready to go. Hope you find everything you need.

Enjoy!

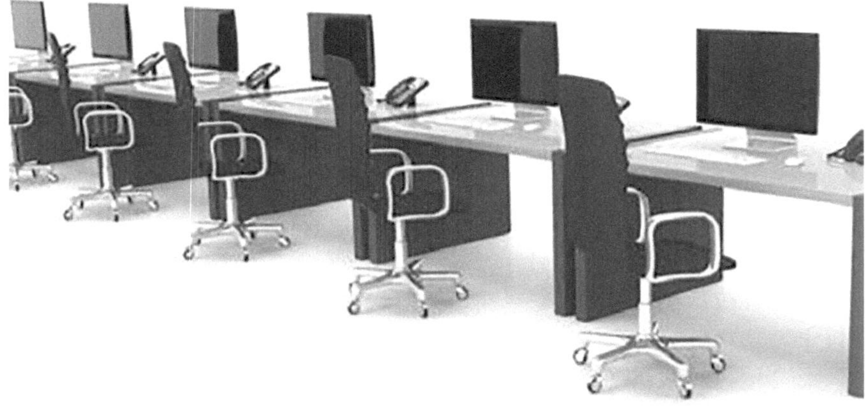

Your phone is ringing, answer it!

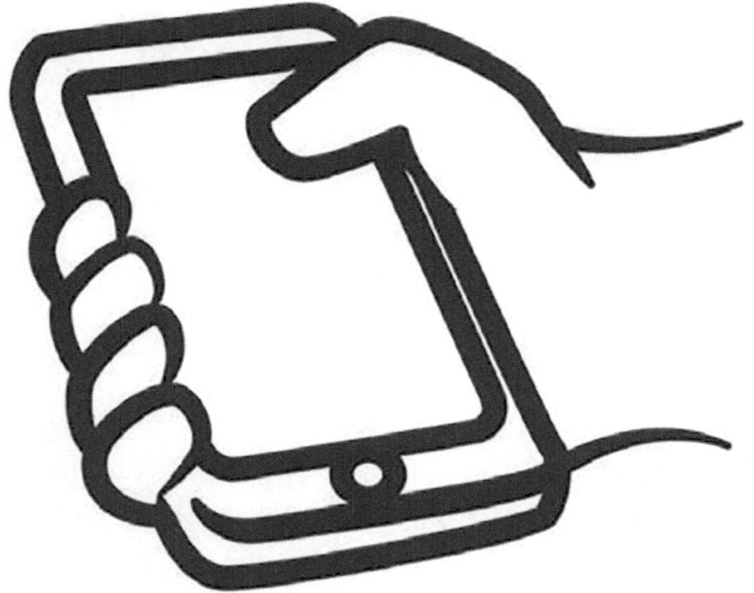

 Miss Asondra StarN'air

Hello, this is Jesus! I just want to say hello and remind you who you work for. Caregivers, you work for me. Although you can't see me, I am always watching you. I am with you always.

If you run into a problem—be it at work or in your everyday life—turn to my Word. It has the answer to everything!

Remember you're serving the King! And "Yes", I can help you with anything!

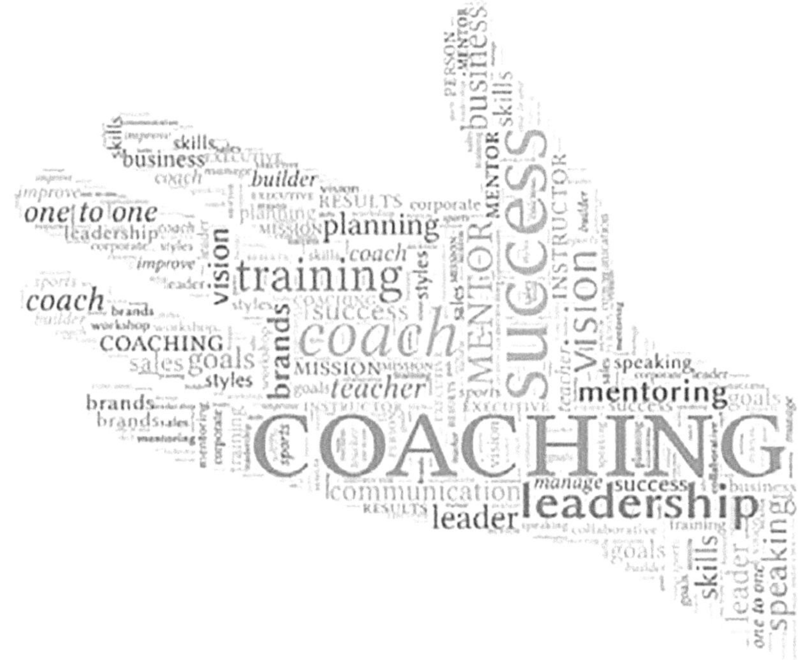

Caregivers Business Prospects

Companies name	Address	Who referred you?
1.		
2.		
3.		
4.		
5.		
6.		
7.		
8.		
9.		
10.		
11.		
12.		
13.		
14.		
15.		
16.		
17.		
18.		
19.		
20.		
21.		
22.		
23.		
24.		
25.		
26.		
27.		
28.		
29.		
30.		
31.		
32.		
33.		
34.		
35.		

 Miss Asondra StarN'air

Get Your Résumé Ready.
Time To Go On Interviews.

Acrylics off, nails short and professional.
Lose the fancy hairdos; be conservative.
Wear business attire or nearly new scrubs.

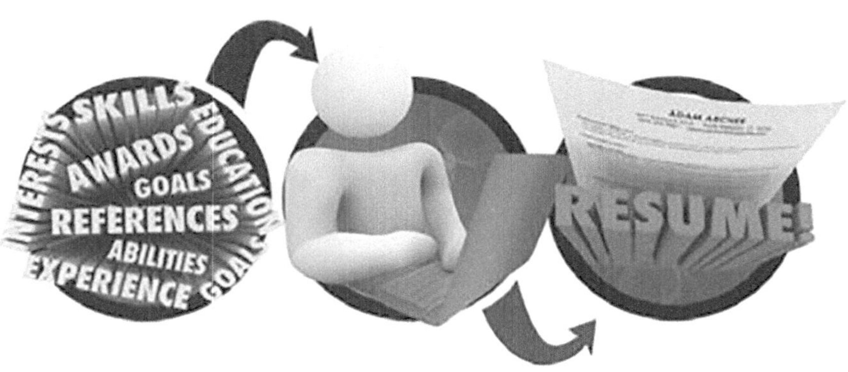

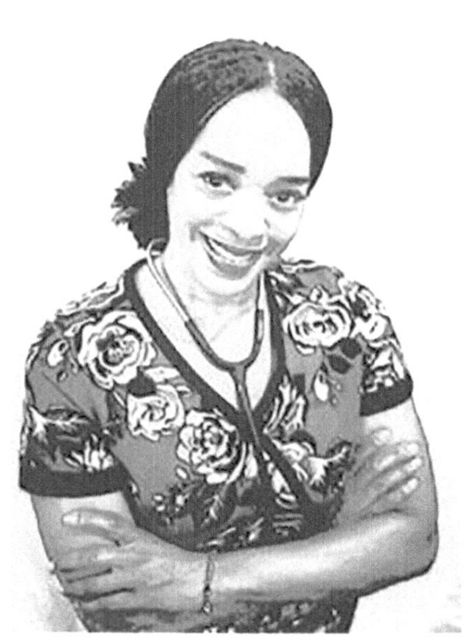

Business Tips

Mail off some thank you letters or send off emails the day after.

Keep this book with you, take it to your interviews, in- side your back office are all your references and interview questions. Ask some of those question. Be proud in a Godly way of course, let them see you have a Caregiver's Bible. I tell you, some will be quite impressed, you don't have to tell them everything that's in your book because this book was written by a caregiver, for caregivers not for employers, or bosses yet they will reap the results. **"Greatly!"** Simply put, **"Growth" and Development is the key.** Along with my burning desire to build and uplift **"Caregivers"** Worldwide. This has brought me joy. I left something behind. Your *Caregiver's Bible To Excellence* book is also a self- love book for those who are not ashamed of the gospel, nor ashamed to be *Caregivers For Christ!*

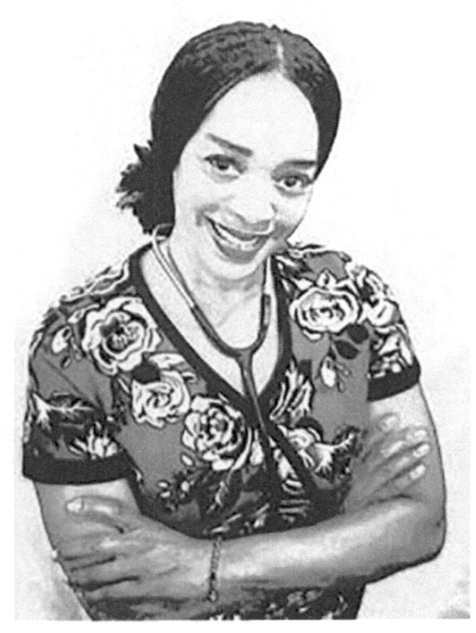

   Miss Asondra StarN'air

Ask Questions, Write Yours!

1. What makes your company /agency different from the rest? Why should I work here?
2. What's your policy on overtime?
3. How many caregivers work for your establishment? How many of them are **STNAs** and are there pay differentiation between **HHA** and **STNAs**—if not, why?
4. What is your idea of an excellent caregiver?
5. Are you a franchise? Do you have other affiliates and multiple locations?

More Questions, Write them below!

6. ____
7. ____
8. ____
9. ____
10. ____

Always, always ask intelligent questions; it indicates you are serious about your profession and that you too are being selective. Remember You are not an aide, you are a **'Professional Caregiver'** with a promise, that you will provide excellent services. Employers must pay for quality caregivers now or pass on the job. Shake the dust off your feet and go to more interviews. **"New Day Caregivers"**, YOU must **"Stick To Your Guns,"** don't give in, wait it out, **"Trust God!"** For **"We"** are not the aides of the past generation, oh no, on the contrary, *'A Caregiver's Bible To Excellence'*, has given you all something that will last, **"JESUS!"**

And with him on our side, *Caregivers All Over the World Shall Rise!*

Say **"No"** to **"Poverty Wages"** or **Crumbs.**
Your Freedom Has Just Begun!

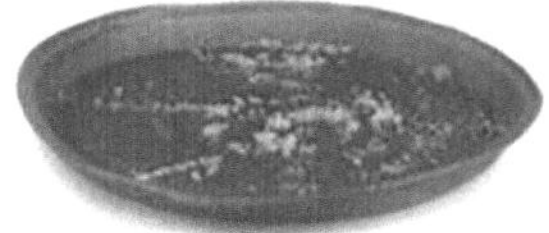

No More Crumbs!

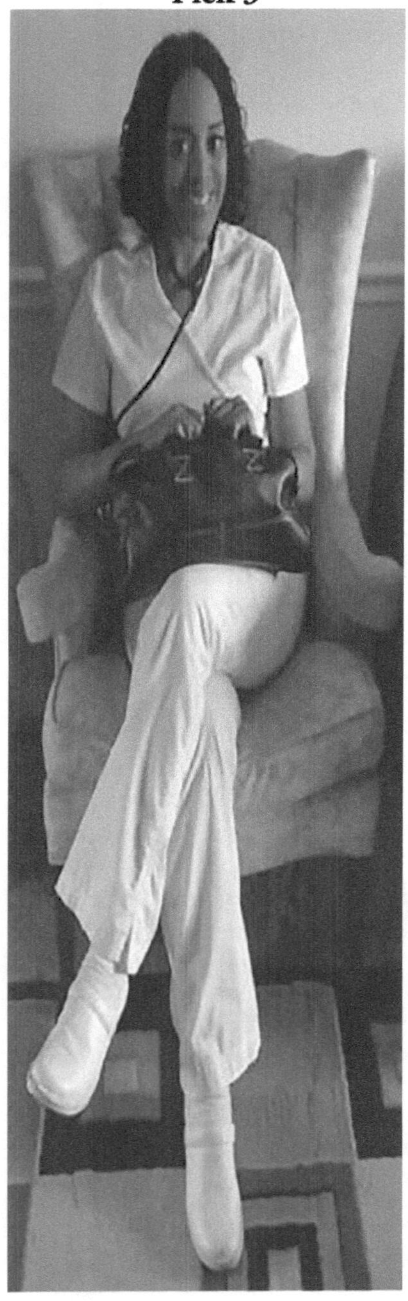

Caregivers Questions

- Why should I choose your agency over your competitors?
- Does your establishment offer professional benefit packages for caregivers?
- Is it okay that I'm called by my name or "caregiver" as opposed to being called an aide?
- Why do you like working for this company/agency?
- Do you have a policy put in place that stops workplace bullies? If so, what are they?
- Do you have affiliates? If so, who are they?
- What about fund-raisers? For example, breast cancer drives, Red Cross, etc.
- Are there any opportunities for advancement/paid tuition?
- What's your company percentage turnover of caregivers each year, and is it stabilizing?
- Why do you think caregivers are leaving? What changes are being implemented to help decrease instability so the company can reach its economic goal, and does that goal include yearly raises for caregivers?
- What's the overall vision and goals for this company/agency?

The Biggest Question of All!

What is your offer and does it include medical and paid vacations?

'No More Crumbs!'

Sample Cover letter

Your name

66346 Dover Avenue, Cleveland Ohio 44125, Email: Jane Doe@Gmail.com
Phone: 216-261-8865

July 15, 2018

Linda Crawford
First Place Homecare Agency
1656 Beachwood Ohio 44127

Dear Hiring Manager,

I am writing in response to your ad seeking a Professional Certified Nursing Assistant. Your job posting states that you are in search of a skilled Certified Nurse Assistant with experience which describes me exactly.

My professionalism and positive attitude along competence, makes me a great candidate for this position. I take ownership of task quickly with confidence that I will succeed beyond expectation. Plus I am creative and a good problem solver and know my scope of implementation. Very friendly and team oriented too!

I believe I'm just what you are looking for and can be an access to your team.

Sincerely,

(Sign your name)

Sample Resume

CAREGIVER

Professional Summary

Skills

*   *

*   *

*   *

*   *

Education:

Qualification:

Work History:

Address, Phone Number, Email Address

   MISS ASONDRA STARN'AIR

Sample Thank You Letter

66346 Dover Avenue, Cleveland Ohio 44125, Email: Jane Doe@Gmail.com
Phone: 216-000-0001

July 15, 2018

Linda Crawford
First Place Homecare Agency
1656 Beachwood Ohio 44127

Dear Linda Crawford,

It was a pleasure to meet with you this week. I really appreciate you taking time out of your day to speak with me about the Caregivers position. I was especially impressed to hear that your agency is opening a second location soon. Congratulations!

During the interview, you asked, what makes me different from other caregivers and why I think I would be a great fit for your agency?

Well I'm sure you have some wonderful caregivers however there is only one of me, what makes me different is my work ethics' and flexibility. Plus I have over a decade of field experience. I understand too that teamwork makes the dream work and I am a team player.

There is no doubt in my mind that I'm what you need and looking for. I am positive I would be a great addition to your team and am excited at the prospect of joining your agency. If you have any other concerns or questions feel free to call me anytime.

Thanks again for your time and consideration.

Sincerely,

(Your Name)

Get Your House In Order!
(Be human resource–ready at all times.)

Caregiver, make sure you are up-to-date and current on the following:

- CPR
- First aid
- Nursing certifications and licenses
- Physical
- TB Shots
- Med Pass (optional)
- Yearly in-service requirements/ education
- Car Insurance
- Owner's Permits/ License Renewals
- Updated Résumés and Cover Letters
- Foster and Daycare Yearly Requirements
- All Other Important Documentations
- Daycare Childcare Records
- Shot Records for each Pet
- Post Updated Daycare State License
- Update All State Licenses
- Update changes in address, telephone numbers and name changes.

Forget- me -nots ,write them down below. This is your workstation, not mine.

-
-
-
-
-
-
-
-
-
-
-

Business References

Name	Occupation	Email	Phone No.

Personal References Name

Name	Email	Phone No.

Previous Employment List and dates

Company	Dates	Supervisor's name	Contact number or Email

Caregiver Referrals List

Hey caregivers did you know that many companies and agencies have a **'Caregiver to Caregiver' Referral Program?** Well they do. All you have to do is refer other quality caregivers like yourself and get paid. Each organization may be different so ask and find out what you need to do. But make sure **YOU** do all the documentations on who, what, when and where otherwise, you may find yourself having to prove you referred that person, I'm just sayin' people forget.

Below is a referral list for you to write in the names, companies and dates etc.

Full name of referred Company/Agency Person you talked to date of referral

1. ____

2. ____

3. ____

4. ____

5. ____

6. ____

7. ____

8. ____

9. ____

10. ____

11. ____

12. ____

13. ____

14. ____

15. ____

16. ____

17. ____

18. ____

19. ____

20. ____

Happy Birthday List

Name   Birthday

Important Numbers

Name   Number

          Miss Asondra StarN'air

Tax Write-Offs List

Items   Services

Caregiver's Notepad

Caregiver's Notepad

Caregiver's Notepad

 Miss Asondra StarN'air

Caregiver's Notepad

Caregiver's Notepad

Caregiver's Notepad

Business Prospects

Company / Agencies	Address	Contact Person	Referred By

Standard Questions For Each Potential Employer

- What is your idea of an excellent employee?
- Do you have affiliates—other companies you are connected with? If so, who are they?
- Are there opportunities for raises and advancements?
- What makes your company/agency different from the rest?
- What's the turnover rates of caregivers? What do you think is happening?
- Is there a benefit package for caregivers?
- How many Aides vs State Tested Nurse Assistance do you have, and is there a pay differentiation? If not, why?
- Does your company offer incentives, and bonuses?
- Are employees capped at forty hours a week? Can we do overtime?

Caregivers you can add your own set of questions these are some of mine. but you have to start asking important question especially if you want to be taken seriously and paid fairly. The bible says "You Have Not Because You Ask Not" **James 4:2**

March With Me! **They Want Quality Caregivers, We Want Quality Pay!** If they won't give it to us, walk away, nothing else to say! Tell them bye-bye, have a nice day! **NEXT...**

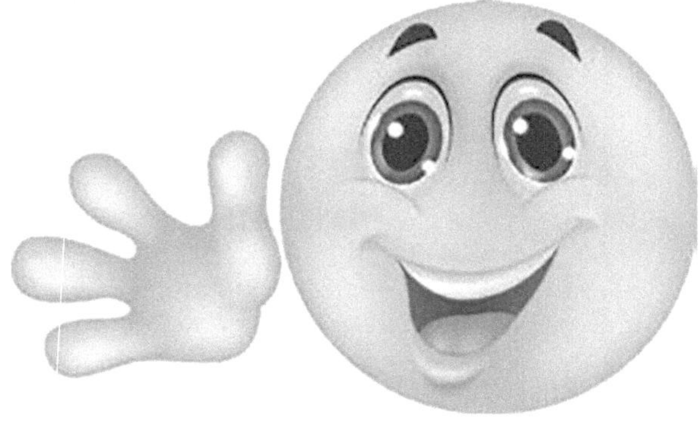

We work For Jesus, Not Man!

Colossians 3:17 And whatever you do, in word or deed, do everything in the name of the Lord Jesus, giving thanks to God the Father through him.

Colossians 3:23–24 Work willingly at whatever you do, as though you were working for the Lord rather than for people. Remember that the Lord will give you an inheritance as your reward, and that the Master you are serving is Christ.

Corinthians 10:31 Whether therefore ye eat, or drink, or whatsoever ye do, do all to the glory of God.

Romans 12:11–12 Never be lazy, but work hard and serve the Lord enthusiastically. Rejoice in our confident hope. Be patient in trouble, and keep on praying.

Don't talk about it; be about it. Walk the walk of excellence.

Proverbs 14:23–24 All hard work brings a profit, but mere talk leads only to poverty. The wealth of the wise is their crown, but the folly of fools yields folly.

Philippians 2:14 Do everything without grumbling or arguing.

Diligent hands and hard work always pay off in the end—always.

Timothy 2:6–7 And hardworking farmers should be the first to enjoy the fruit of their labor. Think about what I am saying. The Lord will help you understand all these things.

Proverbs 10:4–5 Lazy hands make for poverty, but diligent hands bring wealth. He who gathers crops in summer is a prudent son, but he who sleeps during harvest is a disgraceful son.

Proverbs 6:7–8 Though they have no prince or governor or ruler to make them work, they labor hard all summer, gathering food for the winter.

Proverbs 12:24 Diligent hands will rule, but laziness ends in forced labor.

Proverbs 28:19–20 A hard worker has plenty of food, but a person who chases fantasies ends up in poverty. The trustworthy person will get a rich reward, but a person who wants quick riches will get into trouble.

There is a difference between working hard and overworking yourself. Listen to your body—work, rest.

Psalm 127:1–2 Except the LORD build the house, they labour in vain that build it: except the LORD keep the city, the watchman waketh but in vain. It is vain for you to rise up early, to sit up late, to eat the bread of sorrows: for so he giveth his beloved sleep.

Ecclesiastes 1:2–3 "Everything is meaningless," says the Teacher, "completely meaningless!" What do people get for all their hard work under the sun?

Work, help others. Life is not about us—it's about caregiving to others.

 Miss Asondra StarN'air

Acts 20:35 I have shewed you all things, how that so labouring ye ought to support the weak, and to remember the words of the Lord Jesus, how he said, "It is more blessed to give than to receive."

Don't be lazy; work is what we are here for. It gives us meaning and a sense of accomplishment.

Proverbs 13:4 Lazy people want much but get little, but those who work hard will prosper.

2 Thessalonians 3:10 While we were with you, we gave you the order: "Whoever doesn't want to work shouldn't be allowed to eat."

2 Thessalonians 3:11–12 We hear that some people in your group refuse to work. They are doing nothing except being busy in the lives of others. Our instruction to them is to stop bothering others, to start working and earn their own food. It is by the authority of the Lord Jesus Christ that we are urging them to do this.

Proverbs 18:9–10 A lazy person is as bad as someone who destroys things. The name of the LORD is a strong fortress; the godly run to him and are safe.

Proverbs 20:13 If you love sleep, you will end in poverty. Keep your eyes open, and there will be plenty to eat!

Working for the devil is sure to send you to hell! We must make our living honestly.

Proverbs 13:11 Dishonest money dwindles away, but whoever gathers money little by little makes it grow.

Proverbs 4:14–17 Don't take the path of the wicked; don't follow those who do evil. Stay away from that path; don't even go near it. Turn around and go another way. The wicked cannot sleep until they have done something evil. They will not rest until they bring someone down. Evil and violence are their food and drink.

Motivation

Philippians 4:13 For I can do everything through Christ, who gives me strength.

Revelation 2:2–3 I know your deeds, your hard work, and your perseverance. I know that you cannot tolerate wicked people, that you have tested those who claim to be apostles but are not, and have found them false. You have persevered and have endured hardships for my name, and have not grown weary.

1 Corinthians 4:12–13 We work wearily with our own hands to earn our living. We bless those who curse us. We are patient with those who abuse us. We appeal gently when evil things are said about us. Yet we are treated like the world's garbage, like everybody's trash–right up to the present moment.

Genesis 29:18–21 Jacob loved Rachel. And he said, "I will serve you seven years for your younger daughter Rachel." Laban said, "It is better that I give her to you than that I should give her to any other man; stay with me." So Jacob served seven years for Rachel, and they seemed to him but a few days because of the love he had for her. Then Jacob said to Laban, "Give me my wife that I may go in to her, for my time is completed."

How are we doing so far?

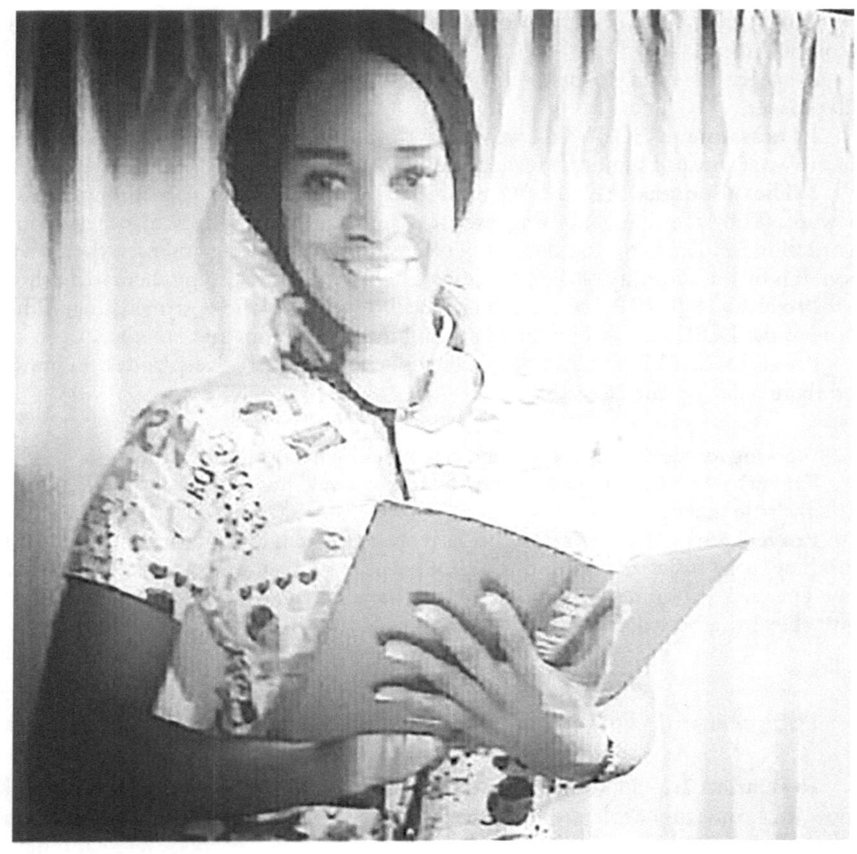

Hope you like your office.
It's a pleasure serving all of you!

**I also added a few more things you need to stay aware of
Keep turning the page, there's more...**

"SMILE"!
Your SMILE is Your Logo

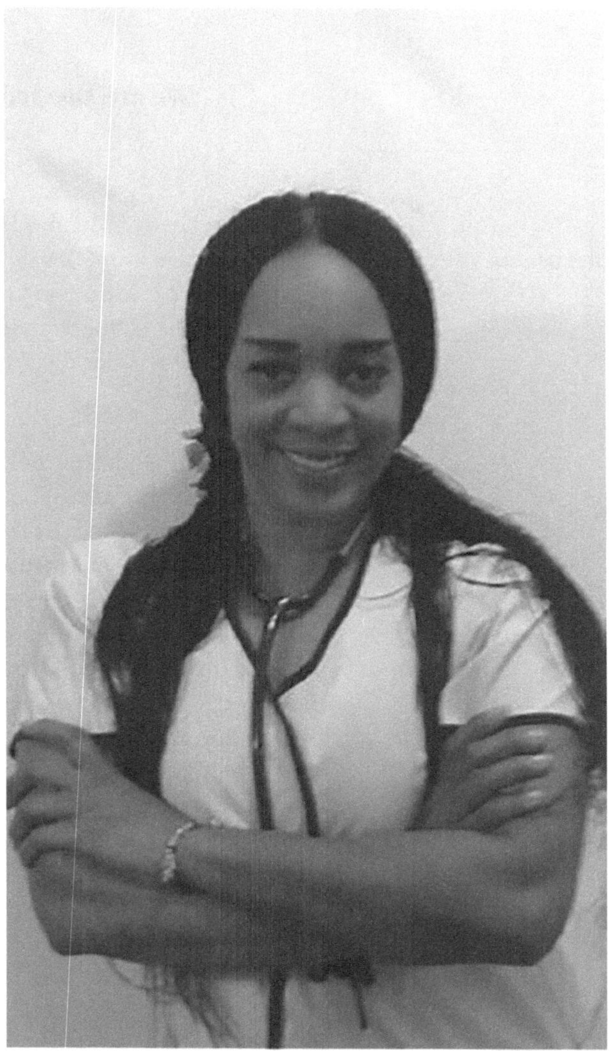

Your **PERSONALITY** is your Business Card,
How you leave others feeling after they have met
you becomes your **TRADEMARK so, "SMILE"!**

C. A. R. E. G. I. V. E. R. S.

Christ

Almighty

Reaches out to

Everybody, everywhere

Gives

Individuals

Varieties of gifts

Each

Received

Something Special

We are Blessed!

Caregivers, God has a plan for each and every one of us. There is no need to be jealous or envious of others. What is for you is for you. Nothing can stop God's plan for your life. **Isaiah 14:27.**

Get with God, let him love on you and make you whole. God has given his children special gifts, perhaps more than one. But it's up to us to use it, and do something with it, you see, we are more than caregivers. Caregivers we are dream builders too and I'm here to tell you God has big plans for those that are hardworking, faithful and true. The kind of caregiver you want to be is your choice it's up to you but as for me and my house we shall serve the **LORD**, I'm with **JESUS!** The Greatest Caregiver of All!
**Everybody's Got a Gift
If You Look Inside You'll Find It!**

Caregivers

Don't forget, when you are having troubles Jesus is on the main line call him up and tell him what you want or what you need. He loves you, and He cares for you, "YES", **"The Lord"** will help you!

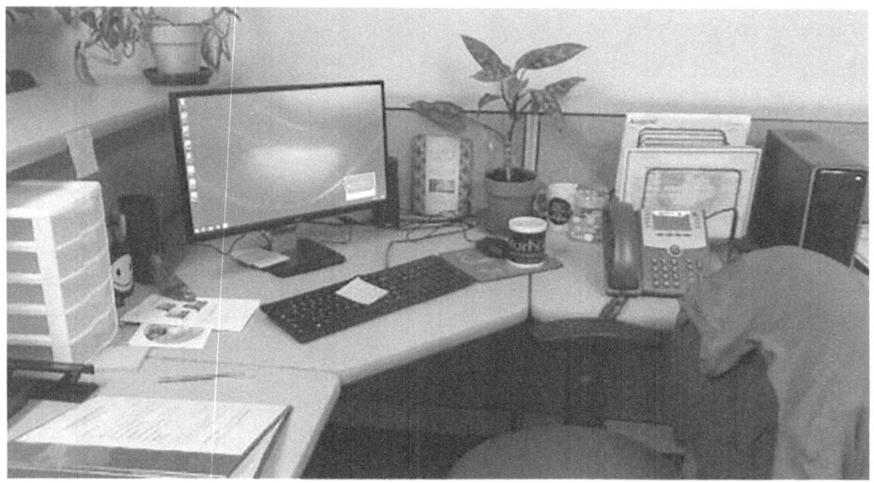

There is nothing God won't do
for those who obey and love him,
Absolutely Nothing!

Emergency Numbers for Caregivers

When your heart is troubled	call	John 14
When you feel abandon and alone	call	Psalms 23
When God seems far away	call	Psalms 91
When you are being set up or attacked	call	Psalms 27
When you are bitter and want to get even	call	Ephesians 4:31
When you are overwhelmed	call	Isaiah 40:28
When you're being tempted	call	James 1:13-18
When you need help	call	Psalms 46: 1-2
When you are worried	call	Philippians 4:6-7
When you are weak and need strength	call	Isaiah 41:10
When you need love	call	Jeremiah 31:3
When you need a Prosperity	call	Malachi 3:10
When you need wisdom	call	Proverbs 1-31
When you need rest	call	Psalms 127:2
When you need answers to life questions	call	Ecclesiastes 3:2
When you need a Friend	call	Proverbs 18:24
When you need a new life	call	Colossians 3:10 & 4:16
When you lack patients	call	Galatians 6:19
When you need peace	call	Philippians 4:6
When you are worried	call	Matthew 6:25-34
When you are lied on, slandered and persecuted	call	1 Peter 4:12-14 & John 15:18
When you are Afraid	call	Isaiah 41:10
When you are betrayed	call	Proverbs 19:5 & Ephesian 6:10-18
When you are sick	call	James 5:14-14 & 1st Peter 4:19
When you are down and out	call	Matthew 11:28-30
When you need "JOY"	call	Romans 12:12 & James 1:2-4

 Miss Asondra StarN'air

Abuse Pledge for Caregivers

- I will not allow those in my care to hit me.
- I will tell them **"It's Wrong"!**
- I will asks the individual to stop.
- I will not provide personal care until abuse stops, this is for my own protection and theirs.
- I will reassure the person that I am going to take excellent care of their needs and help pro- vide a safe environment for both of us but abuse is not allowed.
- I will take the necessary breaks in between to help bring balance to the situation.
- I will ask management for instructions on how to handle the situation when those in my care are abusive.
- If the abuse does not stop, I will no longer care for that particular person. Abuse of any kind is **WRONG** and must be dealt with spe cialist by the management team. Caregivers don't come to work to get punched, hit, kicked or spit on.
- My environment has to be a safe place for me to work in at all times.
- I will love and pray for those who hurt other people, but I will not be a victim anymore.

Bottom Line

'Abuse is Abuse' and anyone who does it must be stopped. No one should have to go to work and get abused, especially the caregiver, enough is enough!

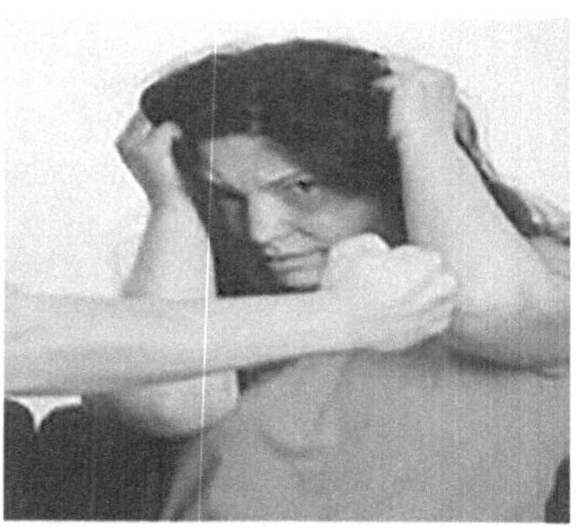

CAREGIVER ABUSE

1. Don't argue with the person.
2. Shift the conversation
3. Ask, how can I please you?
4. Show me how you want it done.
5. Excuse, yourself if it's safe to do so, take a bathroom break and breathe, ask God to help, go back out and start again.
6. Wait, let them talk, you listen. Be humble.
7. Come up with something creative to do with them.
8. If nothing is working, just do your work, give them space and time to cool down.
9. Don't ever take it personal. But report it.
10. Ask for help from your company or if you are a family care provider, take a break, use respite care.
11. Document the behaviors times and dates.
12. If the caregiver abuse does not get resolved come off that assignment and contact your ombudsman.

"Caregivers Matter"!

21st Century CareGivers, It's A New day!

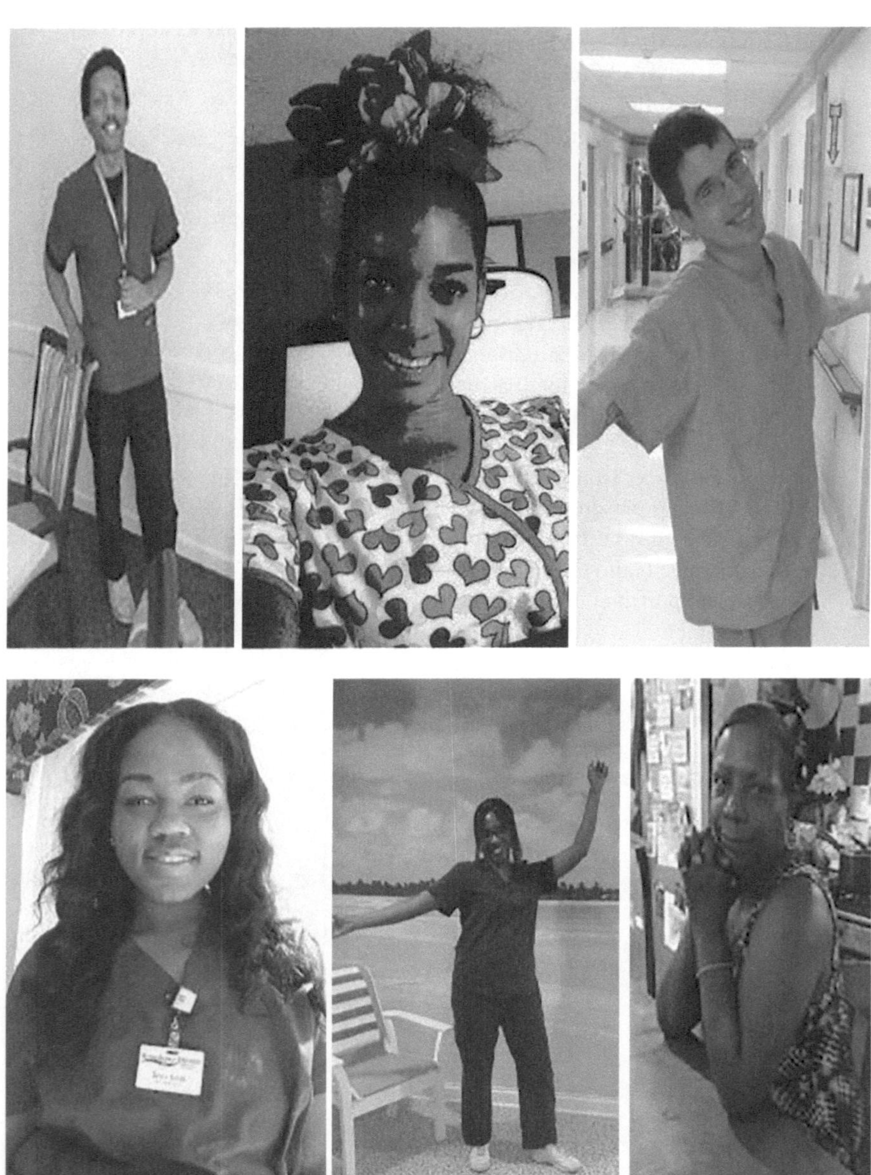

The New-Day Caregivers

When it comes to finding a job in the health-care industry, it is very important caregivers choose the right company or agency. It's not just about landing a job; it's about landing the right one. Ask yourself what does this company have to offer me and my family? Today's caregiver must not settle; we must begin to set high standards for ourselves. If the employer doesn't offer adequate wages and benefits, move on.

Trust in God! He is our main source; our daily bread comes for him. He will provide everything we need while we weed out employers who just want to keep us "aides" down and out. There are plenty of other options out there for us. Research shows caregivers are in such high demand. That's power in our hands, so let's stop settling for crumbs. Keep interviewing until you find the right fit. Keep asking questions too. It looks good on you, 'Yes it Does!'

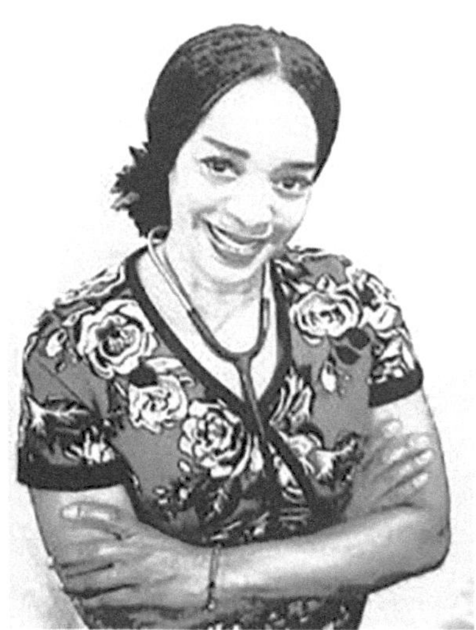

We Are New Day Caregivers "We Deliver"!

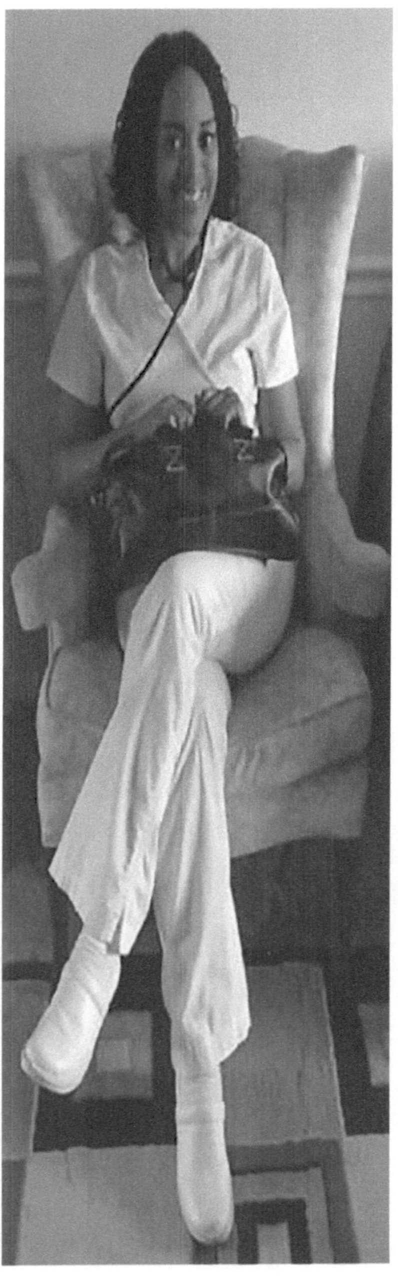

Caregivers Questions

- Why should I choose your agency over your competitors?
- Does your establishment offer professional benefit packages for caregivers
- Is it okay that I'm called by my name or "caregiver" as opposed to being called an aide?
- Why do you like working for this company/agency?
- Do you have a policy put in place that stops workplace bullies? If so, what are they?
- Do you have affiliates? Who are they?
- What about fund-raisers? For example, breast cancer drives, Red Cross, etc.
- Are there any opportunities for advancement/paid tuition?
- What's your company percentage turnover of caregivers each year, and is it stabilizing?
- Why do you think care givers are leaving? What changes are being implemented to help decrease instability so the company can reach its economic goal, and does that goal include yearly raises for caregivers?
- What's the overall vision and goals for this company/agency?

The biggest question of all!

What is your offer and does it include medical and paid vacations?

'No More Crumbs!'

Management

Developing a good management team is very important to running a successful organization. Managers must know how to manage and understand the qualities that make up good management. **Caregivers, look out for "YOU" too!**

These are some of the qualities we need to look for in management before we join the team:

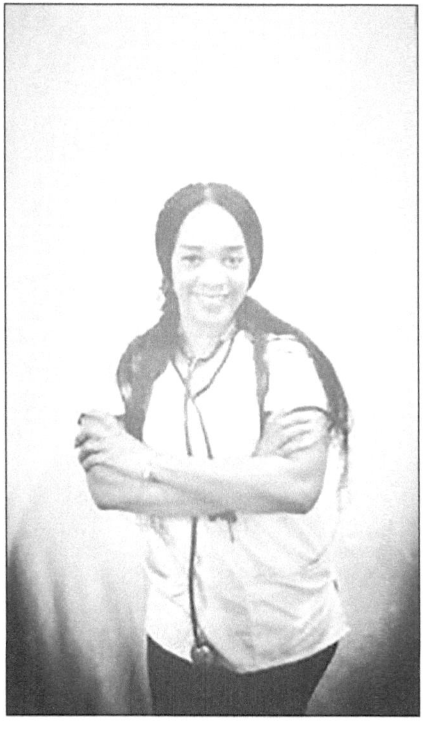

1. Appreciation of employees
2. Provide adequate and updated resources!
3. Be good listeners and are fair at making good decisions.
4. Empathetic and caring toward employees
5. Professionalism and kindness.
6. Great and honest leadership, no favoritism.
7. Easy and fair employee evaluations.
8. Offer incentives
9. Hospitality Management Skills.
10. Team Builder.

High Quality Management Matters!

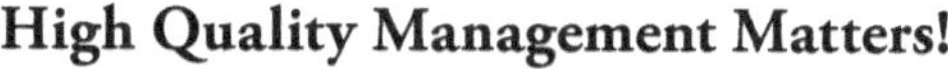

Hey Caregivers!

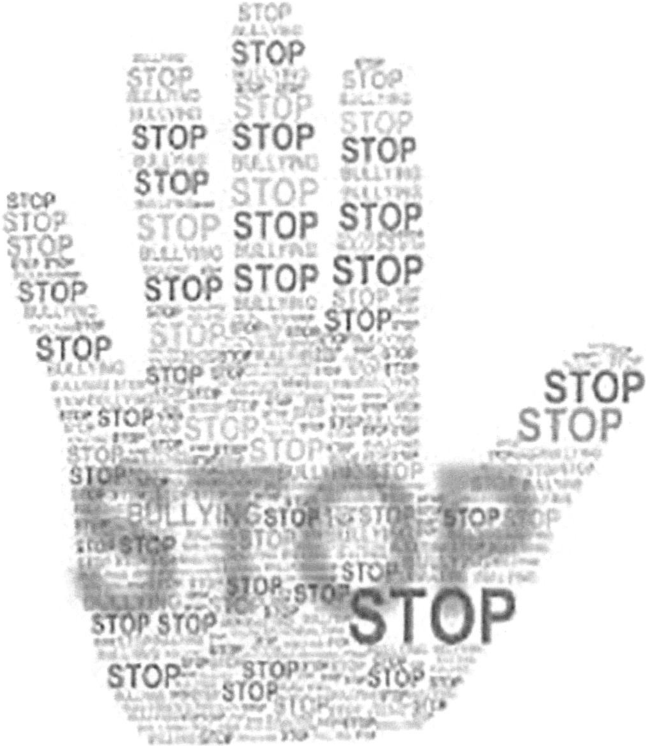

Should **"You"** Be doing That? Should **"You"** Be Wearing That?

 MISS ASONDRA STARN'AIR

The Interview

- Never ever wear jeans to an interview.
- Arrive at least fifteen minutes early.
- Make sure your cell phone is turned off.
- Stand until asked to be seated.
- Have a business greeting. Example, you can say some thing like this: "Hello, my name is _______________. Thank you so much for this interview. I am so glad to be here."
- Don't forget to SMILE!
- Let the interviewer lead, not you.
- Limit your response, but make it an excellent one.
- If asked, if you have any questions, say yes.

It is very important you show some deep interest in the organization you'll be working for. I always ask a few questions—just a few, two or three. For example, "Are you a franchise, or do you have other affiliates you partner with? What is your company's policy on harassment/bullying in the workplace?" Here's another one: "Do you welcome new ideas, and are their opportunities for advancement?"

WHAT TO BRING

- Résumé and cover letter.
- Three business references.
- Three personal references.
- Certifications.
- Driver's license.
- Social security card.
- Car insurance.
- Current physical and TB record (within 4 to 6 months) of current year.
- Void check for direct deposit.
- Emergency contact persons.
- Professional Email address.
- CPR/First-aid certification.
- Other Certification.
- Copy of recent background checks. They may or may not accept; bring anyway.
- Antibody Titer Test if you plan on working in acute care (Hospitals).
- Take caregivers bible too; it has all your numbers and references and so forth in it, plus impressive tools and resources you can show off during the interview. This book will help show others you are serious about the business of caregiving.

Don't Leave Home Without It!

Those are some examples of mine. You can ask other questions, but have some. Intelligent individuals always have questions because we understand that we are not just going for a job but establishing relationships of understanding and respect—a partnership. Just like they have an expectation of us, the caregiver, we also want to be assured we will have an overall good experience working for them as well.

- Carry an organized business case of some sort that has copies of everything I listed over there to the right, in your tool box.
- Have an 'Exit Greeting'. The first and last impression seals the job!

Sample Exit: "I can't tell you enough how grateful I am that you took the time to see me. I really love being a caregiver, and I hope you can tell as well. I like what your agency/company has to offer. I would love to work for you, and hope the feeling is mutual. It was a pleasure meeting you. Again, thank you for seeing me today. Enjoy the rest of your day!"

That's mine. You can use this one or your just 'Exit' well!

Beauty Tips For Caregivers

Appearance says a lot about us!

It is very important that "Caregivers" realize the importance of good appearance, individuals in our care, appreciates it more than they can say, people like seeing caregivers look fresh and vibrant, pretty or if you are a guy, well groomed too.

Caregiver who take pride in how they look tend to be the ones who are more professional, at least that what I've noticed.

Therefore, caregivers look the part, I tell you, there is absolutely nothing wrong with loving what you do and looking good too! But remember, dress for success, how we look says a lot about us.

If you want to be taken seriously dressed appropriately.

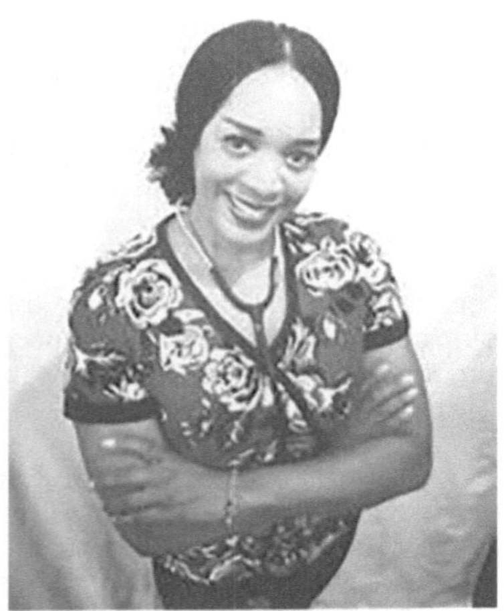

Tools You Can Use!

Looking Good is, Good!

Beauty Tips For Caregivers!

- Wear nice and neat work apparel that match well together.
- Add a flower in your hair why not?
- Wear a 'Smile'!
- Wear professional work shoes
- Keep your hair well groomed.
- Short, unpolished, clean hands and nails.
- Conservative makeup/or none at all but moisturize your wonderful face.
- Professional work bags.
- Clean work badges
- Wear love in your heart!
- Wear Jesus 24/7 it does wonders for the mind body and soul!

Caregiver Star

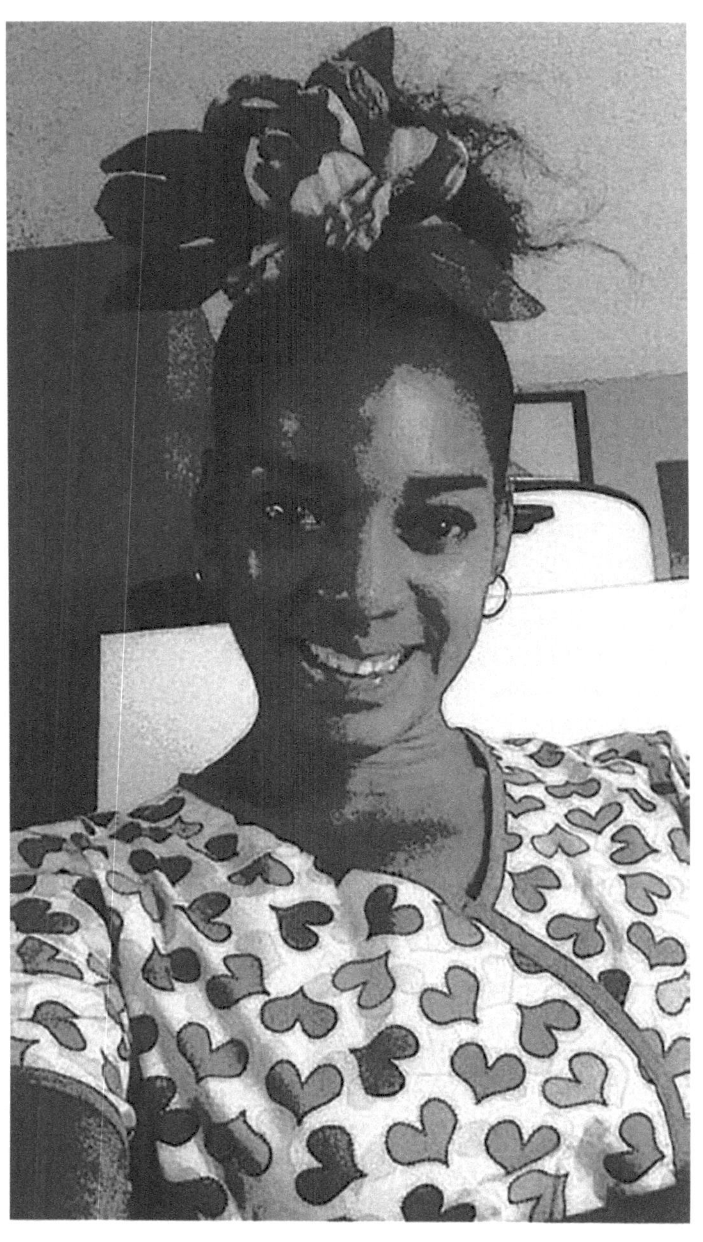

Appearance

The day of your interview it is very important that you are prepared and looking you're very, very best.

It's certainly true **"First Impressions Means Everything"** and I want to make sure Caregiver's are ready and looking fantastic! The way you look matters.

Do not wear Jeans on an interview, period. Orientation, maybe, but not on during the interviewing stage.

You want to look fresh, professionally posed and polished.

Be smart, use the tips in this book, dress for success not for the streets and carry a business bag or tote. Make sure you have writing utensils and a notepad. Employers should not have to find you those important items.

And please, please, please, please ladies, leave the wild colors and extreme hairstyles out. Don't show up to work like that, I know times are changing but still, how we look still matters especially if you want to land a good job. I'm just saying'! Watch what you wear too!

We are **"New day Caregivers"**, we have to look the part too. If you don't have the right clothes for the interview just wear a nice pair of scrubs. Employers love that, it shows you are ready to start right away! That's what I wear mostly to healthcare interviews, nice scrubs.

Lastly, smile, don't worry, be happy, you got this!

New Day Caregivers on the Rise!

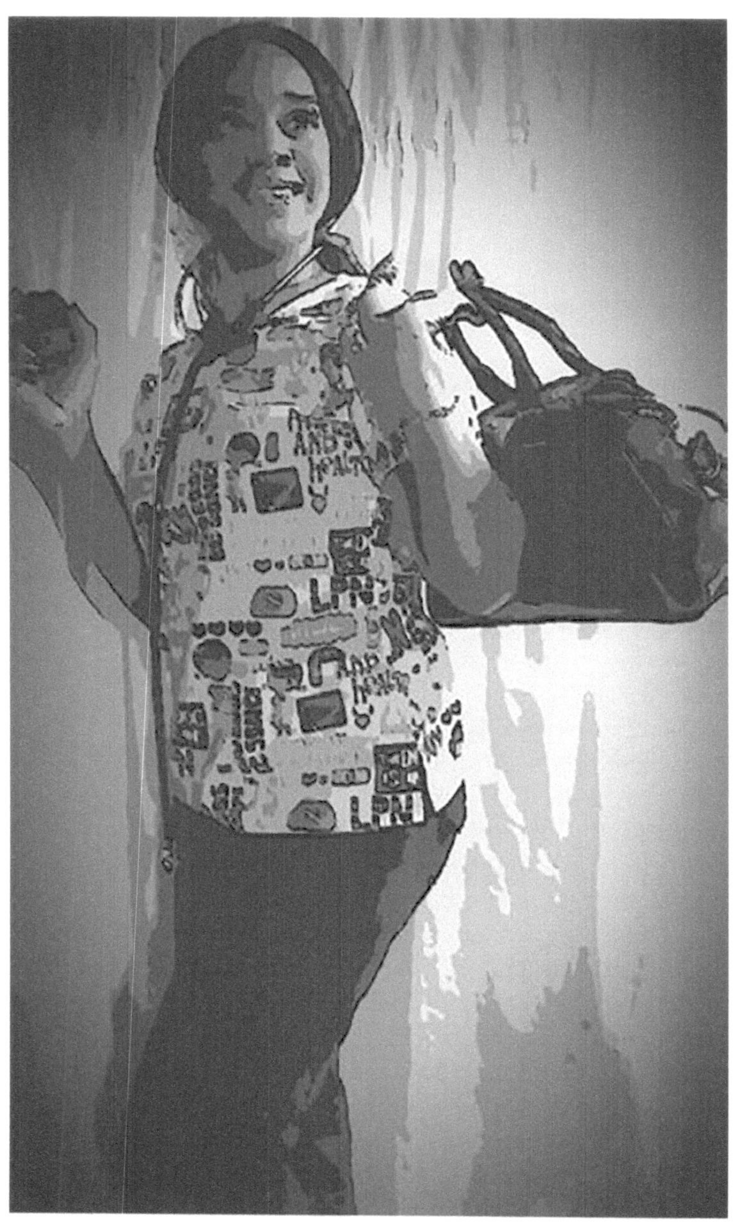

Caregiver's Closet

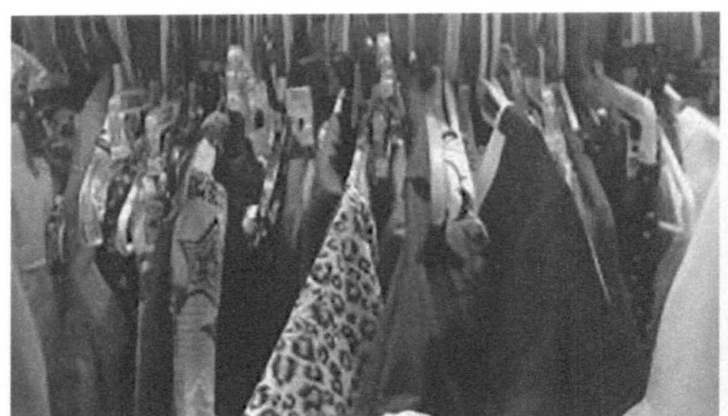

If You Want Success, Invest!
Tips

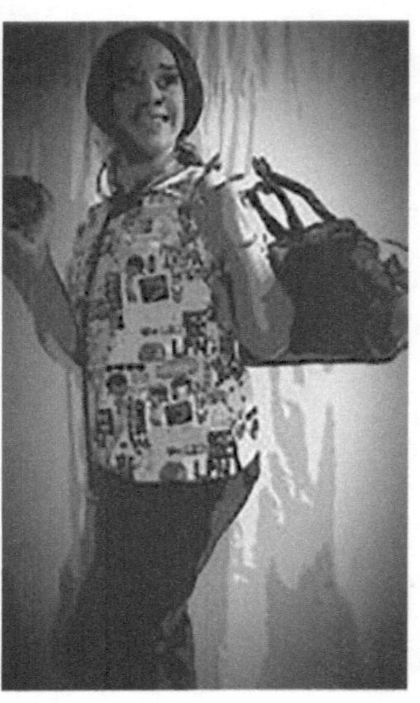

'She's Got It!'

'She's Hired Too'!

- Have lots of variety it make going to work fun and exciting!
- Pull back your hair, keep it out of your face.
- Don't over-do make up, keep it light and simple.
- Don't wear jewelry, work watch is ok.
- Get a Florence Nightingale work bag (**FNB**).
- Purchase pairs of professional and comfortable work shoes.
- Reframe from wearing tight fitting clothes to work, make sure you can bend and move without splitting you apparel.
- Spandex and yoga pants are totally out, don't even think about it!
- Place all you work gear in your caregivers closet, if you don't have a separate one make one, purchase an instant closet for just your work belonging. Why? Because it's smart and keeps you organized.
- Caregivers you should not be looking for scrubs when it's time to go to work or your shoes. Keep everything in one place no excuse to be late.
- And please don't forget your ***Caregiver's Bible To Excellence*** book without it you can get lost or back into your old ways of doing things and we don't want that. **"We Want Excellence, We Want Growth"**!

Foot Care for Caregivers

Being on your feet all day can be harmful to your feet. When your feet hurt, you hurt!

Caregivers we need to be mindful of good foot care and make it a priority as part of a daily routine to take better care of our feet.

By addressing the problem early we can decrease the chances of a more serious condition that sometime require injections or surgery.

Caring for the feet is relatively simple, it starts with wearing the right shoe and foot care on a regular bases.

TLC FOOT CARE

13. Don't wear cheap shoes.
14. Avoid wearing flat shoes.
15. Wear special work shoes designed for comfort and arch elevation.
16. Sit while you chart, if possible.
17. Sit on your breaks, take a load off
18. Pray over your feet ask God to heal them.
19. Soak and pamper your feet at least three times a week.
20. Relax on your off days, Keep your feet elevated, feet up, read your bibles. Have a cup of tea!
21. Wiggle your toes and feet daily for stretching and circulation.
22. Keep toenail cut low.
23. Do foot massages regularly.
24. See a Podiatrist, to find out the underlying problems if these tips are not helping.

In your tool box over to right, I have provided you with some tips on how to tender love and care for your feet, something we don't do enough of, until we are in pain, or hurting and forced to see a doctor.

We don't have to let it get that far, if we began now, early, our feet can do what Jesus did, ***"Walked"*** Yes, ***"Jesus walked" and so MUST "WE"!***

God Bless You!

Our Feet Are The Foundation Of Our Bodies

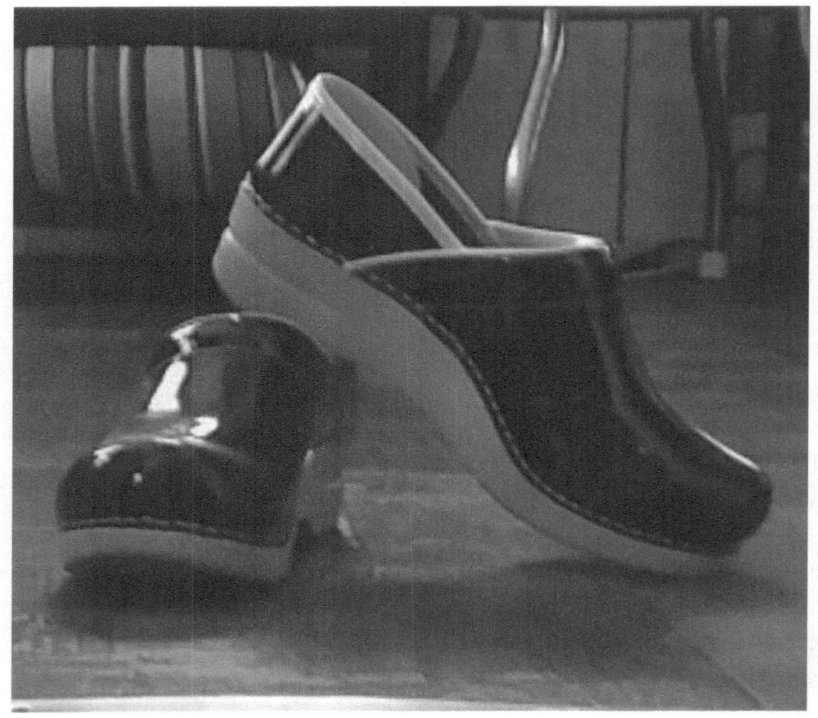

Go Cheap and Reap "Bad Feet"!

 Miss Asondra StarN'air

Acrylic Long Nails

N- Not
A- Allowed
I- In
L- Long-Term Care or Facilities
S- Settings.

Clean hands are the single most important factor in preventing the spread of germs.

Wearing artificial fingernails increases the risk of germs because pathogens now have a place to hide—under the nails.

Good Nail Hygiene!

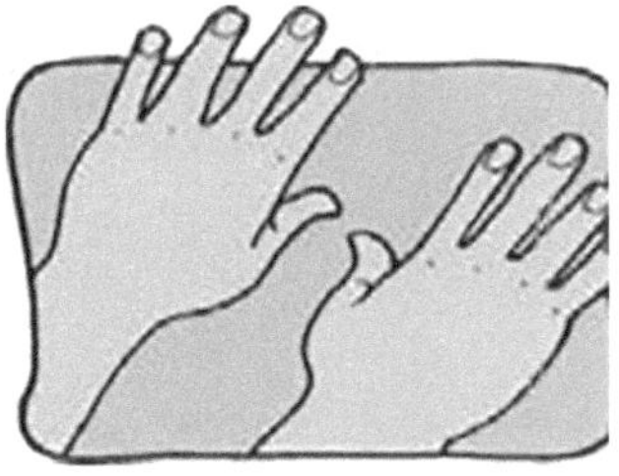

Professional Caregivers do not wear artificial nails and keep their real nails trimmed low.

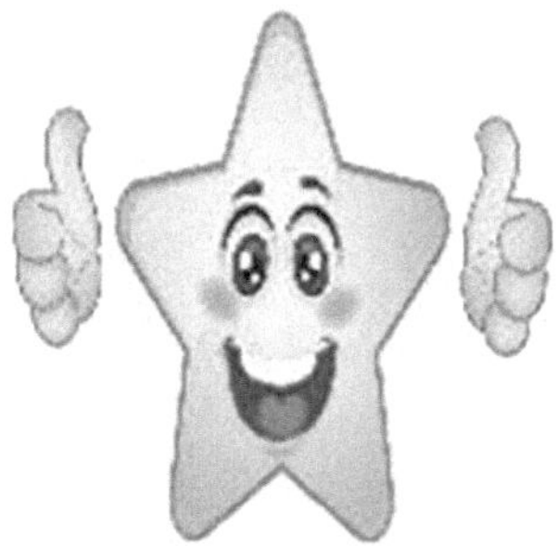

Way to go!

Male Caregivers

Men you are a welcome addition to a field predominantly ran by women. Having Male Professional Caregivers is very much need today. The more the merrier!

You men bring something totally different and unique to the floor, a kind of strength that women don't possess, residence notices too. With your strength and male know how it could prove to be just what the doctor order to help boost life right back into male patients that are in need of support and understanding, or just another man to talk too. Again welcome aboard!

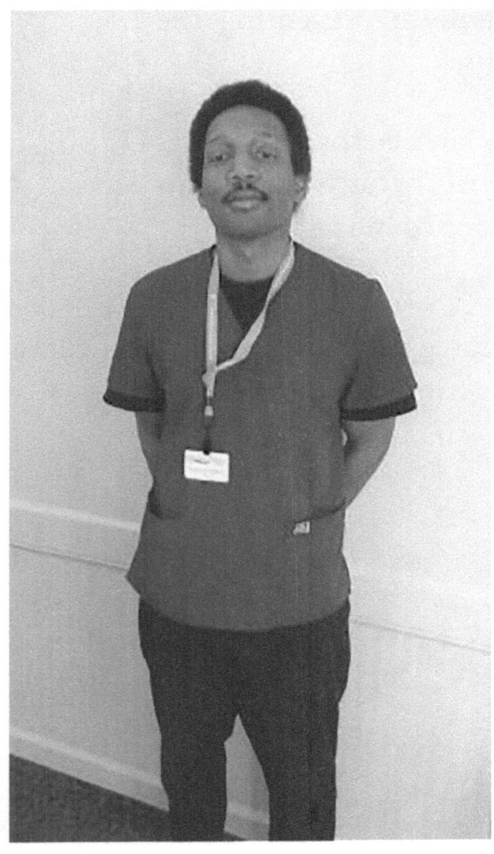

 Miss Asondra StarN'air

Twenty-Five Affirmations for Caregivers

1. I am an excellent caregiver.
2. I am a professional.
3. I am smart and intelligent.
4. I am so blessed.
5. I am doing something about stress; I'm getting rid of it.
6. I am patient and kind.
7. I am prosperous.
8. I am faithful to God.
9. I am sorry for my sin. I shall repent and not do it again.
10. I am a child of the Most High.
11. I am developing into what God wants me to be.
12. I am thankful.
13. I am learning something new every day.
14. I am becoming a nicer, more loving person.
15. I am a team player.
16. I am staying away from strife from now on.
17. I am changing, getting closer and closer to God.
18. I am starting to read my Bible every day now.
19. I am going the extra mile. Love does not depend on two hearts; it depends on one (mine).
20. I love my **Caregiver's Bible To Excellence** *book* and telling everyone I know about it.
21. I am an empathetic, understanding, passionate, reliable, loving caregiver.
22. I am ready to do whatever God calls me to do without murmuring or complaining
23. I am starting to seek God's will and purpose for my life.
24. I am dying to self so Jesus can come and live inside me.
25. I am giving my life to Christ; I want to follow him now.

Daily Affirmations for CareGivers

I am a professional caregiver.
I am beautiful in every way.
I am successful; I love being a health-care provider.
I am learning new and useful skills.
I am a competent caregiver.
I am supportive of other caregivers.
I am a team player.
I am taking better care of myself.
I am making smarter food choices.
I am exercising more now.
I am starting to drink more water.
I am saying no to junk food.
I am always on time to work.
I am a positive person.
I am done with negativity.
I am minding my own business from now on.
I am done with gossiping.
I am welcoming change, growth, and development in every area of my life now.
I am a child of God, and it shows in my behavior.
I am happy.
I am full of gratitude.
I am starting to rest more. I realize getting a good night's sleep is very important.
I am changing in a great way. I have lots of love and respect for my bosses and coworkers.
I am finding more time to spend with God and his word now.
I am starting to read the Bible a lot more, and I see the difference in my life. I have more peace of mind. I feel like I can do all things in Christ, who strengthens me. **'I Feel Brand New!'**

Don't Go There!

Conversations Caregivers Should Avoid

1. **Your personal beliefs,** It can result in backlash if the other person doesn't agree.
2. **Private information**—it can make things awkward moving forward for both you and the other person.
3. **Gossip of any kind,** Close your mouth!
4. Discussing subjects like religion and politics is taboo. Don't go there, period.
5. **Controversial dialogue** is a debate waiting to happen; don't go there either.
6. **Avoid "Office Grapevine"** with you as the primary focus. Shift the conversation quickly. "Oh, look at the time, I need to finish up my paperwork" would be a great exit.
7. **Avoid disagreements;** call the office if you need professional advice.
8. **'The Tongue'** talk less, listen more, do your chores!
9. **Avoid getting in lengthy conversations, period.** Aren't you supposed to be working? **"Hello"!**
10. **Leave your opinions out, you're asking for it!** Instead focus on caregiving and excellence!
11. **Leave your opinions out, you're asking for it!** Where is your lunch box? **"Bring it!"**
12. **Practice 'Professionalism'** don't give out your number.

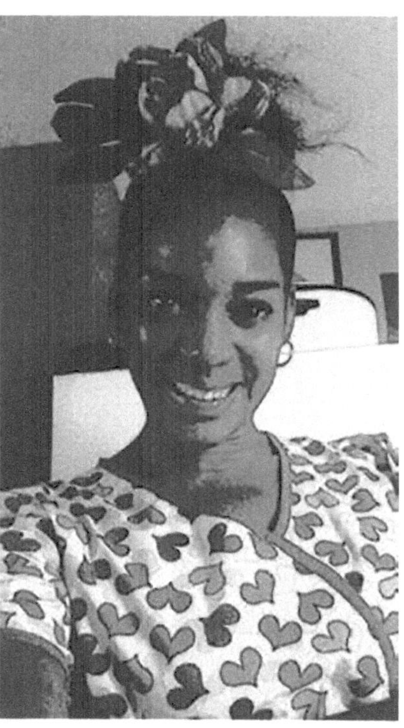

Be Excellent, Be A Light!

Team Player

Be a team player, help each other out!

We all need each other, we are a team, and no one is successful alone. Together we're strong!

Miss Asondra StarN'air

Together we are one.

Everybody matters.

Always be ready to help out.

Meet each other's needs.

Practice kindness and generosity.

Love like sisters and brothers.

Answer when called upon.

Yield to strife and negativity.

Eat smartly!

Run the race **"TOGETHER"**!

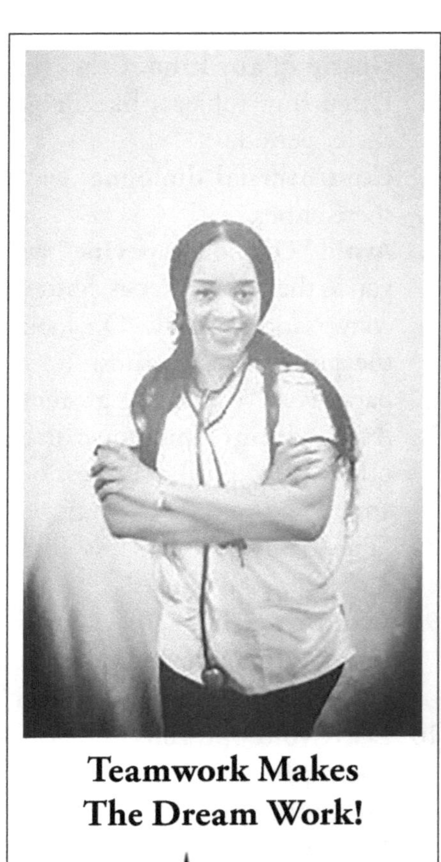

Teamwork Makes The Dream Work!

N'air

Workplace Cliques

Workplace Cliques every place have them. If the leader is positive and has the organization best interest in mind get with this group see what you can bring to the table too. The more the merrier I say because positive people help set a great precedence for overall staff camaraderie. It feels good to work in an environment that embraces ideas and togetherness.

However if the leader in the click is a negative person, the entire group can become toxic spreading poison throughout the organization.

Therefore caregivers you must choose your water cooler friends carefully, if you are a following of Jesus Christ like some of you say you are, you have a responsibility to look out for the innocent. Bad cliques do bad and cruel things to others they bully and create hostile environments. Worse, they lie and get innocent people fired. If you see something, say something.

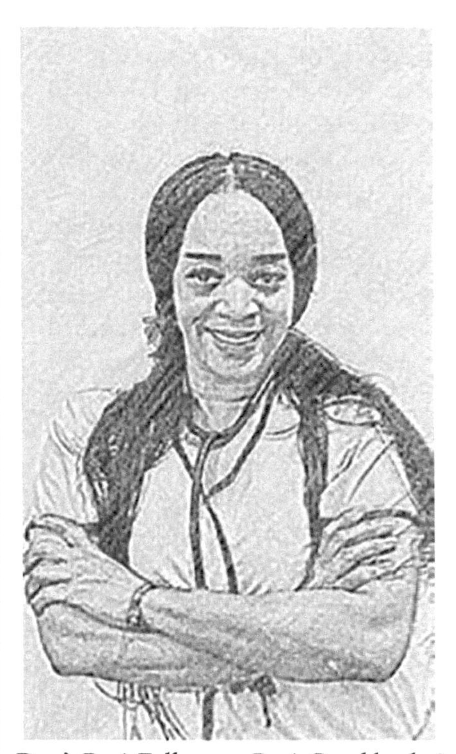

Don't Be A Followers, Be A Good leader!
- Respect your job, **"Phones Off".**
- Say No to Gossip and Negativity.
- Hangout with Jesus, not with Haters.
- If You See Something, Say Something!

You Become What You Hangout With!

Sabotage

'For everyone who does evil hates light (excellent caregivers) and does not come to the Light for fear that his /her deeds will be exposed. **John 3:20** People we mightiest well face it, we have some wicked and evil workers among us that hates excellence, and boy don't I know, I have been targeted most of my caregiving career, I have been knocked down too many time to count but I never got knocked out, I'm still here and standing. We don't fight like the world fights, we fight with the word of God that's our sword. And Jesus is our LORD! Sabotage is what people do who hate God and themselves, inside they are evil and dark, jealousy and hatred is how they make their mark.

But like Jesus, Light is Stronger than darkness!

So if there is any caregivers out there suffering loses from evil doers, sabotaging all your good hard work and falsely accusing you, don't retaliate, ***"WAIT!"***

The scriptures says something like this: Those who dig a hole for others, will fall in it themselves.

Forgiver them like Joseph in the bible he forgave his brothers who left him for dead, they dull a hole too but one

Tips on how to deal with workers of iniquity

- Act like Jesus stay focus on His Father's business 'Excellence'
- Defend yourself without being defensive.
- Pull that person aside and try to see eye to eye.
- If that doesn't work, report it to your boss.
- Forgive Them, Remain Positive!
- Document and Keep a running record with times and dates Document.
- Find Scriptures that strengthen you during this time.
- Meet with your boss regularly.
- If the problem is coming from your boss or higher up, put it all in Jesus hand. Pray for that fallen man/woman.
- Stay in constant prayer.
- Always do **'GOOD'** to those who hate you. Love no matter what.
- Don't' leave the 'Love Position'!
- Offer your services to them, e.g. can I help you with this? Would you like me to … etc.
- Ask God to take over the situation you can't handle it.
- Stop caring about what's happening to you and focus on God. Perhaps God, like He's doing with me is using it all for his **GOOD**. Lord knows what his people go through.
- Lastly, after you have done all you can do **'STAND'** and wait on the salvation of 'The **LORD'**!

day they all feel in one, they needed Joseph to help save them and their land. **Genesis 37:18-36**

A lot of haters dug holes for ***"Me Too"*** but I'm about to make history! *A Caregiver's Bible to Excellence* is going to help set 'Aides' /Slaves all over the world free and out of poverty, not me but **GOD** gets the **VICTORY!**

Therefore faithful ones, press on in excellence, sabotaging co-workers will have their day, continue to let *Jesus Lead The Way!*

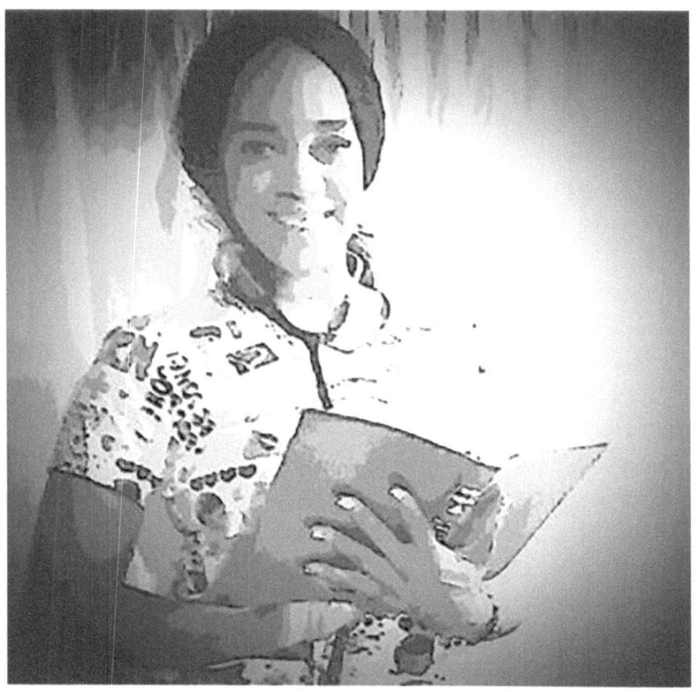

**Look At Me
"I'm Still Standing!"**

Caregiver's Leftovers

Don't taste good,
do your job like you should!

What are caregiver leftovers? Glad you ask, it's when a caregiver has a job to and do not do it. They leave their leftovers on purpose for others to do. Here's the thing caregivers, those working in home and private care especially if you work a 8 to 12 hour shift, there is absolutely no reason why you can't get all your work done and laundry too. Mediocre workers many times play silly and foolish games and it time that stops. A Caregiver's Bible to Excellence is to help make you just that **EXCELLENT!** We don't leave leftovers. We go in and do Jesus work, we leave no stones unturned. Who cares if the next person has nothing to do when they get there, Caregiving is more than doing chores and perhaps now that other caregiver has time to come up with creative ideas to get that person up and engaged in activities or more time to be with them. And too, it shows that other caregivers what an excellent Caregiver looks like, **"YOU"** so hopefully it will rub off on them too. Besides 'Excellent Caregivers' the ones Jesus is raising up, We don't leave 'Leftovers' (work). No, we don't get caught up on who does what, our minds are set on Jesus and quality care, we know some don't play fair but who cares? We strive for excellence, again we don't play those silly games all the love and hard work we do is in Jesus name.

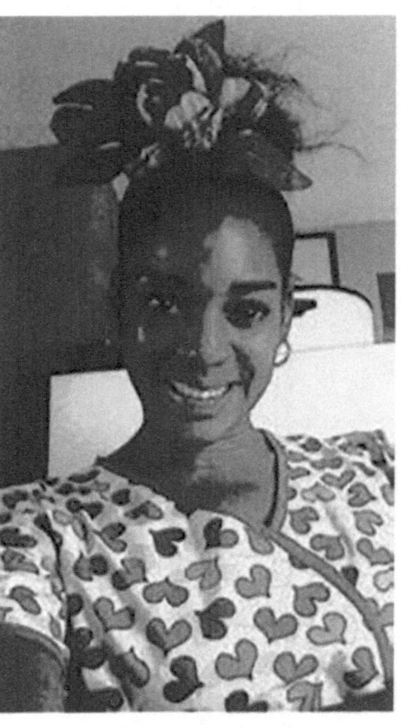

Caregiver Leftovers

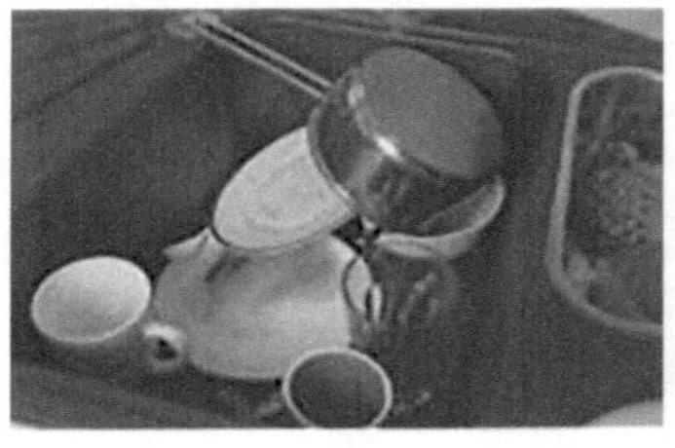

And to the facility workers, you are not off the hook, stock your own rooms, stop talking and texting and get back to the business of caregiving. Nobody wants leftovers all the time, complete all your work **'Shine'!**

Pride vs. Pride

Caregivers did you know there is a things called good pride and bad pride? Well there is and sometimes we get caught up. It is one thing to be excellent and take lots of pride in what you do that's the good pride. However when no one can tell you or show you anything because you know it all, and think you can't be shown new ways of doing things then you are caught up in the bad pride. You are not being humble at all, but that's when we fall!

The scriptures says that God hates the proud people who think they don't need God or anybody telling them how to live or what to do.

Here's my message, **"Be Excellent, Be Great** but also, **'Be Humble Too!"** Allow others including other caregivers to lead and show you new ways of doing things. Don't be so full of the bad pride that you lose out on new growth and development, thing are always changing, nothing stays the same but **'GOD'**. So , moving forward, be full of the good pride so that we can help bless lives.

But I guess the choice is up to you
Pride vs Pride, 'You' Decide?
As for me and my house we
shall serve the Lord!

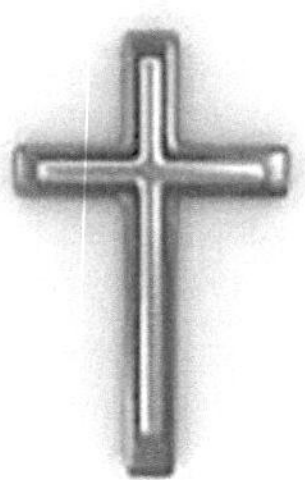

Good Pride, Bad Pride

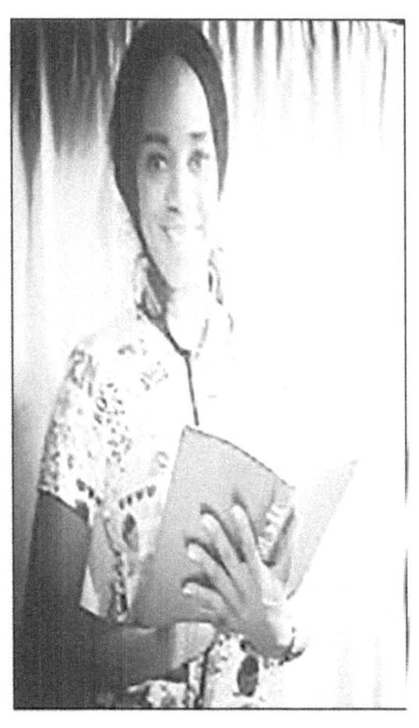

Pride brings a person low,
but the lowly in spirit gain honor.
Proverbs 29-23

Do nothing out of selfish
ambition or vain conceit,
Rather, in humility value
others above yourself.
Philippians 2;;3

"Stay Humble"!

Caregivers
For-Get–Me – Not's

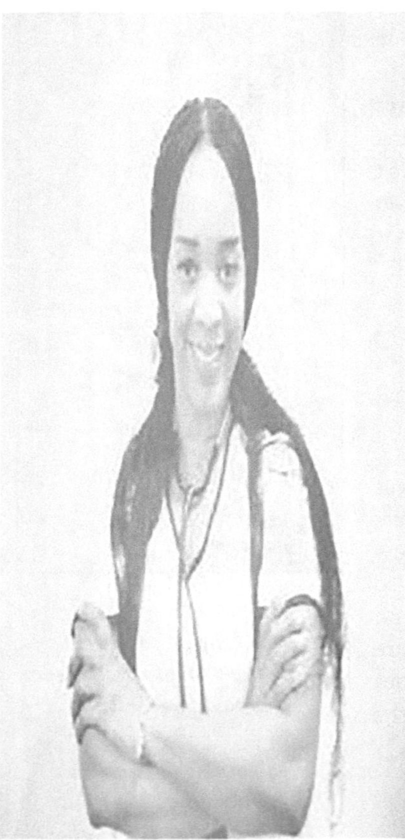

Sometimes a day at work can be so overwhelming and full of unanti cipated problems or unexpected guest that we forget to do what we normally do. So I have prepared some **For-Get-Me-Not's** for you.

Forget–Me–Not's

- Wash your hands coming and going
- Take out the garbage
- Sign In -Clock out
- Unplug the coffee pot
- Finish your documentations
- Grab your FNG work bag
- Put more gas in your tank
- Eat smart
- Bring your own food and drink
- Feed the pet
- Water the plants
- Stock your rooms
- Shopping Receipts
- The clothes in the dryer
- Wash and put up the dishes
- Lock up
- Turn off the lights
- Pick up prescriptions
- Call in prescriptions
- Report signs and symptoms
- Cut your Cell phone off/vibrate
- Texting can wait
- Don't be late
- Stop at the store after work
- Monthly breast exams
- Tithe
- Grab your Caregiver's Bible
- Carry your Holy Bible
- Pick up your child from school
- Workout today
- Leave caregivers notes
- Cleanup behind yourself
- Call if you are going to be late
- Teamwork makes the dream work
- Clean the bathroom mirrors
- Follow & complete the care plan
- Praise and thank the LORD
- Do a random act of kindness
- Do excellent work today
- Love, laugh, **Live for Christ!**

Overboard

When it comes to caregiving of course we want to give those we are caring for our all. We want to make sure all their needs are meet. However, sometimes we go **"Overboard."** We do things that are not required trying to win that person over but we don't realized that not every caregiver is going to do what you do. For example **'Meal Time'**, you go in and make fancy dishes like you are their personal chef making things like sauté veal and shrimp and homemade pound cake supreme, this is extreme and going overboard. Other caregivers are not going to do that nor am I, unless I'm paid for that additional service. And don't let your agency tell you it's your job unless they give you 80 percent of what they are taking in on that case. If they what a personal chef they have to pay for it! And some will.

That was just one example, here is another, hooking up their cable and programing their devices, this is not what we do, you are such a sweetheart, but you are going overboard and asking for trouble. What happens if you tell them one day **"NO"**, you may have to go? Caregivers I tell you from experience don't start something you can't finish, stick with the care plan.

What's Overboard?

- Filling Pill boxes, knowing you are not supposed to.
- Cleaning out closets, that's for merry maids.
- Cooking chef type meals that's for chefs, we are there to make simple and easy foods, until family arrives.
- Computer and office work.
- Assembling store bought items
- Full time house cleaning, we are supposed to do only light housekeeping.
- Shovel Snow, **NO!**
- Haul all the garbage cans out, no we are not aides/slaves we are healthcare professionals
- Polish all their silver and remover all the china from the cabinet.
- Playing the lottery for them
- Purchasing cigarettes and alcohol.
- Lying for them
- Cooking for the entire family
- Cursing in their car, going away from where you are supposed to be.
- Trying to be their best friend.
- When you dump your money and bills problems on them.
- When you ask to borrow money.
- When you bring your child to work.
- When you don't follow the Care plan.
- And when you don't follow Christ

You've Gone Overboard!!! Look to the Lord, don't Go Overboard!

Get The Care Plan, Stick with the Care Plan!

Stick With The Care Plan! Because when we don't other caregivers behind you don't have a chance because you have spoiled that customer rotten, and they will reject other professional caregivers who know not to go **"Overboard"**, We are there to **Stick To The Care Plan!** Don't take matters in your own hands. Last time, **Stick To The Care Plan!**

Besides you are not being fair or professional when you manipulate your way into people lives by going "Overboard." **"Stop It"!**

Excellent Caregiver Look to the LORD

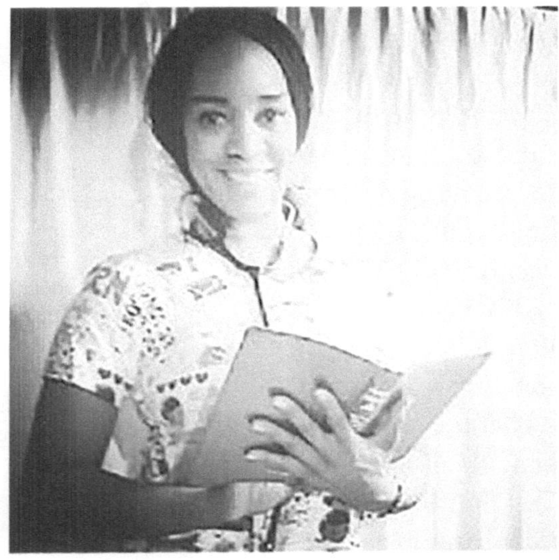

For Our Reward!

FILL -INS,

Fill –INS, also known as fill-it in's.

Caregivers doing fill –Ins' doesn't give us the right to do nothing when we get there. If you are going to be a caregiver care. Care about the full time job that day, take out the trash, and treat that fill –in case as if it's your one and only case. Do all the fundamentals of care.

Too many caregivers who do fill –in's

Get lazy and think it's a time to make easy do nothing money, you're wrong honey!

Fill –In's is a time to shine, a time to let others see how excellent you are, be that star, God will take your career far.

FILL–INS, Go Out and Win!

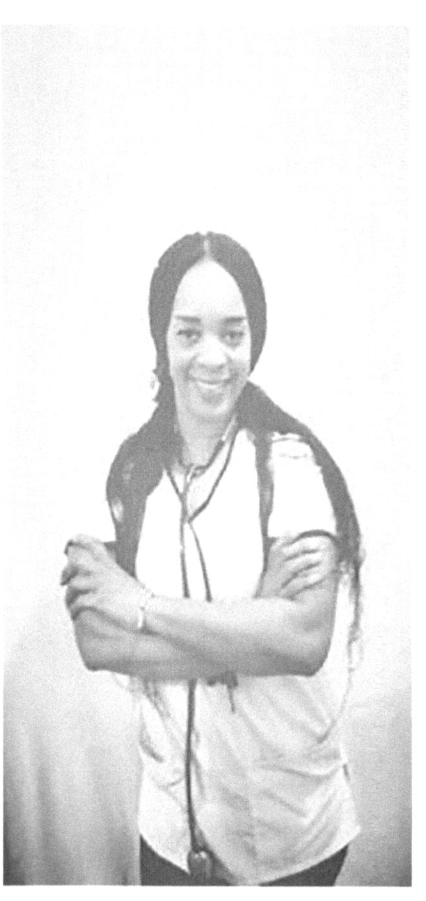

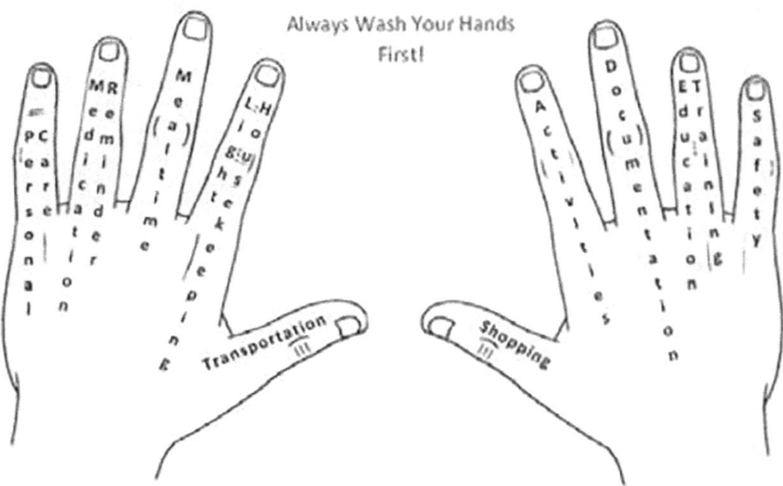

Professional   **Tender Loving**

Hands on Care

WOW!

Ten More Caregiving Tips Inside Your Hands

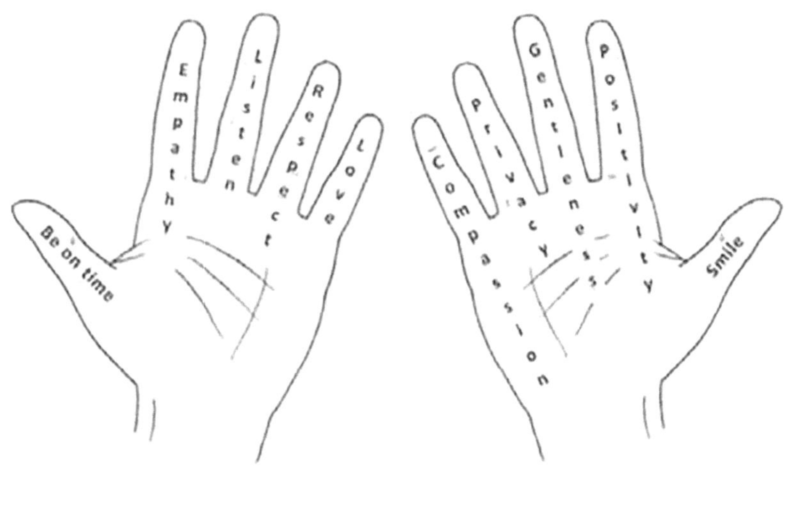

New   **Day**   **Caregivers**

Delivers, We Rock!

Protect Yourself!

Just like our senior have rights, caregiver have rights too. Unfortunately there have been a lot of false accusations, accusing caregivers of mistreating or just not giving adequate service when in fact, they have.

Sometimes the ones we are caring for, cares nothing for us, no matter what we do. And because too of all the stereotypes, prejudice behavior and hatred toward **"Aides"**, all over the world. Caregivers everywhere get abused, used, set up and lied on all the time. Sometimes even by their own employers if they think they are about to lose **MONEY**, they call it damage control, I call it slavery hold. Like what I'm saying or not, this page is important caregivers 'Protect Yourself'!

Here's How:

1. If you are a working caregiver in a facility setting and you are caring for a trouble maker do not go in their rooms alone, have another caregiver or nurse go in with you. They can stand by the door to witness or help you. **"Protect Yourself"**!
2. If you are a working caregiver in a home care setting, document the repeated behavior, call the management team, expect changes or give appropriate notice and come off that case, don't allow anyone to abuse you anymore. **'Protect Yourself'**!
3. If the abuser is a co-worker or boss keep a running record of what's happening with all the dates and times handy. Next, schedule a meeting with their superiors. After you've done that and things don't change or get worse, **"Resign."** *God will have you back working in no time.* Don't work where you are mistreated and disrespected anymore. Trust Jesus like I do, he will open a new door! **"Protect Yourself"**!
4. Cast all your cares on Christ. He knows and sees everything that going on, God neither slumber nor sleep. Trust him, He is a righteous God, He will deal with each according in his own time. Remember Caregivers the battle is not ours it's the **Lords!** *2 Chronicles 20:15*
5. I'll say this again, always, always forgive those who mistreat or hurt you. Pray for them, love them still. Never stop being an excellent person. Know that no weapons formed against you shall ever prosper.

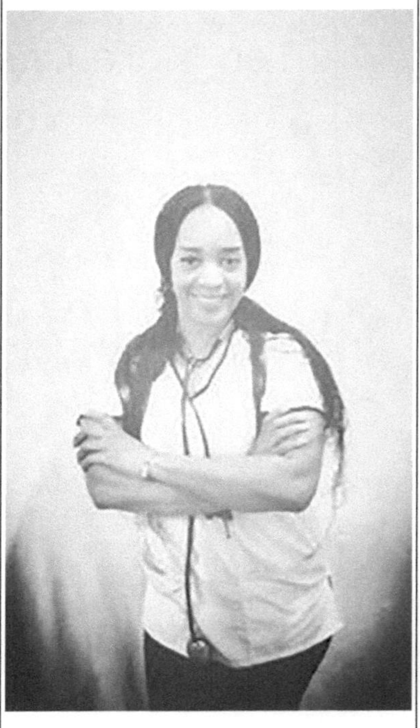

Protect Yourself!

 MISS ASONDRA STARN'AIR

I Don't Care, Caregiver's

I don't care, caregivers, unfortunately, there out there everywhere all over the world! But these are not real caregivers, they are counterfeits. But some of them have to go out and get a job to keep 'county quite', if you know that I mean, (I think you do) and being an **"Aide"** does not require a college degree, anybody can be a caregiver so they say but that's a lie.

See, if they don't have that good heart, Jesus is looking for, no matter if they can do the job or not, they are **"high risk"** to everybody, including the facility or company that hired these counterfeits.

How then, can we weed them out? Glad you asked. First by what comes out of their mouths when the boss is not around. And next by their care-giving attitude, are they there for fun or for the customer? Do they care about being on time and when they do get there how do they look? Are they tired and hung over? Things like that matter, The bible says you will know them by their fruits. But as some of you already know Counterfeits come in places like the real thing, for example resumes.

FAKE CAREGIVERS

- They go after good caregivers.
- They don't care about being on time, or showing up for work.
- They are **NOT** team players.
- They are trouble makers.
- All they do is complain.
- They handle patients recklessly. They don't care!
- In facilities, long term care especially, they hide off in places to avoid helping other co-workers.
- They are always text messaging or on their phones, care -giving is not top priority.
- They are not professional.
- They break a lot of rules.
- They are manipulators, they win over management staff and feed them all kinds of lies.

Anybody can pull off a great resume these days but it is written in *Numbers 32:23* your sin will find you out. Here's another one *Luke 8:17* for all that is hidden will be revealed, be brought to the open, and everything that is concealed will be brought to light."

These **'Fake Caregivers'**, counterfeits get hired in and once comfortable, **"Turn"**, their real self and evil deeds emerges. Over in the text box are some of the negative attributes of **"Counterfeit Caregivers"** be advise everyone, be on the lookout! **"They're Everywhere!"**

Be The Real Deal Or Get Out Of This Field!

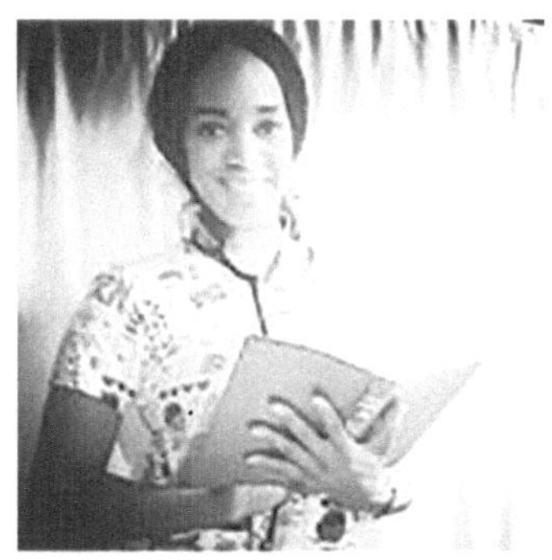

Obesity

Obesity is a problem, obesity is bad!

There is just no other way to describe it, we must get the weight off and keep it off. Otherwise you are playing a dangerous game with your life.

You're fooling yourself if you think, it's ok to be overweight! It isn't, nor is it healthy.

Being overweight, leads many times to obesity, once that happen you are in real trouble, real big trouble.

Being out of shape or obese is a major health risk. Obesity and overweightness can cause many complications like the following:

- **Hypertension**
- **Type 2 diabetes**
- **Coronary Heart disease**
- **Stroke**
- **Sleep Apnea**
- **Gall Bladder disease**
- **Respiratory problems**
- **Dyslipidemia**
- **Depression /low -self esteem**
- **Negativity, Jealousy and Insecurity**
- **Hatred toward healthy/fit successful people.**
- **Poor Job Performance**
- **Body aches and pains**
- **Laziness and poor teamwork**
- **Causes accelerating aging**
- **Unusual tiredness, chemical imbalances/sometimes body odor**
- **Gradual physical decline**

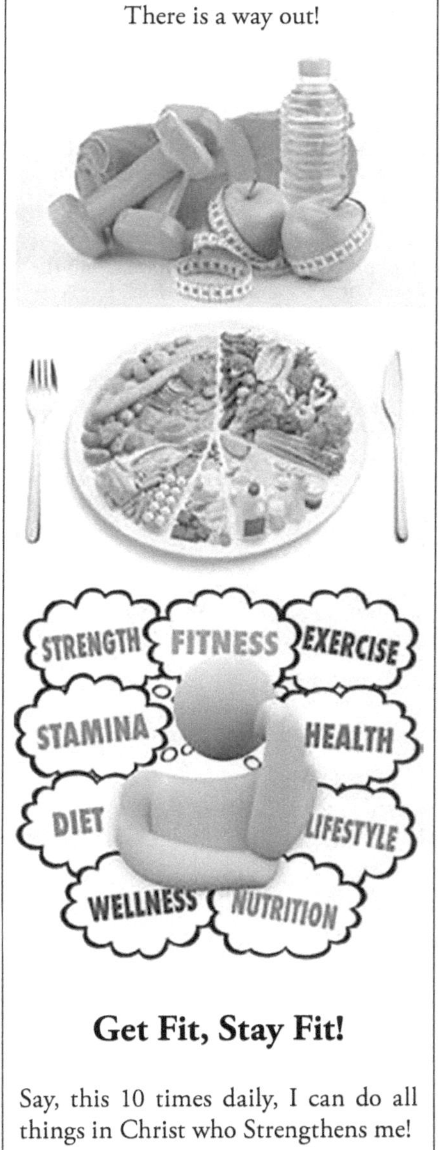

Get Fit, Stay Fit!

Say, this 10 times daily, I can do all things in Christ who Strengthens me!

Philippians 4:13

Say No To Overeating!

Pardon me but, I'm sorry that I could not find anything positive about overweightness and obesity. If you finds something positive, post it, let us all know, otherwise see you at boot-camp! You can do it, you MUST do it!

Get The Weight Off And Keep It Off!

Now before I get off the subject of obesity let me make it crystal clear that it is not my intention to offend the overweight population, not at all. I am here to help, you already know it is not healthy to go on this way, your doctor has also told you this. Over eating and not exercising is not good period, it does affect job performance, not only that it effects your entire life and other who will have to care for you later on.

Obesity is NOT Good!

It's true obesity or being overweight is not good but today you can change all that, I do believe if you keep doing my boot camp and asking God for help, plus stay in his word, you'll be able to get the weight off and keep it off. It won't be easy, it's going to take at least a year to see major results but it will be well worth it in the end I promise you. Just stay committed and focus you can do it I know you can, look to Jesus He's the man with the real fitness plan!

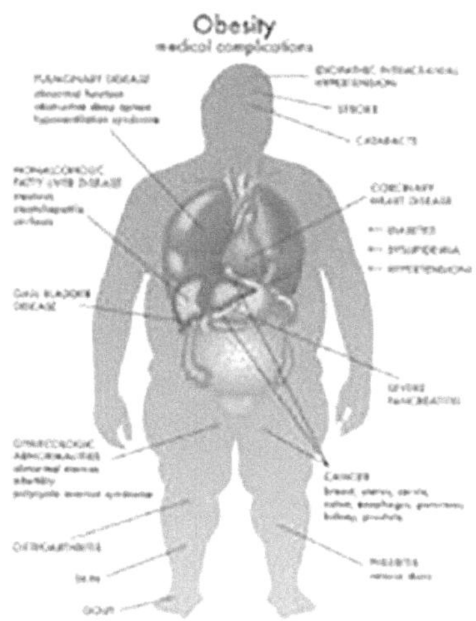

Obviously Yours Is Not Working!

Staying Active Matters!

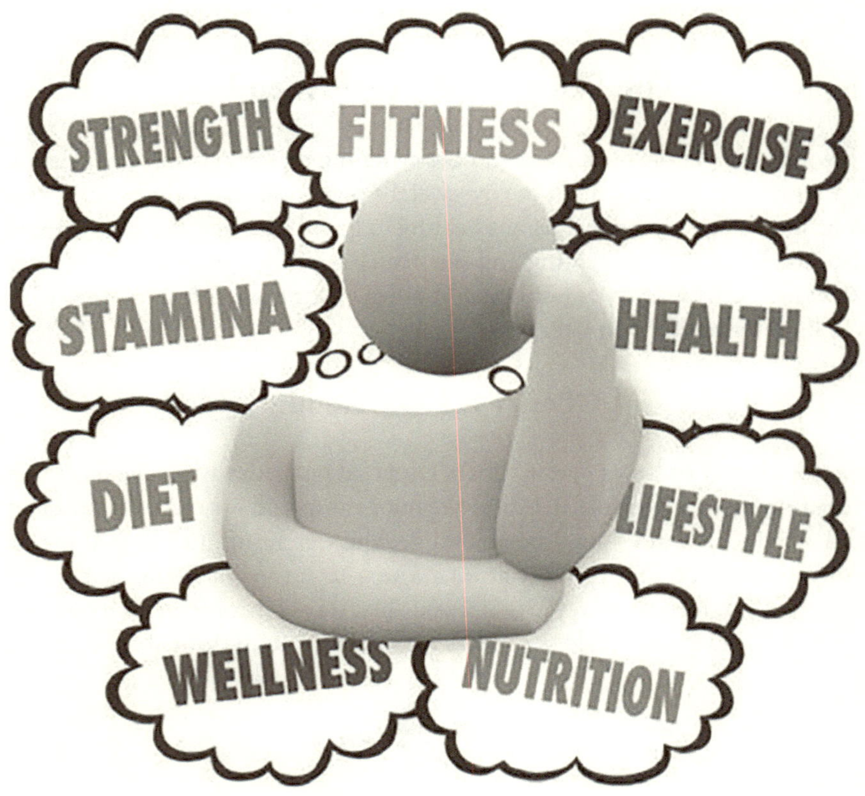

Eating The Right Foods does Too!

Caregiver Call OFF's

Caregiver Call Offs are a huge problem in the healthcare industry especially in homecare and some nursing homes.

When a caregiver waits to the last minute and calls off everyone suffers especially the person who needs the care. What are we going to do about it caregivers? We are going to **"Stop It."** We are moving toward *'New Day Caregivers'* we don't do that. Now for a minute just imagine if it was us or one of our loved ones who got stranded without care, how would we feel? Not Good I'm sure, so from now on let's do some things different, let's be more responsible and professional shall we. There is nothing like being a caregiver everyone can count on while you're making those changes *"Get Reborn"* become Caregivers for Christ!

Look I know we are human like everyone else we get sick or have emergencies too, and unexpected things happen in our lives that may cause us some problems, I get that, me too, I'm a caregiver, me too but, here's the thing, it's how you handle life situations that says if you are a professional or not. If you know

Go To Work!

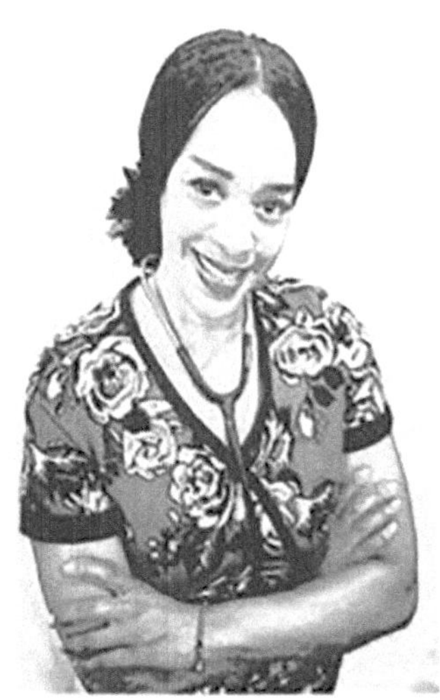

We all have stuff to deal with, work and everyday life can be challenging and painful too sometimes. But we must not forget our obligations and commitments. If you work, you still have a job to do. Go to work, show up, do your job, God will fix it, whatever is wrong, but don't leave a helpless person or your team members stranded and alone.

Things You Can do:

- Sick, Call Quick
- Schedule time off
- Seek help with personal problems, talk to GOD first
- Have your own emergency work plan, a list of co-workers numbers that can help you out.
- Live righteously and stay healthy.

you have a sick person waiting for you and not enough time to get them another caregiver, here's what you do, **'GET OFF YOU'**, don't think of yourself, get up and go to work. No that God will take care of you and your situation, keep your commitments, stay true and loyal to your job.

And if you are ill, or suddenly got sick of course you can't go to work, you can make that person sick too but what you can do is pick up your phone and **"Call Quickly"**, the second you feel sick not wait to the last minute. The rule of thumb in this book for home care providers mostly because we are all that person has today there is no other staff, we are it! The 'Rule of Thumb' is this: Unless it's a 'Documented Emergency.'

Show up, Show up, Show up!

GET UP, GET DRESS, GET TO WORK!
A Prayer Couldn't Hurt!

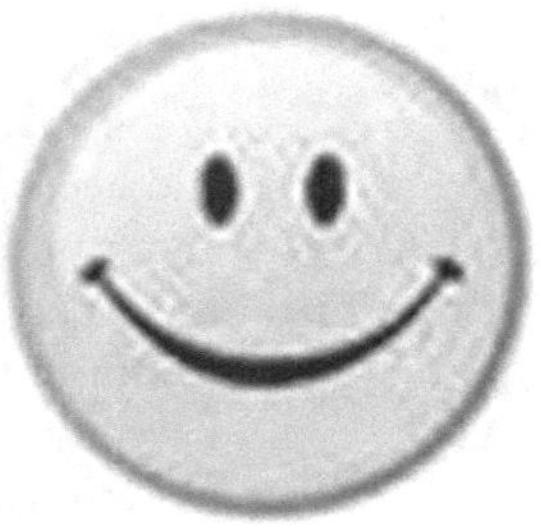

   MISS ASONDRA STARN'AIR

'ALL-IN' with Jesus!

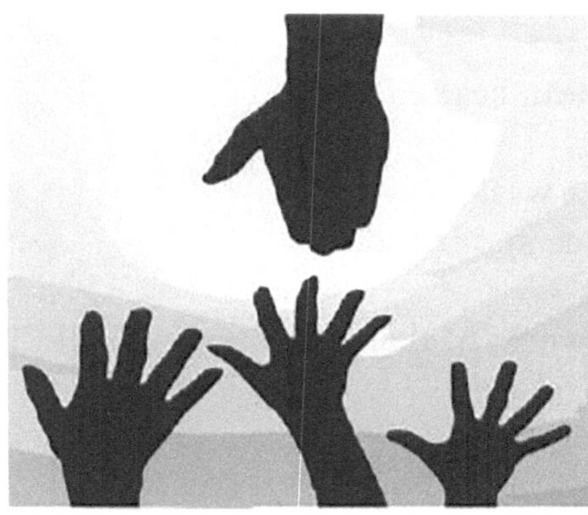

Be Caregivers for Christ
for the rest of your life!

- Be **ALL-IN** with Diversity!
- Be **ALL-IN** with Perfect Attendance!
- Be **ALL- IN** with **Bibles Study**
- Be **ALL-IN** with **Holiness!**
- Be **ALL-IN** with doing the right thing!
- Be **ALL- IN** for economic equality for caregivers nationwide.
- Be **All- IN** for high quality care.
- Be **ALL-IN** for **CHANGE!**
- Be **ALL-IN** with maintaining a fit and healthy body!
- Be **ALL-IN** with lifting the glass ceiling! **"Higher Pay"**
- Be **ALL-IN** with denouncing sin!
- Be **ALL-IN** when Jesus calls you!
- Be **All -IN** with "Rest" so we can put out our best.
- Be **ALL-IN** say, **Jealousy and 'Bullying Must End!'**

'All-IN'

Hey caregivers out there, do you want to join a winning team? Do you want to fulfill all your hopes and dreams? Well if you do you've come to the right place. Jesus is reaching out to anyone who wants to join his winning team, and what's great about his team is that you do not have to be a LeBron James a former player of the Cleveland Cavaliers or any other sports star, no sir, no ma'am, all you have to do is believe like Abraham. Believe that our God can get us to the promise land, be **'ALL-IN' And Together Let's Win!**

Take His HAND!

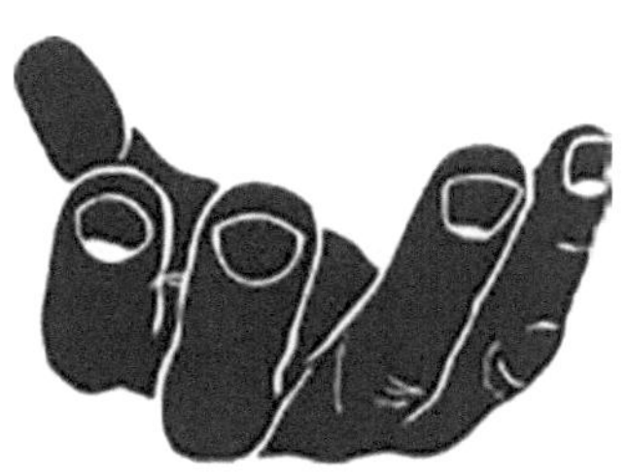

"STAY ALL-IN"

- Be **All- IN** finish what you started.
- Be **ALL-IN** don't be cruel or mean hearted.
- Be **ALL -IN** don't leave, stay!
- Be **All -IN** and let Jesus lead the way!
- Be **ALL-IN** with a lifetime coach and friend!
- Be **ALL- IN** with Excellence!
- Be **ALL-IN** remember, **"Teamwork, Makes The Dream Work"!**

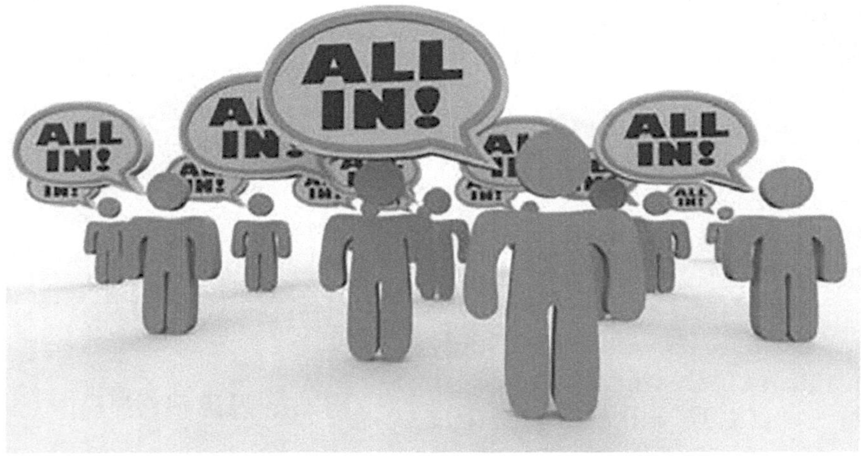

- Be **All- IN** for **"Change!"**
- Be **ALL-IN** for Debt free living.
- Be **ALL -IN** with tithing and giving.
- Be **All -IN** "You see something, Say something!
- Be **ALL-IN** with the sabbath
- Be **ALL- IN** with breaking bad habits.
- Be **ALL-IN** with *'A Caregiver's Bible To Excellence!'*

Every Part of "YOU" Matters!

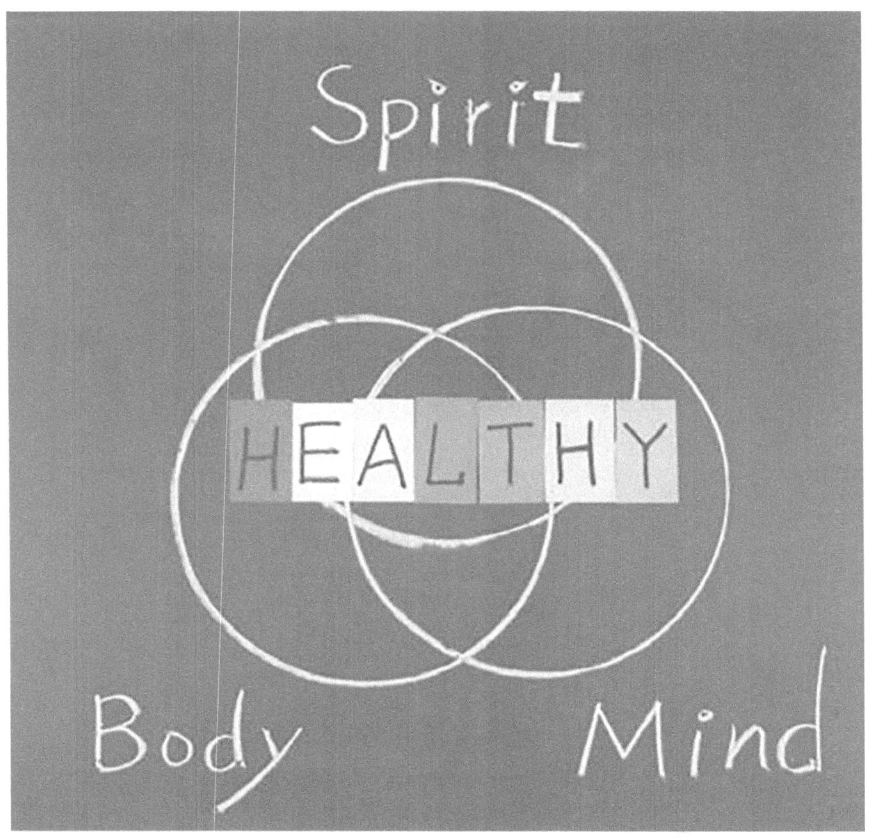

Get To Know Yourself Better!

Maslow's Hierarchy Of Needs

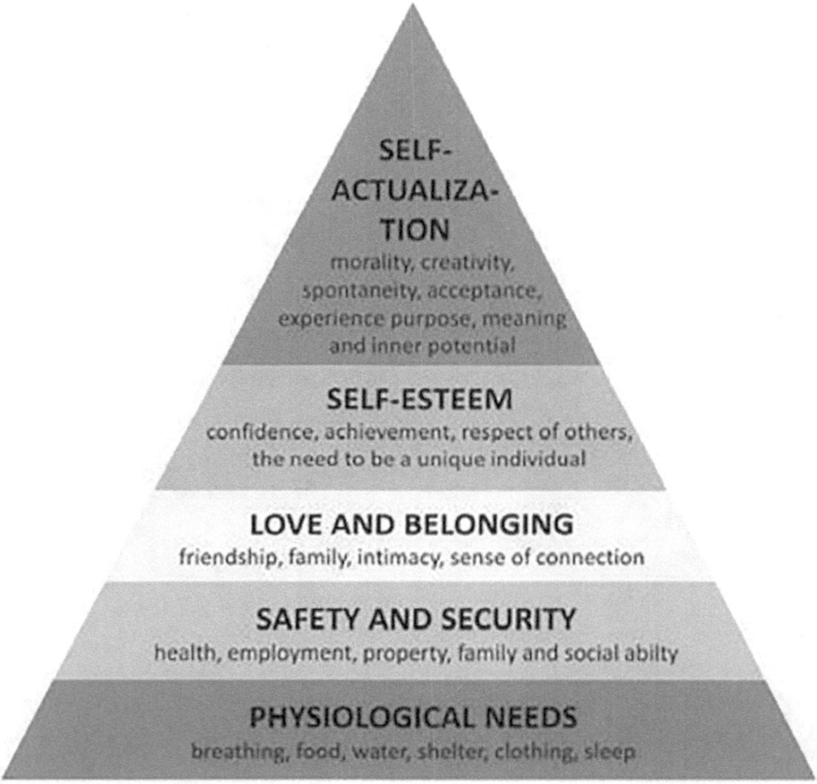

Read His Word, Stay Focus!

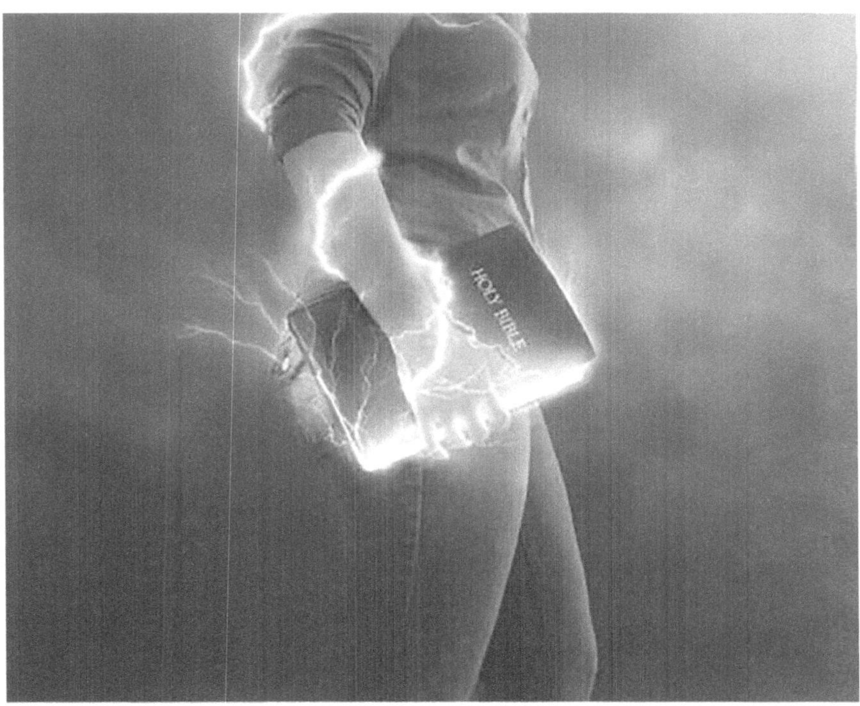

Keep saying every day, I can do all things in Christ who gives me the strength, to lose weight, go back to school, handle everyday situations, get out of toxic relationship, become debt free, you name it, it's true **"YOU"** can do all things in Christ so, **"Just Do It!"**

Phil 4:13

SMART PHONE, Here We Go Again!

Is your Smart Phone really smart? No it is not if you put it before your other responsibilities, your phone calls and texting can wait.

Go see about your residence, patients or clients. Get your priorities straight!

Hey, I'm just the messenger, don't get mad at me. But I do agree cell phones are becoming a nuisance in the work place. That's why this cellphone is up in your face! Turn it off, get back to work, Jesus is calling, that phone call can wait!

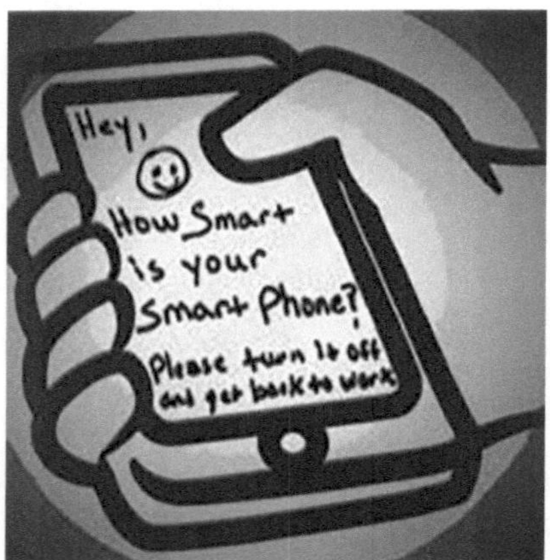

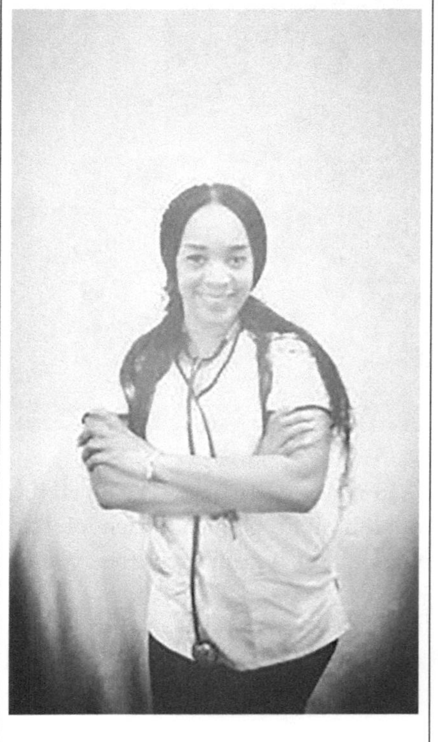

 Miss Asondra StarN'air

"Stop And Notice"

Have you noticed any changes today with the persons you are caring for?

Seems different than usual
Talks less, than usual, "quite"
Overall, just not with it, some confusion
Puts off doing activities, use to love it

Ate and drank very little or not at all
No interest in anything, food, activities or socializing etc.
Don't seem to have any enthusiasm or energy or care anymore

Note: caregivers, are there any bruises, rashes, bed soars or skin tears
On and off their daily routine, unable to get up or remember things.
Tract infection (**UTI**) urine cloudy, dark, bloody, strange smelling etc.
Is weak and disoriented
Calling out for help more often than usual or not calling for help at all
Elimination: off a bit, diarrhea, constipation, not voiding at all.

"Tell Your Nurse!"

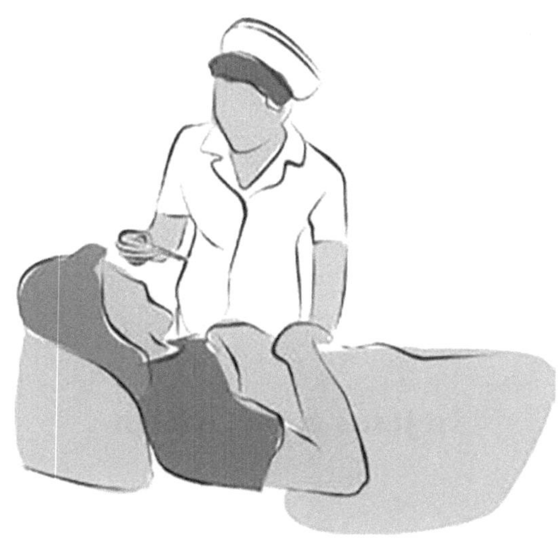

S O A P

Serve those in need.

Obey God's word.

Apply what you read.

Pray for understanding.

Once we do all that, "Our hands" will really be clean!

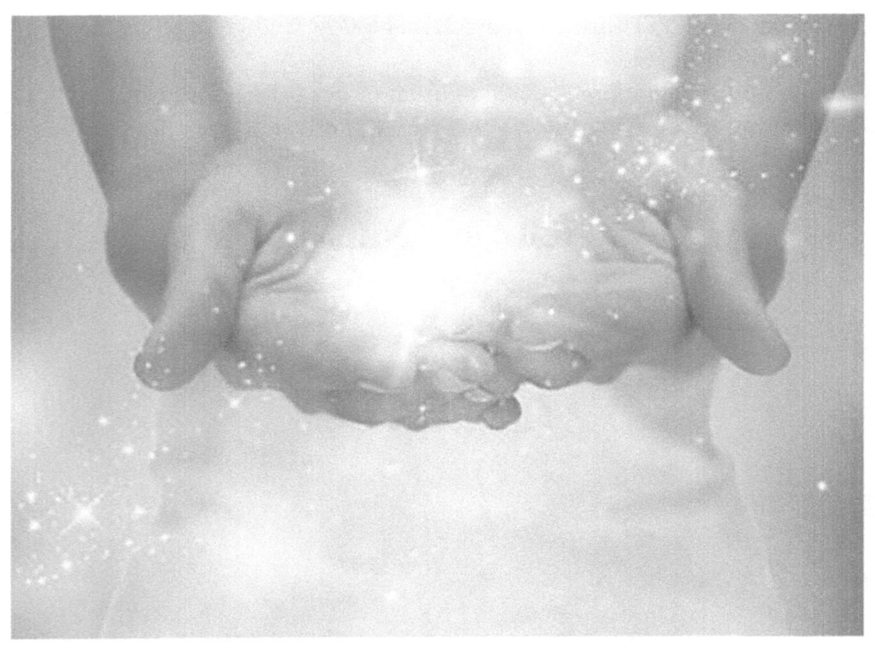

In Jesus name, Amen!

 Miss Asondra StarN'air

Stay In The Know

Normal Vital Signs

Blood Pressure:
Adults: defined with 2 measurements on 2 different dates at least 2 weeks apart
Normal BP <120/<80 mmHg
PreHTN: 120-139/80-89 mmHg
HTN Stage I: 140-159/90-99 mmHg
HTN Stage II: $\geq$160/$\geq$100 mmHg

Children:
Birth (12 Hr, <1000g): 39-59/16-36 mmHg
Birth (12 hr, 3 kg): 50-70/25-45 mmHg
Neonate (96hr): 60-90/20-60 mmHg
Infant (6 mo): 87-105/53-66 mmHg
Toddler (2 yr): 95-105/53-66 mmHg
School Age (7yr): 97-112/57-71 mmHg
Adolescent (15yr): 112-128/66-80 mmHg

Heart Rate:
Adults:
Female: 55-95 bpm
Male: 50-90 bpm

Children:
Neonate: 100-180 bpm awake   80-160 bpm asleep
Infant (6mo): 100-160 bpm awake   75-160 bpm asleep
Toddler: 80-110 bpm awake   60-90 bpm asleep
Preschooler: 70-110 bpm awake   60-90 bpm asleep
School-aged child: 65-110 bpm awake 60-90 bpm asleep
Adolescent: 60-90 bpm awake   50-90 bpm asleep

Respiration Rate:
Adults:
12-18 breaths per minute

Children:
Infants: 30-60 breaths per minute
Toddlers: 24-40
Preschoolers: 22-34
School-aged children: 18-30
Adolescents: 12-16

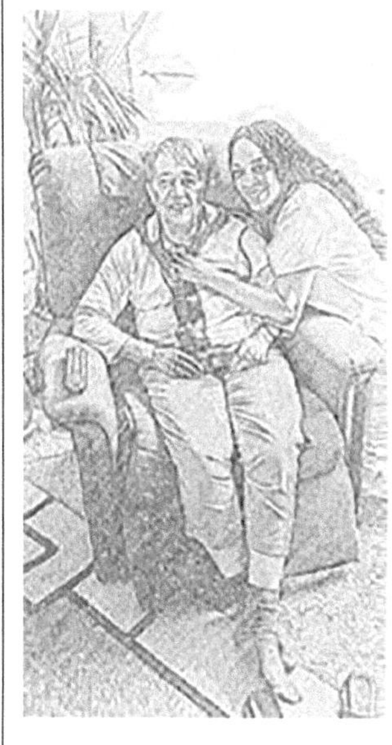

Vitals

The Four components of a set of vitals include:
1. Blood Pressure
2. Pulse
3. Respiratory rate
4. Temperature

Sample Care Plan

Clients Name: _______________________
Month _______________________
Week of ______/______/______ to ______/______/______

Wash your hands, Coming! Hello   ## Homecare Provider

	SUNDAY	MONDAY	TUESDAY	WEDNESDAY	THURSDAY	FRIDAY	SATURDAY
	DATE	DATE	DATE	DATE	DATE	DATE	DATES

Personal Care   /   Wash your hands

Bed bath/Shower
Skin care/shave
Oral hygiene/brush teeth
Denture Care/cleaning
Assist w/dressing & undressing
Prepare for bed/transfers.

Nutrition   Wash your hands
Prepare meals
Breakfast
Lunch
Dinner
Assist w/feeding
Encourage Fluids

Homemaking   Wash your hands
Make bed/change Linens
Laundry/ put away
Clean kitchen/bathroom/main room,
vacuum /trash removal/disinfection/
handwashing

Elimination   Wash your hands

Incontinence care/barrier cream
Position, report skin marking…. sores
Assist w/ toileting, standing, wiping

Circle all that applies   Wash your hands
Other /specialties /pet and plant care
Medication reminder, oxygen, vitals
Grocery shopping, transportation
Duties, assist w/ making phone calls
Emergency , 911, incident report

Client's Signature_______________________ Date_______________________
Caregiver's Signature_______________________ Date_______________________

Caregiver's Note Pad & Mini Incident report

____
____
____
____
____
____
____

**Any incidents circle Y or N, if Yes, complete the following:
Briefly describe, tell us what happened?**

____
____
____
____
____
____
____

**Did you call the Office - Family or 911? Circle Y or N and circle who you called.
Write the complete names of all involved and who you contacted below**

(I) Involved   (C) Contacted

______________________   ______________________
______________________   ______________________
______________________   ______________________
______________________   ______________________

Where you injured?   **Did you have to follow to hospital?**
Circle Y or N   **Y or N**

**Prepare to come into the office to fill out full
incident report within 24 hours**

Thank You!

Caregiver's don't do it!

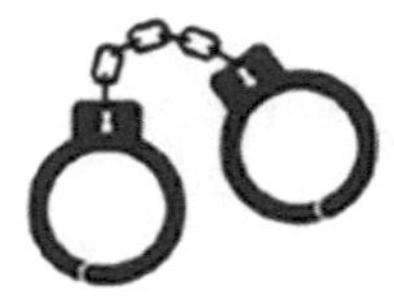

Everyday a number of individuals are caught engaged in some kind of theft and with disappointment, homecare is an area of great concern, so let's address it right now!

Homecare and private duty agencies face theft in clients homes by caregivers more often than reported. This is another form of elderly abuse that mustn't be tolerated.

The service of homecare requires a tremendous amount of trust, so when a care- giver breaks that trust by lying, cheating and stealing it hurts everyone. Yes everyone is affected, the client, the family, owners, management, and other care staff.

Because trust flows from the caregiver that business owner and management will follow through on the commitment made, when a caregiver steals, the company's rep- utation is damaged and some never recover. That's why agencies now have a zero tolerance for stealing, anyone caught steal- ing will be prosecuted, but the good news is 95 to 99 % of Caregivers are honest and upstanding individuals according to my research and that's something to be proud of and the 1% that are not, I wrote a little something for you, check it out!

THEFT

Taking
Has
Eliminated
Future
Trust

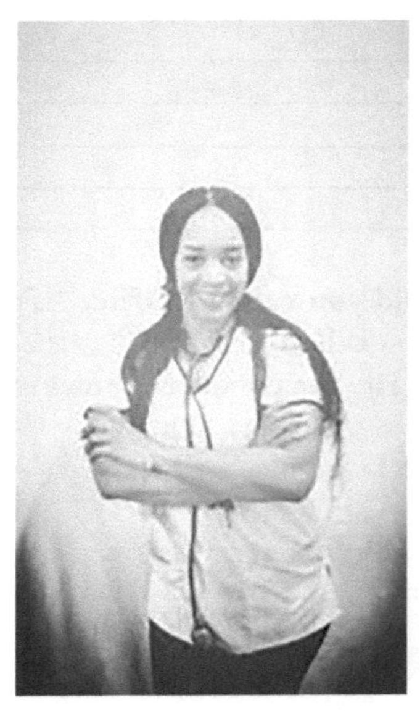

**Don't Steal,
Ask God and it
Shall Be Given!
Mark 7:7**

"If someone seems to be getting away with doing something wrong, trust me it won't be long before their gone

Maybe, God's just giving those a chance to make it all right

For his grace and mercy is new every day, if you need something just pray, you don't have to steal it's not right. Remember God knows and see's everything but if you don't stop stealing your doorbell shall surely ring."

You are under arrest!

You have the right to remain silent

anything you say can be used

against you in a court of law,

you have a right to an attorney

"Warning, warning…

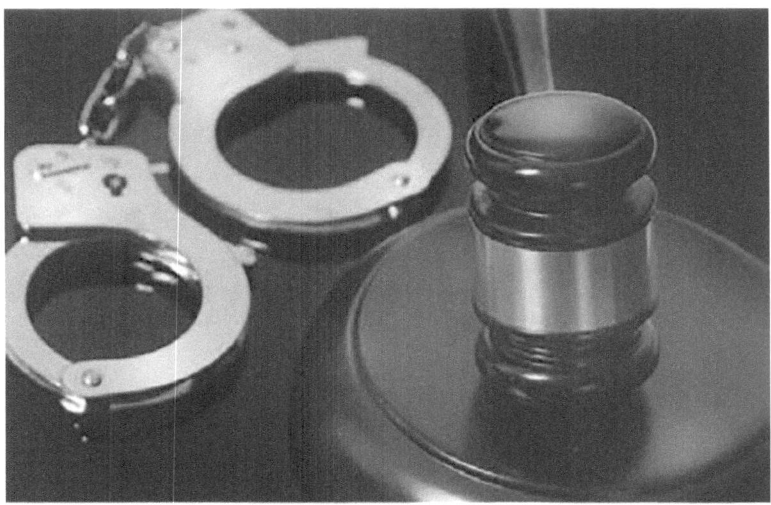

'Caregivers' Don't Do It!"

Stealing!
Caregiver's don't do It, don't Even Think About It!

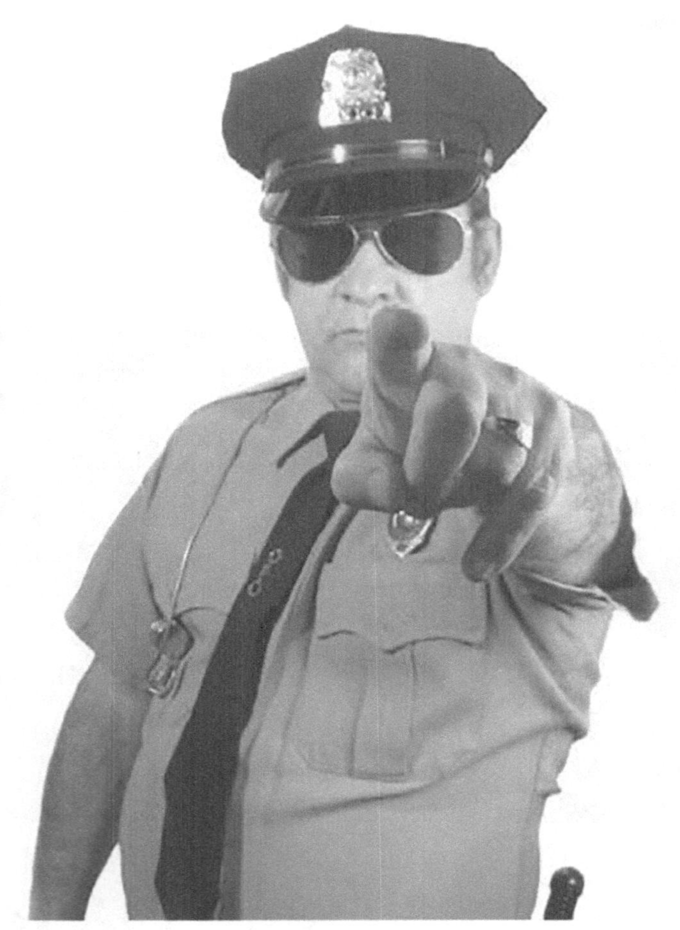

Taking From Others Is WRONG!

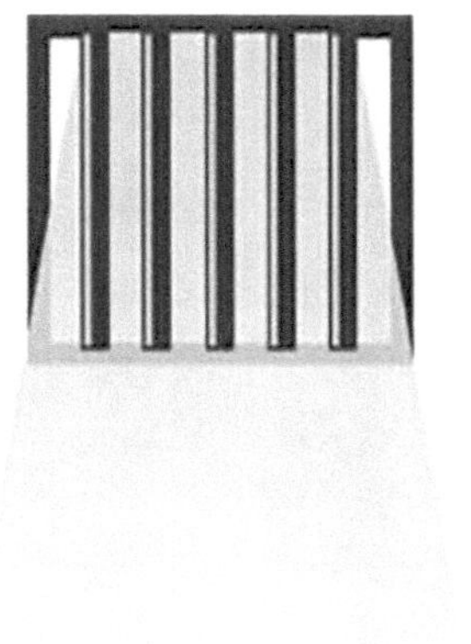

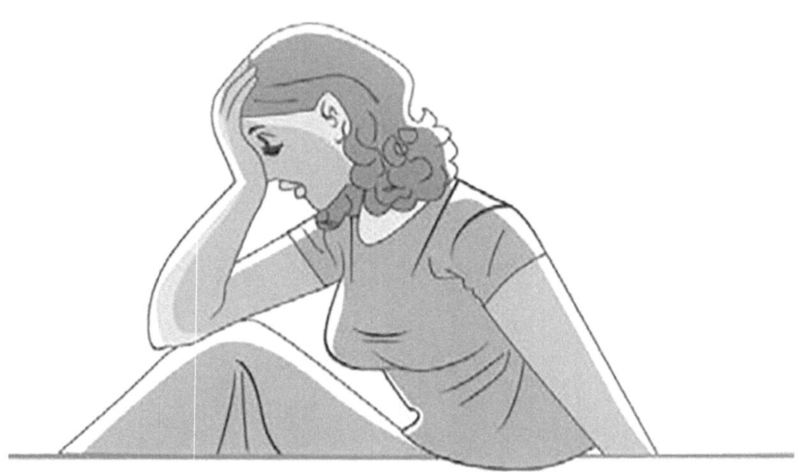

Told You Not To do It!

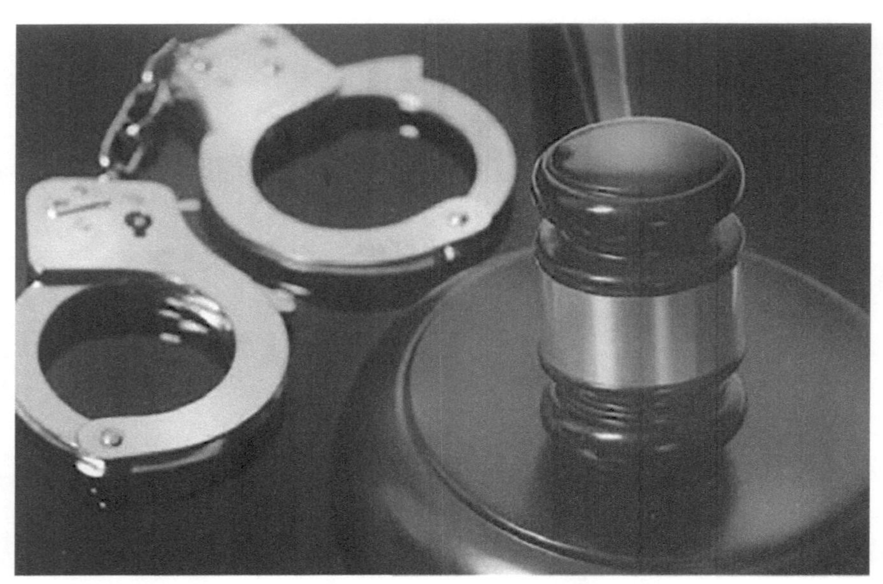

How do You Plead?

"Guilty"!

Now you have plenty of time to read

A Caregiver's Bible to Excellence!

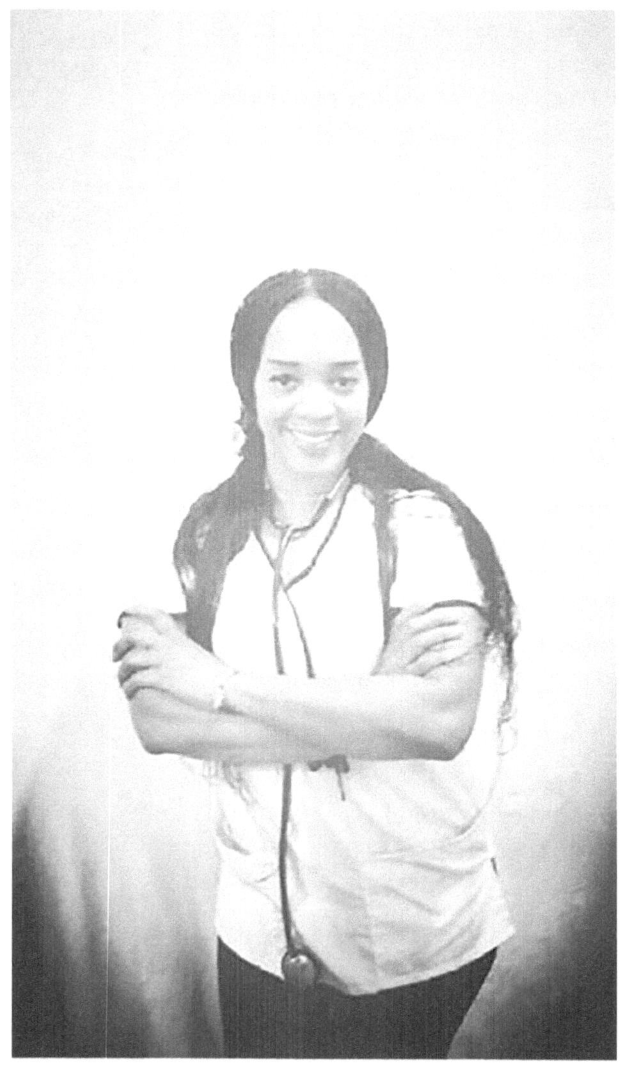

I Will Pray For Your Return!
Everyone deserves A Second Change.

Shopping for Senior's

When shopping for seniors most elderly people already know what they like and don't like, before you go shopping ask them what they would like, don't pick out things you like, stay professional. And for those seniors who don't know what they want and are relying on you to choose for them, choose **'Nutritionally'**. Make sure you are buying all the food groups and make sure you are reading the labels too; and too, watch out for high sodium and high sugar products, start caring about what goes in their mouths. Shop so that they can stay fit and healthy don't load them up with cookies and junk food. Remember **"Fit Not Fat"** 'Smart Eating' is where it's at!

Last few thoughts, if the person in your care loves a certain item why change it? Keep buying that item, stop experimenting on their favorite foods, if you want them to try something new, purchase both items if you can. But if you have to choose between the two buy the one they're used to.

Again most people know what they like and once they like it, they like it! Don't take that choice away from them.

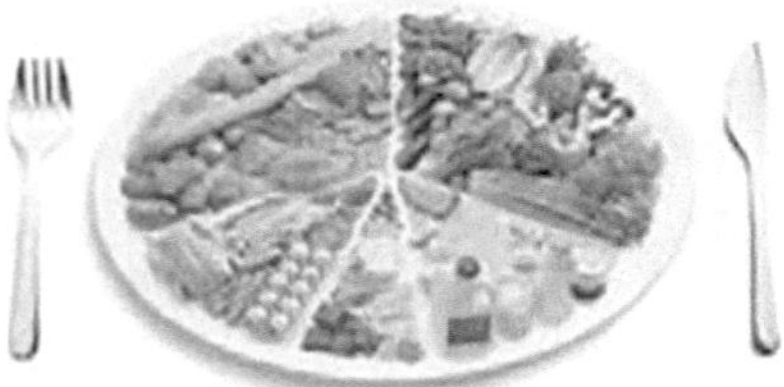

HOW DO YOU KNOW WHEN THEY 'DON'T LIKE IT'!

- They hardly eat it, they say" I'm full already, I can't eat anymore."
- They complain
- When food does not look appealing.
- Meal time becomes nothing to get excited about.
- No variety, Boring!
- Food is rushed, prepared poorly and it's over cook too.
- Food is burnt!
- Tea or Coffee is too hot or cold.
- Their eating table looks a mess and their water glass is not clean. "Hey where are the utensils?"

These kinds of errors can affect a good eating experience for anyone, not just seniors, everybody. So, caregivers let's be mindful and thoughtful during meal times. Let's take our time and do it right maybe they'll eat your food tonight!

Roots

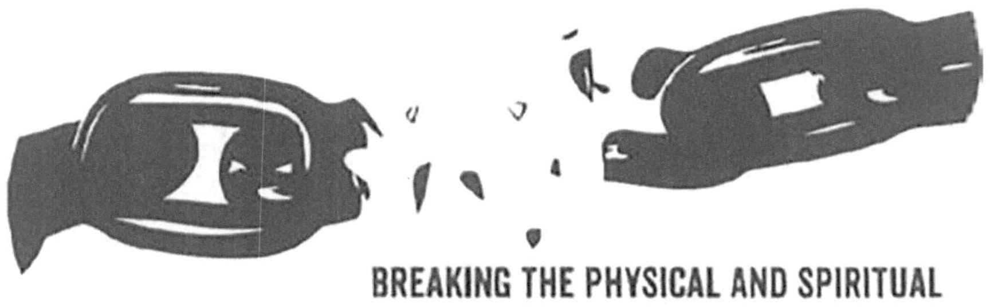

BREAKING THE PHYSICAL AND SPIRITUAL CHAINS OF MODERN DAY SLAVERY

African American's have been working overtime, double hard, ever since we laid foot on American soil. Yes things have gotten better, but our pay as caregivers in particular is insulting. Again we are part of the health care team, yet paid like slaves. Mistreated too if we speak up about the inequality. Well *'A New Day'* is dawning, God is calling people of color especially the black females in this market to fight for change. And all people for that matter who are being oppressed and denied their rights to equal opportunities.

I say, first let's start by giving home health aides a new name. How about **'Home Health Associates'** (HHA) no more Home Health Aides, "No" that's with slaves. The new name has more respectability don't you think? Yes it does, more dignity and love. So, **"FIGHT"** after today, don't let people call you aides anymore, tell them you are a caregiver, not an aide. You are an associate of the healthcare team.

Home Health Associates base rate in 2017 should be at 12.00 an hour or more. State Tested Nurse Assistants (STNA) 15.00 an hour or more. Nevertheless, **"ALL"** healthcare workers should be receiving medical coverage and full benefits too. March with me: **"Some Things Never Change, But Some Things MUST!"**

In God We Trust!

Let's MARCH!

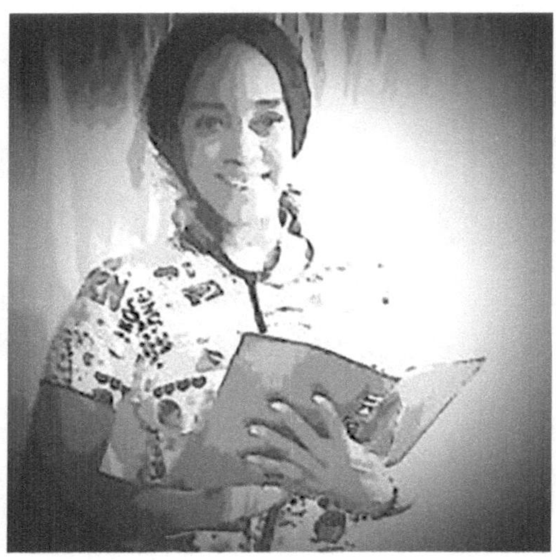

March for freedom and equality, walk together and don't grow weary, we must secure our future not only for us but for our children and their children's children. White supremacy must end on planet earth the very future of humankind depends on it. The world must become color blind until we are

One body in Christ we haven't arrived!

1 Corinthians 12:12

Certification/Training

Caregivers who are serious about their craft should be certified and trained in the following:

- CPR
- First aid
- Alzheimer's and 'Memory Care' training
- Hospice
- Med-Pass when working with DODD
- Certified Nurse Assistant/ STNA
- Hoyer Lift Training
- documentation/communication
- How to take Vitals Signs
- Feeding Tube
- How to change a Colostomy Bag

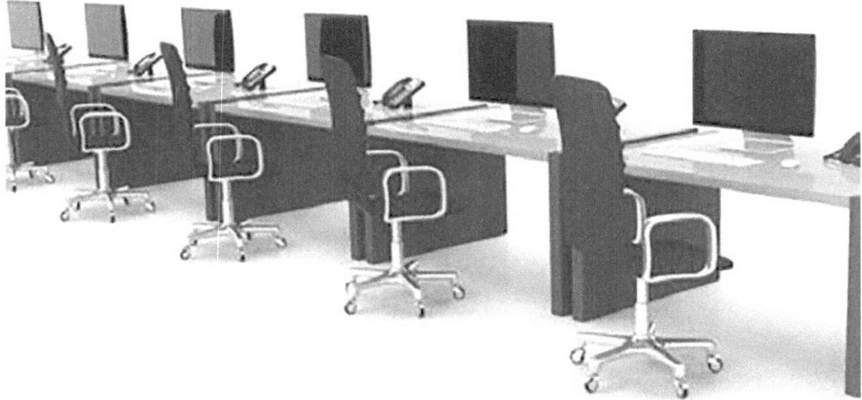

Home Health Aide's Role

Duties of home health aides can vary depending on the agency or the client if it's a private case.

The general duties are:

- Monitors patient condition by observing physical and mental condition.
- Intake and output
- Personal care as needed
- Exercise
- Supports patients by providing light housekeeping and laundry services
- Preparing meals
- Running errands

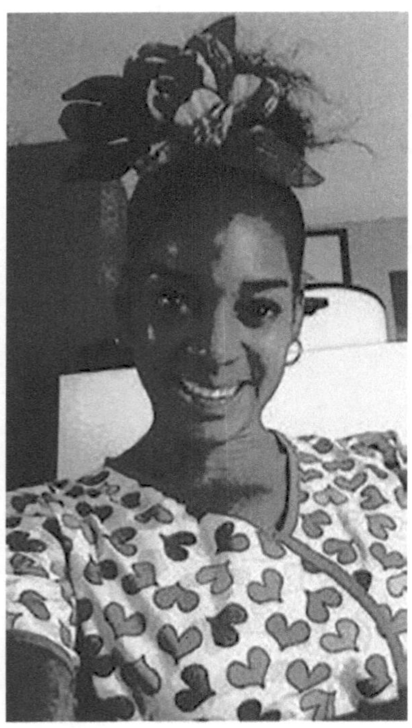

Home health aides' training requirement vary from state to state.

Home Health Aide Training Requirements, 2014

Hours	State	Minimum Training Hours	Minimum Clinical Hours
120+ hours (6 states)	Maine*	180	70
	Alaska*	140	80
	California**	120	20
	Idaho*	120	40
	Illinois	120	40
	Wisconsin*	120	32
76 – 119 hours (10 states)	Kansas**	110	45
	Rhode Island*	100	20
	New Hampshire*	100	60
	Hawaii*	100	70
	Maryland*	100	40
	Montana**	91	25
	Wyoming**	91	16
	Washington*	85	50
	Vermont*	80	30
	New Jersey	76	16
75 hours (34 states + District of Columbia)	Alabama	75	16
	Arizona	75	16
	Arkansas***	75	16
	Connecticut	75	16
	Colorado	75	16
	Delaware	75	16
	D.C.	75	16
	Florida	75	16
	Georgia	75	16
	Iowa	75	16
	Indiana	75	16
	Kentucky	75	16
	Louisiana	75	16
	Massachusetts	75	16

Hours	State	Minimum Training Hours	Minimum Clinical Hours
75 hours (cont'd)	Michigan	75	16
	Minnesota	75	16
	Mississippi	75	16
	Missouri	75	16
	Nebraska	75	16
	Nevada	75	16
	New Mexico	75	16
	New York	75	16
	North Carolina*	75	16
	North Dakota	75	16
	Ohio	75	16
	Oklahoma	75	16
	Oregon	75	16
	Pennsylvania	75	16
	South Carolina	75	16
	South Dakota	75	16
	Tennessee	75	16
	Texas	75	16
	Utah	75	16
	Virginia	75	16
	West Virginia	75	16

*Home Health Aides must be Certified Nursing Aides and have completed the CNA training and competency evaluation

**Certified Nurse Aides may be dual-certified as Home Health Aides with additional training

***Home Health Aides may become Certified Nurse Aides with no additional training provided successful completion of the CNA competency evaluation.

The STNA's Role

STNAs, like orderlies and attendants, aren't licensed care providers in their own right. Instead, they provide care under the direction or supervision of a registered nurse or physician. Their role is to be front-line care providers to the home's patients, attending to their daily needs and monitoring their physical and mental condition. They're the staff members who have the most direct contact with patients and serve an important function as the "eyes and ears" of the trained nursing staff. When a patient's condition deteriorates, the STNAs are the ones who usually notice and bring it to the attention of senior staff.

Basic Personal Care

Much of an STNA's workday revolves around basic personal care, or "bath and bedpan" duty. The STNA helps patients make use of the restroom or bedpan and provides bathing assistance or sponge baths as needed. Patients whose mobility is impaired might also need help dressing and handling basic personal hygiene such as hair washing, tooth brushing, or denture care. At mealtimes, the STNA might help patients to the facility's dining area or bring meals to less-mobile patients and help them eat.

Basic Nursing Care

STNAs also perform a range of basic nursing duties. They reposition bedridden patients regularly to help them remain comfortable and to prevent bedsores. They change bandages and dressings, disinfect catheters, and empty urine drainage bags. STNAs also measure and record the patient's vital signs on a regular schedule, as specified by the nursing or medical staff. They'll measure a patient's pulse rate, temperature, respiratory rate, and sometimes weight, and record that information on the patient's chart. STNAs must be respectful and courteous with residents at all times and be conscious of their rights.

Physical Activity

Staying physically active is an important part of health and wellness for the elderly, so STNAs help with regular exercise and physical activity. They'll assist mobile residents by providing an arm to lean on, or assist them in getting from their bed to the walker. STNAs often lead residents in low-impact exercises designed to preserve or restore their range of motion and overall fitness. For bedridden patients with limited voluntary movement, STNAs manually flex and rotate the limbs to improve circulation and stimulate the muscles.

Training

The State of Ohio specifies a standardized curriculum for STNAs that is available at community colleges, trade schools, or on-site at health-care facilities. Trainees must complete an orientation, followed by the Training and Competency Evaluation Program. The program gives students sixteen hours of classroom training before they're allowed to work with patients, followed by fifty-nine hours of mixed class-room instruction and hands-on supervised clinical experience. The State also specifies that facilities must provide STNAs with a minimum of twelve hours of formal in-service training in the course of each calendar year.

 MISS ASONDRA STARN'AIR

Health Care For Caregivers

Caregivers, things have changed. We no longer have the option of not having healthcare insurance. **"It's The Law."** Everyone must have healthcare insurance or pay penalties. However, it is important too that the caregiver not only be covered but have the proper healthcare insurance too because we are exposed everyday to the dangers involved, such as infections and on-the-job injuries. Therefore, we want to make sure our insurance covers surgeries and hospital stays as well.

But who has the time to look for healthcare insurance? Some caregivers' schedules just do not allow them the time.

Well, I'm here to tell you no worries, there are lots of services online that can make finding health care quick and easy. Or you can just contact "The Healthcare Marketplace "a specialist will help you find coverage right over the phone. They'll even tell you what your new monthly payment will be, and it's based on your income.

Whatever you decide, Listen, hear me **"Caregivers"** out there, **don't delay, or You'll Pay!**

Everyone *Must* have Health Insurance. **"EVERYONE"!**

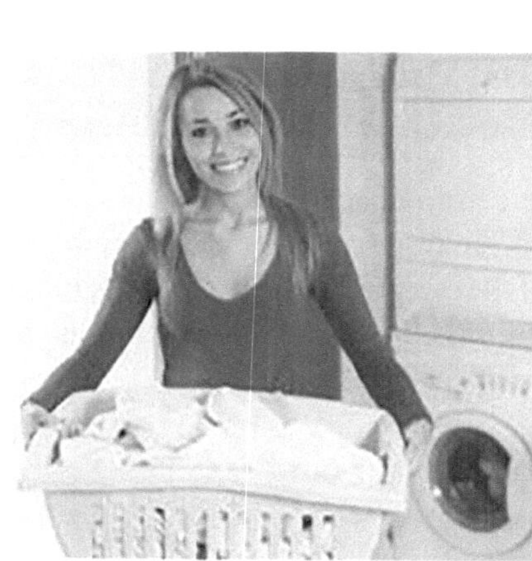

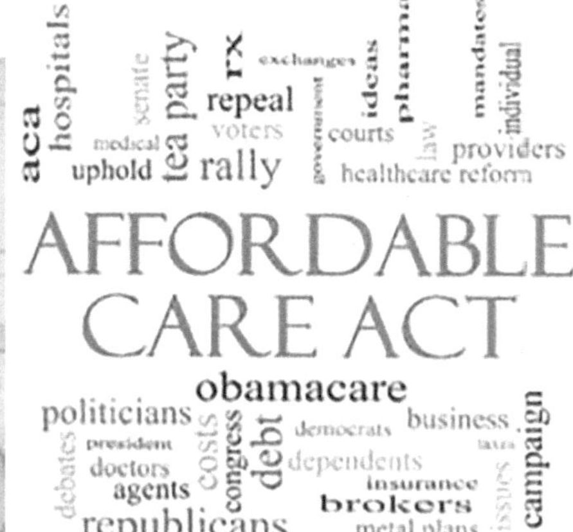

The Private Caregivers

Private caregivers are just that: 'Private' they are self-employed.

These caregivers may or may not be licensed, but many of them have years of experience. These individuals work out their schedule with the family or person they are caring for. They come up with a routine that fits both the client and the private caregiver.

Private caregivers set their own wages. The average rate is $15 to 25 dollars an hour, sometimes more depends on that family. These kinds of cases tend to last for years. In fact, I know someone who worked a private case for twenty-five years.

She worked five or more days a week, plus received bonuses, paid holidays and two weeks paid vacation time. Today these kinds of cases may be hard to come by, but they're out there. Keep looking, however, to find this kind of "Private Case", work of mouth seems to be the best form of advertisement.

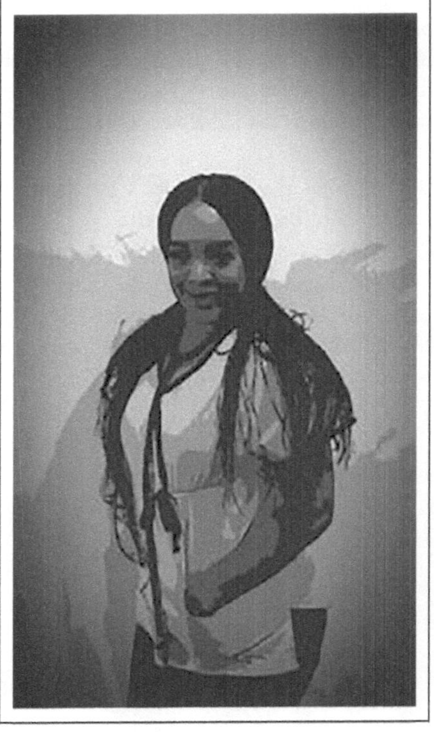

Someone who knows someone who is looking for someone like you.

As far as taxes, it is the responsibility of the caregiver to report their earnings on a **1040-ES, Estimated Tax for Individuals.** For more information, go to **"Self-Employed Individual Tax Center" WWW.IRS.GOV**

You are a private business owner now.
Make a good name for yourself.
Be Professional!

Caregiver's "ME" Time!

Caregivers, celebrate "Your" days off!

- Take a candlelight bath. Have yourself a glass of wine, dark chocolate, or something special.
- Give yourself a spa treatment, facial, soak your feet.
- Next, go out to breakfast, maybe lunch, or make a wonderful meal. You and your family just have a fantastic day; treat yourself well. You deserve it.
- Doll up! Be beautiful today.
- Rest, take a Jesus nap—one full of peace and no worries. Rest is a prerequisite for good health and fitness. When was the last time you put your feet up?
- Go do something fun! Karaoke, dance, bowling, museums, visit a friend. Have fun today!

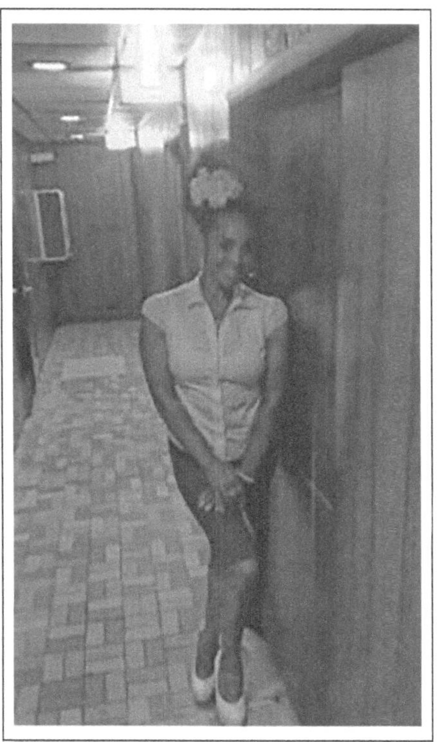

Enjoy Your Days Off!
Use one of your days off as a Sabbath.
Sleep, rest—no work, no nothin'
A perfect day to be with **Jesus!**

Federal Holidays List for Caregivers

- ✓ New Year's Day
- ✓ Birthday of Martin Luther King Jr.
- ✓ Washington's Birthday
- ✓ Memorial Day
- ✓ Independence Day (Fourth of July)
- ✓ Labor Day
- ✓ Columbus Day
- ✓ Veterans Day
- ✓ Thanks Giving Day
- ✓ Christmas Day

In addition, Inauguration Day is also a paid federal holiday. Every four years. It is celebrated on January 20 (or the twenty-first if the twentieth is on a Sunday).

Federal law established these public holidays for **"Federal Employees."** When a holiday falls on a weekend, the holiday usually is observed on a Monday. Note: If it falls on a Friday, Saturday, or Sunday, the holiday is observed on a Monday!

But keep in mind, not everyone gets paid on holidays. Only federal employees are guaranteed these paid holidays; it was set up for them. Private-sector holidays are different; they are not required to close for holidays. Caregivers, you know we work no matter what. The sick needs our service **24/7.**
Not only are private-sector entities not required to close on holidays, they do not have to pay either for holidays or vacations and time off. This is very, very important to remember. So what that means is we much always check with our human resources department to provide us with a list of paid or unpaid holidays.
Never assume—you find out!

The reason for this is what is called the Fair Labor Standards Act **(FLSA)**, which does not require these benefits. One can look at it as a gift, a privilege, or a blessing if you will—but not a right. If you work for a company (and many of us do) that *gives* us these fringe benefits, *hallelujah!*

Regular time—Regular pay
Time in a half—10 plus half would be 15 an hour
Double time—10 plus double time would be 20 an hour
Bonuses are just that "Bonus" and can be monetary in nature or gifts. **"A box of candy!"**

STAR

MISS ASONDRA STARN'AIR
A CAREGIVERS BIBLE TO EXCELLENCE!

CONTACT

Email :
1missasondra@gmail.com

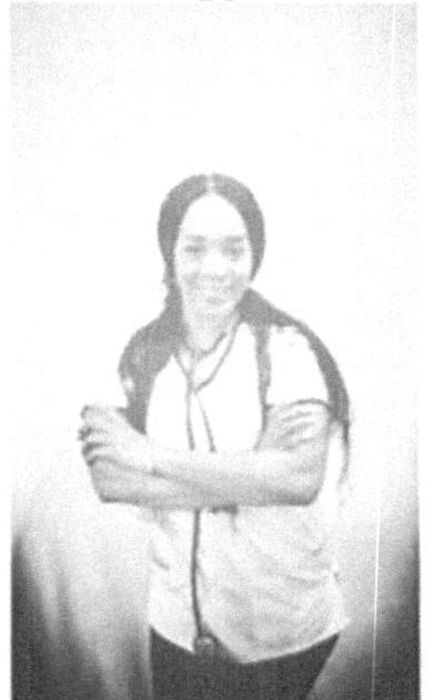

But you are A CHOSEN RACE, A royal PREASTHOOD, A HOLY NATION, A PEOPLE FOR GOD'S OWN POSESSIONS, so that you many proclaim the excellence of Him who has called you out of darkness into His marvelous light for you were once were NOT A PEOPLE, but you are THE PEOPLE OF GOD, you had NOT RECEIVED MERCY, but now you have RECEIVED MERCY.
1 Peter 2.9-10

CAREGIVERS

Dear caregivers, I would like to take this time out to thank all of you for purchasing my book. This book is my gift to all of you. In hopes you become the best caregiver ever, Remember it all starts with Jesus!

Sincerely and with care,
Miss Asondra StarN'air

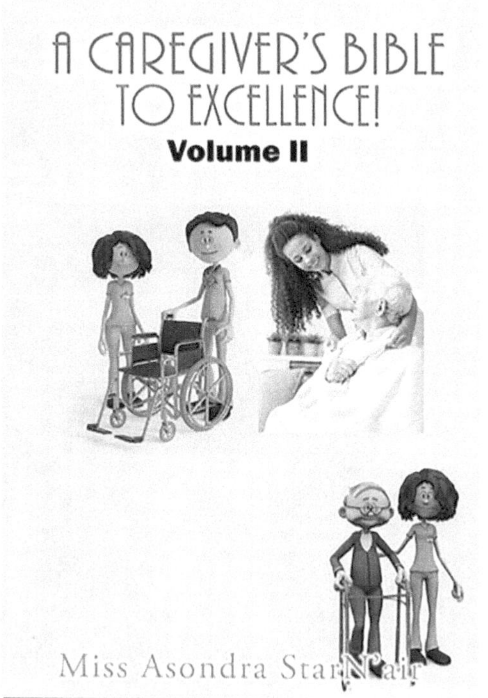

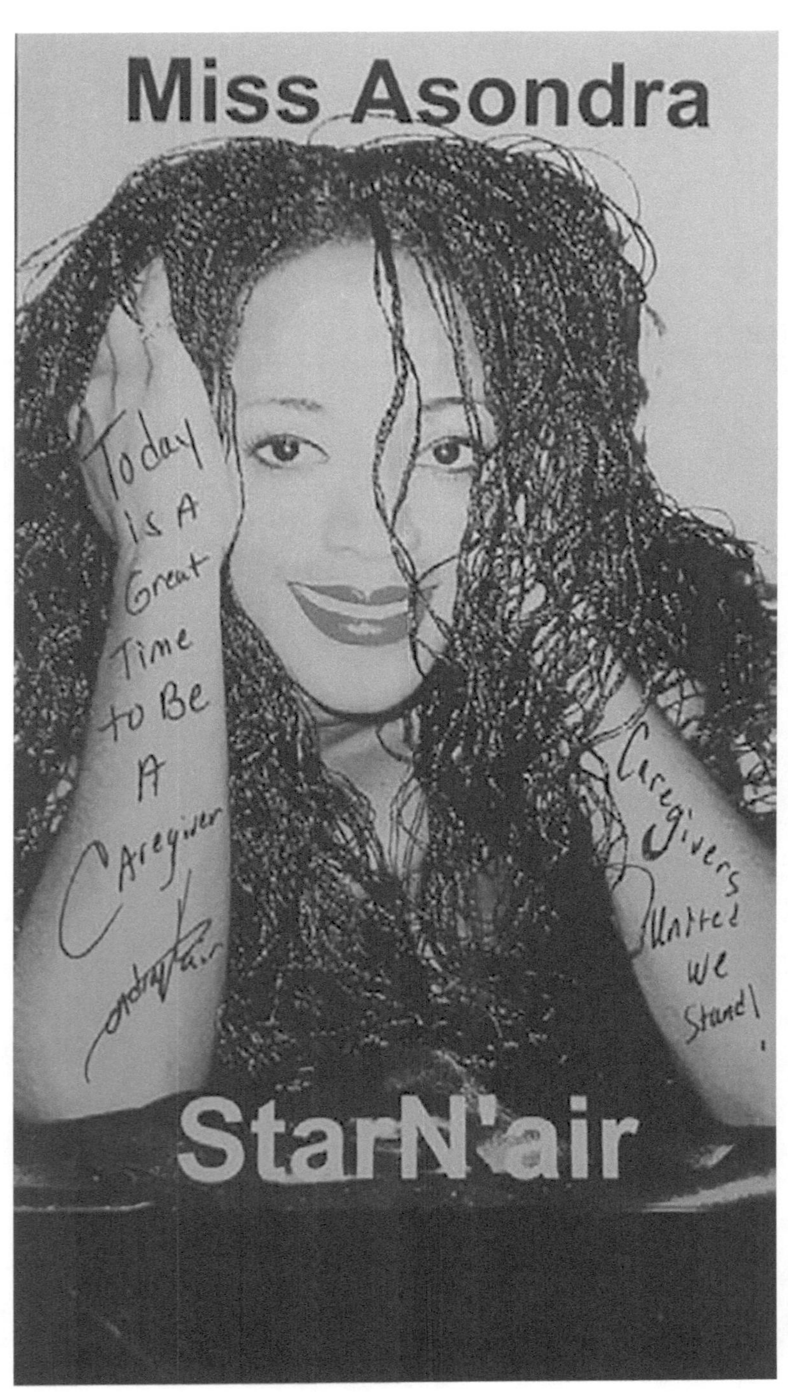

Miss Asondra StarN'air

It's Your Book Now!

A Caregiver's Bible to Excellence is a Transformational Book. You'll never be the same if you do it all in Jesus name! There will be no limits to your greatness!

However, that will not happen if you don't allow the transformation.

Like the Bible, **You** MUST:
Get the Book
Open the Book
Do the Book
Is with you!
Otherwise, you will remain the same ordinary caregiver, nothing special about you. If you are going to be in the care giving business people deserve more than that. **Make that change!**
Be Excellent, Be Transformed! **"Go Out"** light the world up, *A Caregiver "Star" Is Born!*
A Caregivers Bible To Excellence is the **"New Way"** to **High Quality Care Giving and More!!!** Embrace this book and all it has to offer inside. Stop being ordinary get with *Jesus* and become extraordinary. Apply what you have learned through those pages, let it help take you higher than you have ever been. Do it! Reach one heart at a time, you don't need me anymore, now is your turn to shine!

Your Very Own Caregivers Bible

HOW TO USE YOUR CAREGIVERS BIBLE

Get the book

- Take it with you to work every- day, make it part of your **(FNG)** Florence Nightingale work bag.
- Start using your medical terminology section of your caregivers bible when charting and documenting. Doing this will show you have stepped up to high quality care and professionalism. You are no longer an aide, you are a professional caregiver. Keep this book by your side!

Open the book

- Again the more you read your caregiver's bible, the more you transform into a high quality caregiver. Soon you will be on your way to greatness! Allow Jesus to lead the way!

- Write in your caregiver's bibles. It's your book now, not mine. I was just the vessel.

Do the book, and watch what happens, God will bless you like he blessed me.
Let Christ lead!

Be Excellent in Christ!

The CPR of
Creative Personalized Reflections
A Life Worth Sharing!

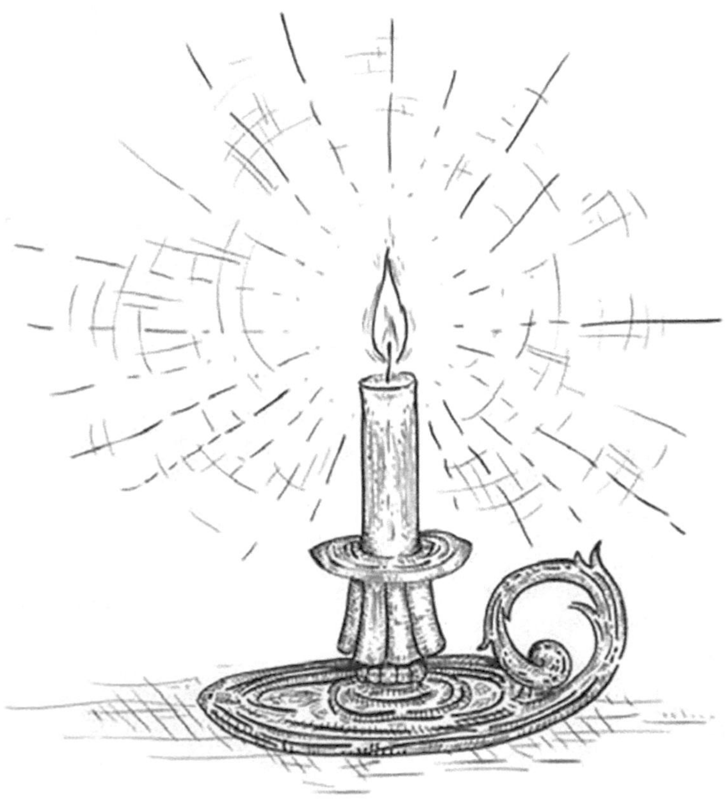

My Caregiver's Memoir

Hello, my name is ____

I was born on ____

In ____

What are you most proud of in your life? _______________________________

____

____

____

____

____

____

What were your biggest accomplishments?

____

____

____

____

____

____

____

What were your biggest mistakes in life, and did you have a chance to correct them?

____

____

____

____

____

____

____

____

____

____

What is your favorite scripture and why _______________________________

____

____

____

____

____

____

____

____

____

What is your dream, and did you ever accomplish it? ___________________

____

____

____

____

____

____

____

____

____

____

Do you think you were successful in life? Why or why not? _____________

____

____

____

____

____

____

____

____

____

____

What were some of your big-ticket item purchases _____________________

____

____

____

MISS ASONDRA STARN'AIR

____

____

____

____

Favorite Foods

____

____

____

Restaurants

____

____

____

TV programs ____________________________________

____

____

____

Books and Authors ______________________________

____

____

____

____

Color ____

____

____

Flower _______________________________________

____

____

Songs and Artist ____

____
____
____
____
____

What are your hobbies? _______________________________

____
____
____
____
____

What was the most exciting thing that ever happened to you?

____
____
____
____
____
____

What hurt you the most? _______________________________

____
____
____
____
____

Do you believe in forgiveness and why _______________________

____
____
____
____

    Miss Asondra StarN'air

Are you a Christian, someone who believes Jesus died for us and is coming back for his people? If you do or don't, tell us in your own words. _________

____

____

____

____

____

____

____

How do you want to be remembered? If you were given the chance to say good-bye to the world, what would you say? ________________________

____

____

____

____

____

____

____

____

____

____

____

____

____

____

____

____

____

____

____

____

____

____

____

____

What advice or wisdom would you offer? _______________________

____
____
____
____
____
____
____
____
____

What would you say to your family? _______________________

____
____
____
____
____
____
____
____
____
____
____
____

Would you want to be cremated or buried? _______________________

____
____
____
____
____
____
____
____
____

How would you like your life celebrated? ___________________________
____
____
____
____
____
____
____
____
____
____
____
____
____
____

Do you have a living will?
____
____
____
____
____
____
____
____

Do you have life insurance? Circle yes or no. If you do, what company? ____
____
____

Would you want to be put on life support? Circle Yes or No Comment ____
____
____

Any ministry donations? If so, what and to who? Circle Yes or No ________
____
____
____

____
____
____

____
____
____

Do you want to Donate your Organs? Circle Yes or No Comments

____
____
____
____
____

What Funeral Home or Church? _______________________
Burial Types (circle one)

Above-Ground   **Underground**   **Cremation**

Finally, your words to those you leave behind. _______________
____
____
____
____
____
____
____
____
____
____
____
____
____
____
____
____

Your Obituary Picture

Find the picture you want on the cover of your Obituary and paste it inside the picture box

Caregiver's Dear Diary pages.

 Miss Asondra StarN'air

 Miss Asondra StarN'air

The Promises of God &
Meditation Room for The Caregiver

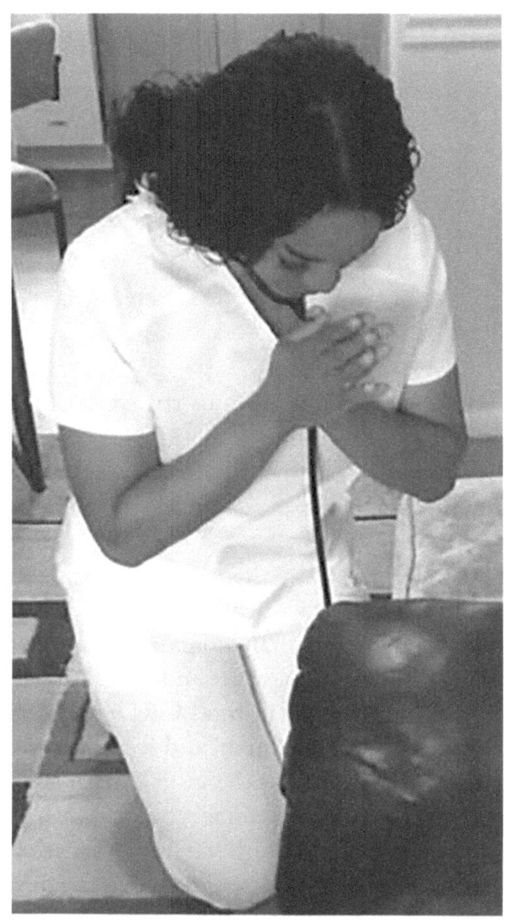

The Promises of God

For all those in need of deliverance and reassurance, no weapons formed against you shall prosper **(Isaiah 54:17)**. Meditate on the promises of God; let this be soothing to your soul.

All scriptures taken from the King James Version of the Bible unless otherwise indicated.

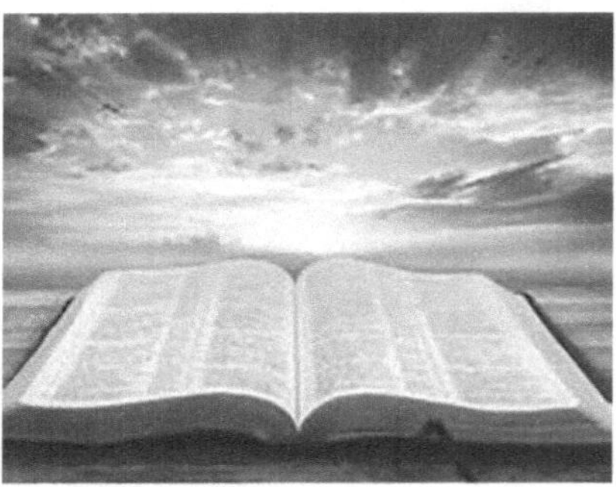

2 Timothy 1:7 "For God hath not given us the spirit of fear; but of power, and of love, and of a sound mind."

Isaiah 58:6 "Is not this the fast that I have chosen? to loose the bands of wickedness, to undo the heavy burdens, and to let the oppressed go free, and that ye break every yoke?"

Isaiah 58:13–14 "If thou turn away thy foot from the Sabbath, from doing thy pleasure on my holy day; and call the Sabbath a delight, the holy of the LORD, honourable; and shalt honour him, not doing thine own ways, nor finding thine own pleasure, nor speaking thine own words: Then shalt thou delight thyself in the LORD; and I will cause thee to ride upon the high places of the earth, and feed thee with the heritage of Jacob thy father: for the mouth of the LORD hath spoken it."

Luke 4:18 "The Spirit of the Lord is upon me, because he hath anointed me to preach the gospel to the poor; he hath sent me to heal the broken- hearted, to preach deliverance to the captives, and recovering of sight to the blind, to set at liberty them that are bruised."

Acts 10:38 "How God anointed Jesus of Nazareth with the Holy Ghost and with power: who went about doing good, and healing all that were oppressed of the devil; for God was with him."

Psalm 91:14–16 "Because he hath set his love upon me, therefore will I deliver him: I will set him on high, because he hath known my name. He shall call upon me, and I will answer him: I will be with him in trouble; I will deliver him, and honour him. With long life will I satisfy him, and show him my salvation."

Joel 2:32 "And it shall come to pass, that whosoever shall call on the name of the LORD shall be delivered: for in mount Zion and in Jerusalem shall be deliverance, as the LORD hath said, and in the remnant whom the LORD shall call."

Jeremiah 32:27 "Behold, I am the LORD, the God of all flesh: is there any thing too hard for me?"

Luke 1:37 "For with God nothing shall be impossible."

Jeremiah 33:3 "Call unto me, and I will answer thee, and show thee great and mighty things, which thou knows not."

Joel 3:10 "Beat your plowshares into swords, and your pruning hooks into spears: let the weak say, I am strong."

Nahum 1:13 "For now will I break his yoke from off thee, and will burst thy bonds in sunder."

Obadiah 17 "But upon mount Zion shall be deliverance, and there shall be holiness; and the house of Jacob shall possess their possessions."

Micah 7:8 "Rejoice not against me, O mine enemy: when I fall, I shall arise; when I sit in darkness, the LORD shall be a light unto me."

Mark 1:25–26 "And Jesus rebuked him, saying, Hold thy peace, and come out of him. And when the unclean spirit had torn him, and cried with a loud voice, he came out of him."

Mark 1:32–34 "And at even, when the sun did set, they brought unto him all that were diseased, and them that were possessed with devils. And all the city was gathered together at the door. And he healed many that were sick of divers diseases, and cast out many devils; and suffered not the devils to speak, because they knew him."

Luke 10:19–20 "Behold, I give unto you power to tread on serpents and scorpions, and over all the power of the enemy: and nothing shall by any means hurt you. Notwithstanding in this rejoice not, that the spirits are subject unto you; but rather rejoice, because your names are written in heaven."

Psalm 91:3 "Surely he shall deliver thee from the snare of the fowler, and from the noisome pestilence."

James 4:7 "Submit yourselves therefore to God. Resist the devil, and he will flee from you."

1 Peter 5:8–9 "Be sober, be vigilant; because your adversary the devil, as a roaring lion, walketh about, seeking whom he may devour: Whom resist steadfast in the faith, knowing that the same afflictions are accomplished in your brethren that are in the world."

John 5:4 "For whatsoever is born of God overcometh the world: and this is the victory that overcometh the world, even our faith."

Thessalonians 3:3 "But the Lord is faithful, who shall establish you, and keep you from evil."

John 14:30 "For the prince of this world cometh, and hath nothing in me."

John 16:33 "These things I have spoken unto you, that in me ye might have peace. In the world ye shall have tribulation: but be of good cheer; I have overcome the world."

1 Timothy 1:18 "This charge I commit unto thee, son Timothy, according to the prophecies which went before on thee, that thou by them mightest was a good warfare."

1 Timothy 6:12 "Fight the good fight of faith, lay hold on eternal life, whereunto thou art also called."

Psalm 41:1 "Blessed is he that considereth the poor: the LORD will deliver him in time of trouble."

Psalm 138:7–8 "Though I walk in the midst of trouble, thou wilt revive me: thou shalt stretch forth thine hand against the wrath of mine enemies, and thy right hand shall save me. The LORD will perfect that which concerneth me: thy mercy, O LORD, endureth forever: forsake not the works of thine own hands."

Psalm 17:3–4 "… I am purposed that my mouth shall not transgress… by the word of thy lips I have kept me from the paths of the destroyer."

Psalm 107:20 "He sent his word, and healed them, and delivered them from their destructions."

Psalm 126:1–2 "When the LORD turned again the captivity of Zion, we were like them that dream. Then was our mouth filled with laughter, and our tongue with singing: then said they among the heathen, The LORD hath done great things for them."

Psalm 34:7 "The angel of the LORD encampeth round about them that fear him, and delivereth them."

Hebrews 1:14 "Are they (angels) not all ministering spirits, sent forth to minister for them who shall be heirs of salvation?"

Isaiah 50:2 "…Is my hand shortened at all, that it cannot redeem? or have I no power to deliver?…"

Jeremiah 1:8 "Be not afraid of their faces: for I am with thee to deliver thee, saith the LORD."

2 Samuel 22:20 "He brought me forth also into a large place: he delivered me, because he delighted in me."

2 Timothy 4:17–18 "I was delivered out of the mouth of the lion. And the Lord shall deliver me from every evil work, and will preserve me unto his heavenly kingdom: to whom be glory for ever and ever."

Romans 8:31–32 "What shall we then say to these things? If God be for us, who can be against us? He that spared not his own Son, but delivered him up for us all, how shall he not with him also freely give us all things?"

Galatians 1:4 "Who gave himself for our sins, that he might deliver us from this present evil world, according to the will of God and our Father:"

Psalm 32:7 "Thou art my hiding place; thou shalt preserve me from trouble; thou shalt compass me about with songs of deliverance."

Psalm 34:4 "I sought the LORD, and he heard me, and delivered me from all my fears."

Psalm 18:2–3 "The LORD is my rock, and my fortress, and my deliverer; my God, my strength, in whom I will trust; my buckler, and the horn of my salvation, and my high tower. I will call upon the LORD, who is worthy to be praised: so shall I be saved from mine enemies."

Psalm 60:11–12 "Give us help from trouble: for vain is the help of man. Through God we shall do valiantly: for he it is that shall tread down our enemies."

Isaiah 41:13–14 "For I the LORD thy God will hold thy right hand, saying unto thee, Fear not; I will help thee. Fear not, thou worm Jacob, and ye men of Israel; I will help thee, saith the LORD, and thy redeemer, the Holy One of Israel."

Proverbs 16:7 "When a man's ways please the LORD, he maketh even his enemies to be at peace with him."

Healing

Let these words be food for the faith of those who are determined to believe God for their healing (whether physical or emotional)! As you read them, ask God to make them alive in your spirit. We encourage you to read them out loud, as it will help your faith. Truly our Lord is a God who heals (Jehovah Rapha).

James 5:13–16 "Is any among you afflicted? let him pray. Is any merry? let him sing psalms. Is any sick among you? let him call for the elders of the church; and let them pray over him, anointing him with oil in the name of the Lord: And the prayer of faith shall save the sick, and the Lord shall raise him up; and if he have committed sins, they shall be forgiven him.

Confess your faults one to another, and pray one for another, that ye may be healed. The effectual fervent prayer of a righteous man availeth much."

Matthew 4:23 "And Jesus went about all Galilee, teaching in their synagogues, and preaching the gospel of the kingdom, and healing all manner of sickness and all manner of disease among the people."

Acts 28:8–9 "And it came to pass, that the father of Publius lay sick of a fever and of a bloody flux: to whom Paul entered in, and prayed, and laid his hands on him, and healed him. So when this was done, others also, which had diseases in the island, came, and were healed:"

Proverbs 16:24 "Pleasant words are as an honeycomb, sweet to the soul, and health to the bones."

Jeremiah 30:17 "For I will restore health unto thee, and I will heal thee of thy wounds, saith the LORD; because they called thee an Outcast, saying, This is Zion, whom no man seeketh after."

Exodus 23:25 "And ye shall serve the LORD your God, and he shall bless thy bread, and thy water; and I will take sickness away from the midst of thee."

1 Peter 3:10 "For he that will love life, and see good days, let him refrain his tongue from evil, and his lips that they speak no guile:"

Isaiah 58:6–8 "Is not this the fast that I have chosen? to loose the bands of wickedness, to undo the heavy burdens, and to let the oppressed go free, and that ye break every yoke? Is it not to deal thy bread to the hungry, and that thou bring the poor that are cast out to thy house? when thou seest the naked, that thou cover him; and that thou hide not thyself from thine own flesh? Then shall thy light break forth as the morning, and thine health shall spring forth speedily: and thy righteousness shall go before thee; the glory of the LORD shall be thy reward."

3 John 2 "Beloved, I wish above all things that thou mayest prosper and be in health, even as thy soul prospereth."

Proverbs 3:7–8 "Be not wise in thine own eyes: fear the LORD, and depart from evil. It shall be health to thy navel, and marrow to thy bones."

Proverbs 4:20–22 "My son, attend to my words; incline thine ear unto my sayings. Let them not depart from thine eyes; keep them in the midst of thine heart. For they are life unto those that find them, and health to all their flesh."

1 Kings 17:21–22 "And he stretched himself upon the child three times, and cried unto the LORD, and said, O LORD my God, I pray thee, let this child's soul come into him again. And the LORD heard the voice of Elijah; and the soul of the child came into him again, and he revived."

Mark 16:18b "They shall lay hands on the sick, and they shall recover."

Mark 11:22 "And Jesus answering saith unto them, Have faith in God."

Matthew 15:28 "Then Jesus answered and said unto her, O woman, great is thy faith: be it unto thee even as thou wilt. And her daughter was made whole from that very hour."

Jeremiah 33:6 "Behold, I will bring it health and cure, and I will cure them, and will reveal unto them the abundance of peace and truth."

Psalm 91:10 "There shall no evil befall thee, neither shall any plague come nigh thy dwelling."

Psalm 105:37 "He brought them forth also with silver and gold: and there was not one feeble person among their tribes."

Psalm 42:11 "Why art thou cast down, O my soul? and why art thou disquieted within me? hope thou in God: for I shall yet praise him, who is the health of my countenance, and my God."

Psalm 103:2–3 "Bless the LORD, O my soul, and forget not all his benefits: Who forgiveth all thine iniquities; who healeth all thy diseases;"

Exodus 15:26 "And said, If thou wilt diligently hearken to the voice of the LORD thy God, and wilt do that which is right in his sight, and wilt give ear to his commandments, and keep all his statutes, I will put none of these diseases upon thee, which I have brought upon the Egyptians: for I am the LORD that healeth thee." (Jehovah Rapha)

Psalm 107:20 "He sent his word, and healed them, and delivered them from their destructions."

Malachi 4:2 "But unto you that fear my name shall the Sun of righteousness arise with healing in his wings; and ye shall go forth, and grow up as calves of the stall."

Acts 10:38 "How God anointed Jesus of Nazareth with the Holy Ghost and with power: who went about doing good, and healing all that were oppressed of the devil; for God was with him."

Luke 17:14 "And when he saw them, he said unto them, Go show yourselves unto the priests. And it came to pass, that, as they went, they were cleansed."

2 Kings 13:21 "And it came to pass, as they were burying a man, that, behold, they spied a band of men; and they cast the man into the sepulchre of Elisha: and when the man was let down, and touched the bones of Elisha, he revived, and stood up on his feet."

Luke 18:38–43 "And he cried, saying, Jesus, thou son of David, have mercy on me. And they which went before rebuked him, that he should hold his peace: but he cried so much the more, Thou son of David, have mercy on me. And Jesus stood, and commanded him to be brought unto him: and when he was come near, he asked him, Saying, What wilt thou that

I shall do unto thee? And he said, Lord, that I may receive my sight. And Jesus said unto him, Receive thy sight: thy faith hath saved thee. And immediately he received his sight, and followed him, glorifying God: and all the people, when they saw it, gave praise unto God."

Isaiah 53:4–5 "Surely he hath borne our griefs, and carried our sorrows: yet we did esteem him stricken, smitten of God, and afflicted. But he was wounded for our transgressions, he was bruised for our iniquities: the chastisement of our peace was upon him; and with his stripes we are healed."

Matthew 8:16–17 "When the even was come, they brought unto him many that were possessed with devils: and he cast out the spirits with his word, and healed all that were sick: That it might be fulfilled which was spoken by Esaias the prophet, saying, Himself took our infirmities, and bare our sicknesses."

Peter 2:24 "Who his own self bare our sins in his own body on the tree, that we, being dead to sins, should live unto righteousness: by whose stripes ye were healed."

Job 33:24–25 "Then he is gracious unto him, and saith, Deliver him from going down to the pit: I have found a ransom. His flesh shall be fresher than a child's: he shall return to the days of his youth:"

Psalm 41:1–3 "Blessed is he that considereth the poor: the LORD will deliver him in time of trouble. The LORD will preserve him, and keep him alive; and he shall be blessed upon the earth: and thou wilt not deliver him unto the will of his enemies. The LORD will strengthen him upon the bed of languishing: thou wilt make all his bed in his sickness."

Psalm 56:13 "For thou hast delivered my soul from death: wilt not thou deliver my feet from falling, that I may walk before God in the light of the living?"

Psalm 116:9 "I will walk before the LORD in the land of the living."

Psalm 118:17 "I shall not die, but live, and declare the works of the LORD."

Joel 3:10 "Beat your plowshares into swords, and your pruning hooks into spears: let the weak say, I am strong."

Galatians 3:13 "Christ hath redeemed us from the curse of the law, being made a curse for us: for it is written, Cursed is every one that hangeth on a tree:"

Galatians 3:29 "And if ye be Christ's, then are ye Abraham's seed, and heirs according to the promise."

Jeremiah 32:27 "Behold, I am the LORD, the God of all flesh: is there anything too hard for me?"

Proverbs 18:21 "Death and life are in the power of the tongue:"

Psalm 84:11 "For the LORD God is a sun and shield: the LORD will give grace and glory: no good thing will he withhold from them that walk uprightly."

Job 5:26 "Thou shalt come to thy grave in a full age, like as a shock of corn cometh in his season."

Numbers 12:13 "And Moses cried unto the LORD, saying, Heal her now, O God, I beseech thee."

Psalm 30:2–3 "O LORD my God, I cried unto thee, and thou hast healed me. O LORD, thou hast brought up my soul from the grave: thou hast kept me alive, that I should not go down to the pit."

John 10:10 "The thief cometh not, but for to steal, and to kill, and to destroy: I am come that they might have life, and that they might have it more abundantly."

Mark 2:11 "I say unto thee, Arise, and take up thy bed, and go thy way into thine house."

Mark 10:52 "And Jesus said unto him, Go thy way; thy faith hath made thee whole. And immediately he received his sight, and followed Jesus in the way."

Hebrews 13:8 "Jesus Christ the same yesterday, and today, and forever."

Acts 3:6–8 "Then Peter said, 'Silver and gold have I none; but such as I have given I thee: In the name of Jesus Christ of Nazareth rise up and walk.' And he took him by the right hand, and lifted him up: and immediately his feet and ankle bones received strength. And he leaping up stood, and walked, and entered with them into the temple, walking, and leaping, and praising God."

Acts 9:33–34 "And there he found a certain man named Aeneas, which had kept his bed eight years, and was sick of the palsy. And Peter said unto him, 'Aeneas, Jesus Christ maketh thee whole: arise, and make thy bed.' And he arose immediately."

Acts 14:8–10 "And there sat a certain man at Lystra, impotent in his feet, being a cripple from his mother's womb, who never had walked: The same heard Paul speak: who steadfastly beholding him, and perceiving that he had faith to be healed, Said with a loud voice, Stand upright on thy feet. And he leaped and walked."

Kings 4:32–35 "And when Elisha was come into the house, behold, the child was dead, and laid upon his bed. He went in therefore, and shut the door upon them twain, and prayed unto the LORD. And he went up, and lay upon the child, and put his mouth upon his mouth, and his eyes upon his eyes, and his hands upon his hands: and he stretched himself upon the child; and the flesh of the child waxed warm. Then he returned, and walked in the house to and fro; and went up, and stretched himself upon him: and the child sneezed seven times, and the child opened his eyes."

Isaiah 61:1–3 "The spirit of the Lord GOD is upon me; because the LORD hath anointed me to preach good tidings unto the meek; he hath sent me to bind up the brokenhearted, to proclaim liberty to the captives, and the opening of the prison to them that are bound; To appoint unto them that mourn in Zion, to give unto them beauty for ashes, the oil of joy for mourning, the garment of praise for the spirit of heaviness; that they might be called trees of righteousness, the planting of the LORD, that he might be glorified."

Isaiah 54:17 "No weapon that is formed against thee shall prosper . . ."

Deuteronomy 28:7 "The LORD shall cause thine enemies that rise up against thee to be smitten before thy face: they shall come out against thee one way, and flee before thee seven ways."

John 15:7 "If ye abide in me, and my words abide in you, ye shall ask what ye will, and it shall be done unto you."

Luke 7:12–15 "Now when he came nigh to the gate of the city, behold, there was a dead man carried out, the only son of his mother, and she was a widow: and much people of the city was with her. And when the Lord saw her, he had compassion on her, and said unto her, Weep not. And he came and touched the bier: and they that bare him stood still. And he said, Young man, I say unto thee, Arise. And he that was dead sat up, and began to speak. And he delivered him to his mother."

Mark 1:30–31 "But Simon's wife's mother lay sick of a fever, and anon they tell him of her. And he came and took her by the hand, and lifted her up; and immediately the fever left her, and she ministered unto them."

Proverbs 9:10–11 "The fear of the LORD is the beginning of wisdom: and the knowledge of the holy is understanding. For by me thy days shall be multiplied, and the years of thy life shall be increased."

2 Kings 5:14 "Then went he down, and dipped himself seven times in Jordan, according to the saying of the man of God: and his flesh came again like unto the flesh of a little child, and he was clean."

John 9:11 "He answered and said, A man that is called Jesus made clay, and anointed mine eyes, and said unto me, Go to the pool of Siloam, and wash: and I went and washed, and I received sight."

Matthew 8:8,13 "The centurion answered and said, Lord, I am not worthy that thou shouldest come under my roof: but speak the word only, and my servant shall be healed. And Jesus said unto the centurion, Go thy way; and as thou hast believed, so be it done unto thee. And his servant was healed in the selfsame hour."

     Miss Asondra StarN'air

Mark 2:10–12 "But that ye may know that the Son of man hath power on earth to forgive sins, (he saith to the sick of the palsy,) I say unto thee, Arise, and take up thy bed, and go thy way into thine house. And immediately he arose, took up the bed, and went forth before them all; insomuch that they were all amazed, and glorified God, saying, We never saw it on this fashion."

Acts 9:39–40 "Then Peter arose and went with them. When he was come, they brought him into the upper chamber: and all the widows stood by him weeping, and showing the coats and garments which Dorcas made, while she was with them. But Peter put them all forth, and kneeled down, and prayed; and turning him to the body said, Tabitha, arise. And she opened her eyes: and when she saw Peter, she sat up."

Acts 28:3–6 "And when Paul had gathered a bundle of sticks, and laid them on the fire, there came a viper out of the heat, and fastened on his hand. And when the barbarians saw the venomous beast hang on his hand, they said among themselves, No doubt this man is a murderer, whom, though he hath escaped the sea, yet vengeance suffereth not to live. And he shook off the beast into the fire, and felt no harm. Howbeit they looked when he should have swollen, or fallen down dead suddenly: but after they had looked a great while, and saw no harm come to him, they changed their minds, and said that he was a god."

Acts 8:6–8 "And the people with one accord gave heed unto those things which Philip spake, hearing and seeing the miracles which he did. For unclean spirits, crying with loud voice, came out of many that were possessed with them: and many taken with palsies, and that were lame, were healed. And there was great joy in that city."

Mark 6:12–13 "And they went out, and preached that men should repent. And they cast out many devils, and anointed with oil many that were sick, and healed them."

Luke 10:1–2 "After these things the Lord appointed other seventy also, and sent them two and two before his face into every city and place, whither he himself would come… Therefore said he unto them… heal the sick that are therein, and say unto them, The kingdom of God is come nigh unto you."

John 9:43–45 "And when he thus had spoken, he cried with a loud voice, Lazarus, come forth. And he that was dead came forth, bound hand and foot with grave clothes: and his face was bound about with a napkin. Jesus saith unto them, loose him, and let him go. Then many of the Jews which came to Mary, and had seen the things which Jesus did, believed on him."

Acts 19:11–12 "And God wrought special miracles by the hands of Paul: So that from his body were brought unto the sick handkerchiefs or aprons, and the diseases departed from them, and the evil spirits went out of them."

Matthew 14:14 "And Jesus went forth, and saw a great multitude, and was moved with compassion toward them, and he healed their sick."

Mark 6:56 "And whithersoever he entered, into villages, or cities, or country, they laid the sick in the streets, and besought him that they might touch if it were but the border of his garment: and as many as touched him were made whole."

Matthew 9:20–22 "And, behold, a woman, which was diseased with an issue of blood twelve years, came behind him, and touched the hem of his garment: For she said within herself, If I may but touch his garment, I shall be whole. But Jesus turned him about, and when he saw her, he said, Daughter, be of good comfort; thy faith hath made thee whole. And the woman was made whole from that hour."

Luke 4:40 "Now when the sun was setting, all they that had any sick with divers diseases brought them unto him; and he laid his hands on every one of them, and healed them."

John 4:50–53 "Jesus saith unto him, Go thy way; thy son liveth. And the man believed the word that Jesus had spoken unto him, and he went his way. And as he was now going down, his servants met him, and told him, saying, Thy son liveth. Then inquired he of them the hour when he began to amend. And they said unto him, yesterday at the seventh hour the fever left him. So the father knew that it was at the same hour, in the which Jesus said unto him, Thy son liveth: and himself believed, and his whole house."

Acts 5:15–16 "Insomuch that they brought forth the sick into the streets, and laid them on beds and couches, that at the least the shadow of Peter passing by might overshadow some of them. There came also a multitude out of the cities round about unto Jerusalem, bringing sick folks, and them which were vexed with unclean spirits: and they were healed everyone."

Mark 5:39–42 "And when he was come in, he saith unto them, Why make ye this ado, and weep? the damsel is not dead, but sleepeth. And they laughed him to scorn. But when he had put them all out, he taketh the father and the mother of the damsel, and them that were with him, and entereth in where the damsel was lying. And he took the damsel by the hand, and said unto her, Talitha cumi; which is, being interpreted, 'Damsel, I say unto thee, arise.' And straightway the damsel arose, and

walked; for she was of the age of twelve years. And they were astonished
with a great astonishment."

John 14:12–14 "Verily, verily, I say unto you, He that believeth on me, the
works that I do shall he do also; and greater works than these shall he do;
because I go unto my Father. And whatsoever ye shall ask in my name,
that will I do, that the Father may be glorified in the Son. If ye shall ask
any thing in my name, I will do it."

SECTION XIX

The Book of StarN'air

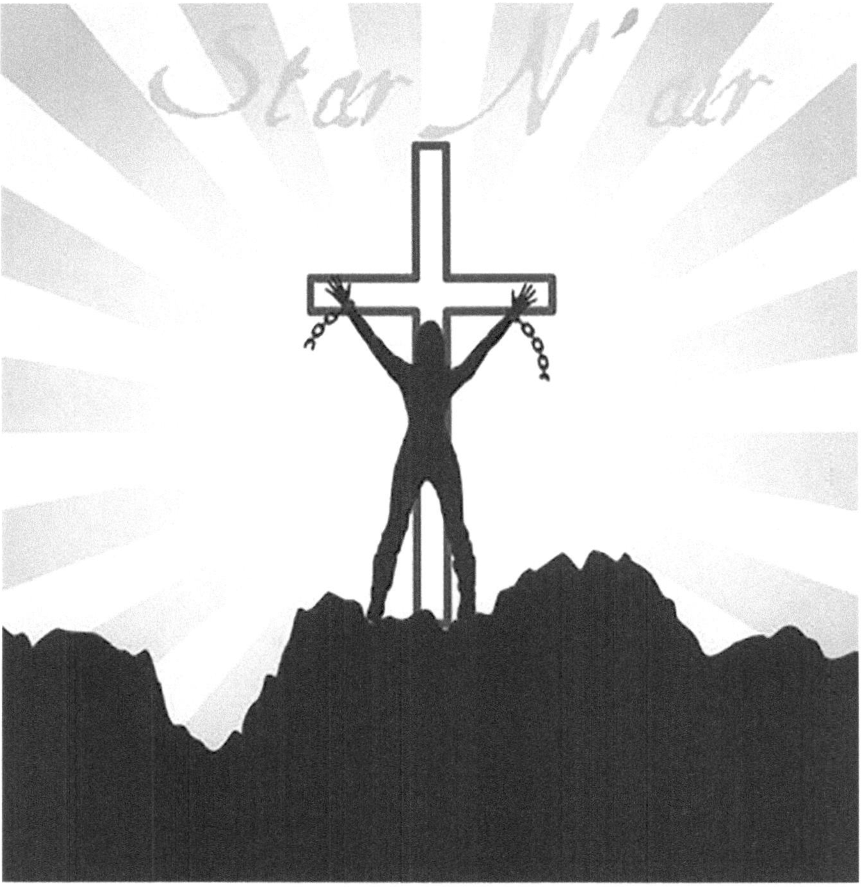

The Book of StarN'air

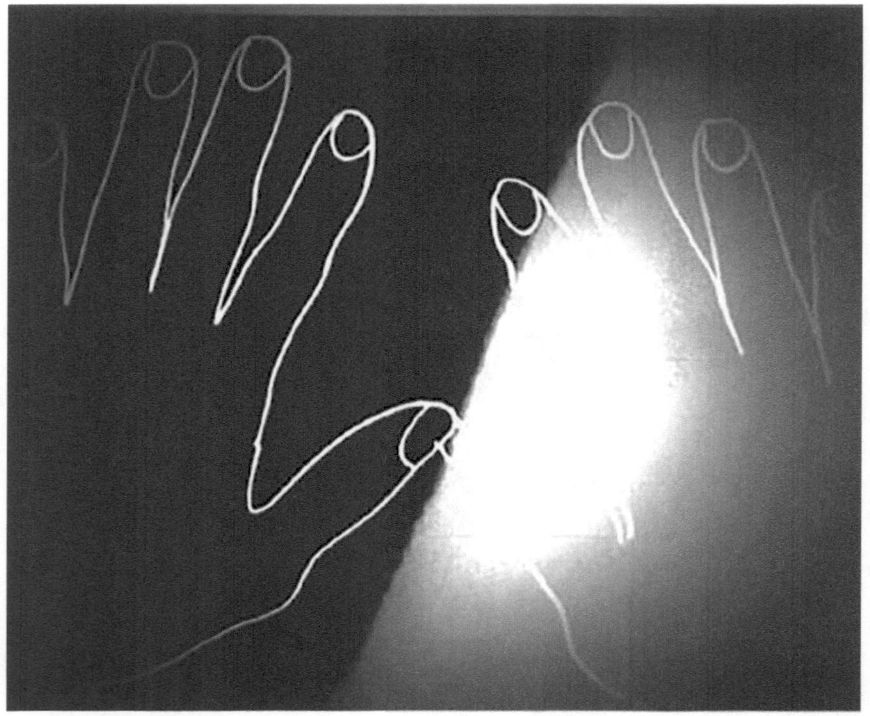

O my Lord, Jesus Christ, son of the Almighty God, The Alpha and The Omega, take me, I'm yours! Can't go on without you. Your word is a lamp to me feet and a light to my path, when Satan tries to put fear in me, guess what? "I laugh!"

Psalms 119:105

Hello World, Welcome To My World!

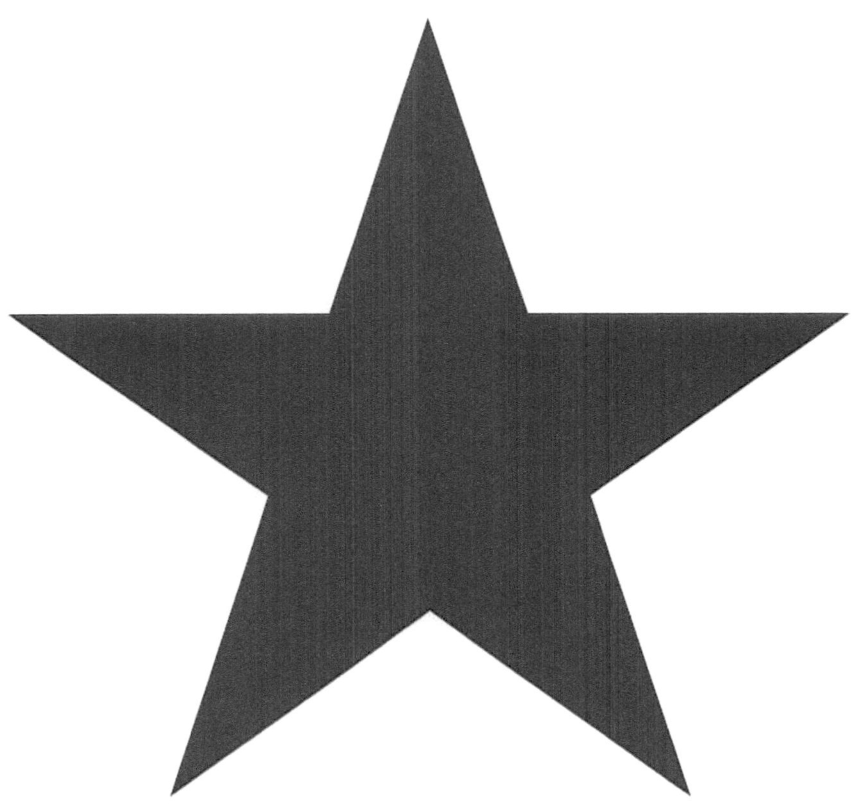

Jesus Christ is **Lord!**

"StarN'air"

World, I am more than a caregiver, I am a child of the most high God! In him I breathe', 'I live', 'I move', 'I sing' and have my being world without him, I'm lost forever. Now, let's talk about the Star N' air, this unique name of mine, well it was given and branded to me, a slave of Jesus Christ, by the 'Holy Spirit' because of my long suffering and obedience to him. No man will come before my God, no man. And let me tell you all something , I may be in the world but not of the world. I'm a forever

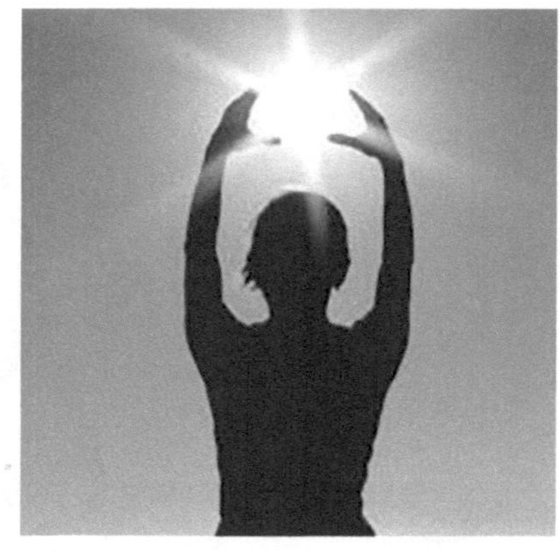

changed girl! And furthermore, there is only one, "True Star" and his name is above all other names, it is by that name, every knee shall bow in heaven and on earth and under earth, and every tongue declare that Jesus Christ is Lord, to the glory of God the father. Philippians 2:8-11

"Jesus" is the ★ and my morning glory, he's the reason why I get out of bed each morning. "I" follow the ★ of Bethlehem, Yes, now you get it, the Star N' air is

'He', not me, that I see! And with him, I shall have the victory!

I am proud and honor to have been given the name StarN'air . You won't find that name anywhere. it's unique and special and I will always remember what it means : I follow the one and only true Star N air Jesus Christ! All The praise and Glory goes to him and him alone. He make me strong!

Don't Hate Me Because I'm...

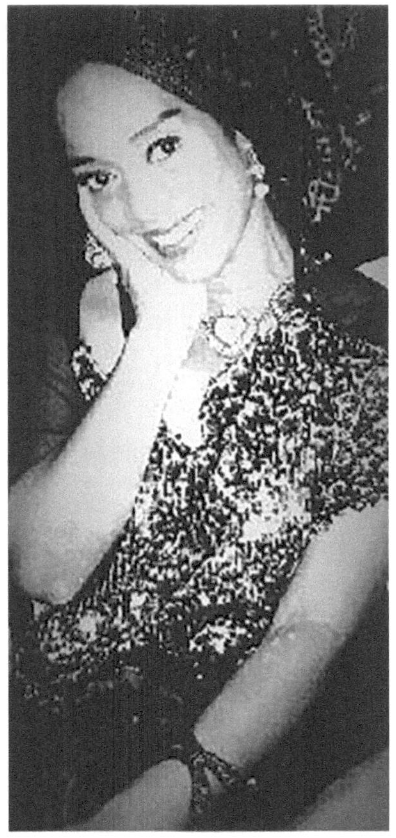

In Love with "Jesus"!

Miss Asondra StarN'air

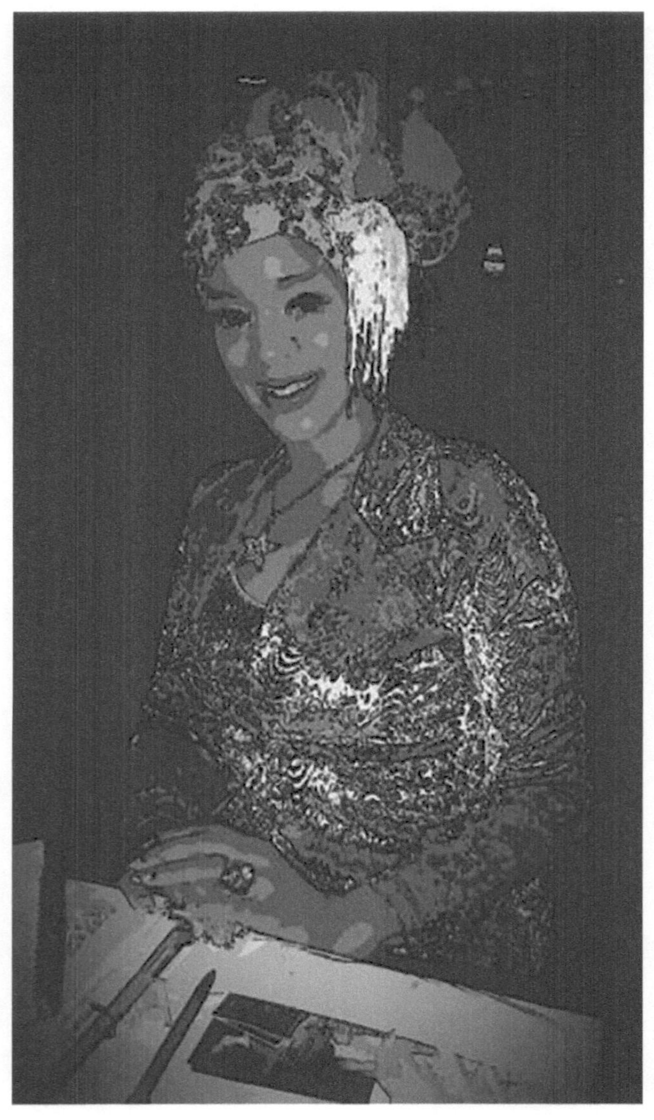

Where I Go, He Goes!

Lord, Why Are They "Trippin"?

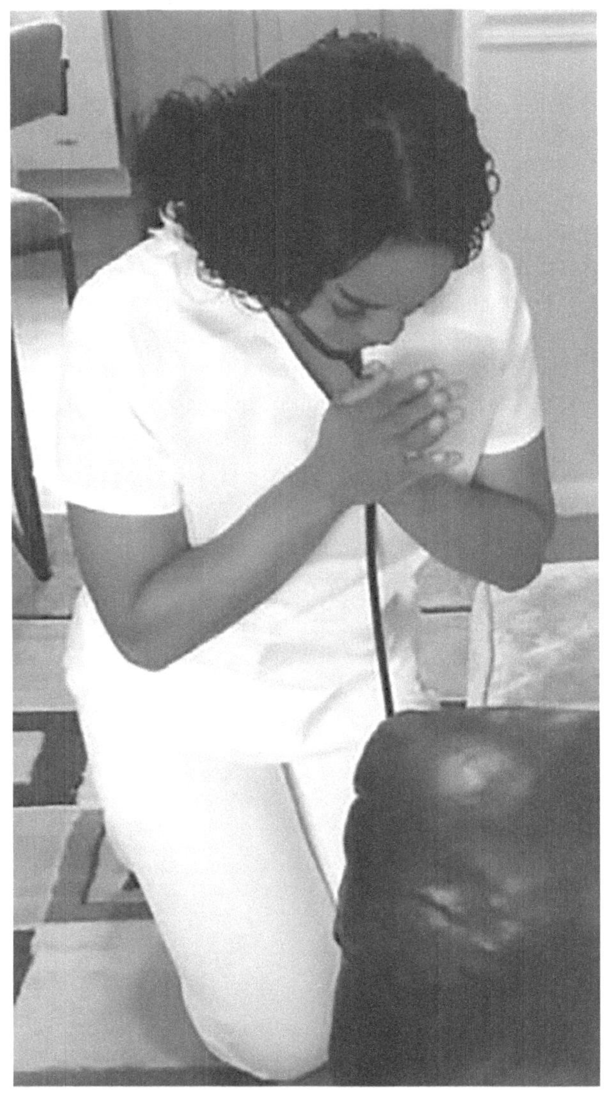

The World Hates the disciples John 15:18–27

"If the world hates you, keep in mind that it hated me first. If you be longed to the world, it would love you as its own. As it is, you do not belong to the world, but I have chosen you out of the world. That is why the world hates you. Remember what I told you: 'A servant is not greater than his master.' If they persecuted me, they will persecute you also. If they obeyed my teaching, they will obey yours also. They will treat you this way because of my name, for they do not know the one who sent me. If I had not come and spoken to them, they would not be guilty of sin; but now they have no excuse for their sin. Whoever hates me hates my Father as well. If I had not done among them the works no one else did, they would not be guilty of sin. As it is, they have seen, and yet they have hated both me and my Father. But this is to fulfill what is written in their Law: 'They hated me without reason.'

The Work of the Holy Spirit

"When the Advocate comes, whom I will send to you from the Father—the Spirit of truth who goes out from the Father—he will testify about me. And you also must testify, for you have been with me from the beginning.

StarN'air Cries

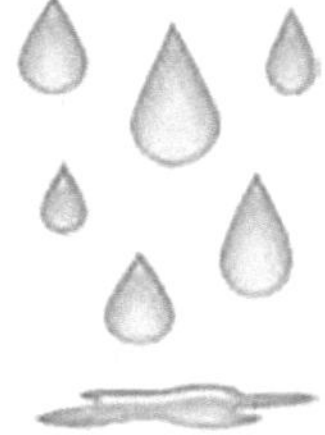

O My Lord, hear my cries, tears has become a real companion of mine. I'm rejected by many and hated too; where are you? **"StarN'air Cries"** it seems there's enemies on every side, Lord where do I hide? No matter the good work I do, their attitudes says StarN'air we hate you.

Come to me, for I'm feeling lonely and blue; I've lost lots of jobs and loved ones too. And not because of anything I've done—it's because of my love, my obedience and devotion to you. I'm rejected! So be it, I say, I shall not be conformed to this dark and evil world. Often times distraught, a welcome face, I'm not. On the contrary, I'm mocked and hated just about everywhere I go, but this my Lord, I know, you know! Nevertheless, whatever the cost, if I perish, I perish. Lord, I don't care, I will follow you anywhere!

Meanwhile, Lord, I'm still here, come quickly, come find me, take me out of my misery. seems like I've been here before, but my name was 'Job'. straight out of biblical times, I'm suffering , but I'll be fine.

Quiet, "Everybody", listen to the sound of the stormy wind, it's dark down here full of hatred and gloom, Lord are you coming soon? Night and day rain drops keeps falling, Lord, my pillows are drenched with tears, hurry, "God" where are you? I'm full of fear!

Oh, ye Wonderful Counselor, Mighty God, Everlasting Father, Peace of Peace, grant me the sun, moon, stars, oh how I long to be where you are, "beam Me Up Scotty" it's time to shine. Lord heal me, rescue me, deliver me from my enemies and empower me, "Holy Ghost", set me free, not only free but, 'Free Indeed!' My life with you Lord is all I need.

Come on, find me, remove these clouds, calm my storms oh how I want to rejoice, praise you, sing and dance like the psalmist David. Lord do for me, what you did for him, and like Joshua, strengthen me, make me stronger, and courageous; powerful, bold! For I am yours, I have already given you my mind, body and soul. Please Lord please, on bended knee, you know my journey's been hard, stretch out your rod, part the sea and come see about me. StarN'air Cries..............

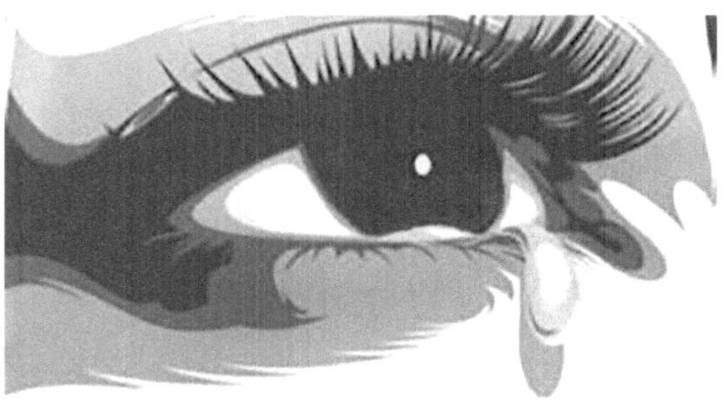

The Excellent Way

And now let me show you a way that is best of all . . .

When I first heard this phrase in the Bible in **1 Corinthians 12:31**, *'The Excellent Way',* something inside of me was **"Ignited"**, and I got **"Excited"**! Without turning the page, I paused for a moment, *"All I Could Think Of Was Love!"*

In my heart, I truly believe *'Excellence'* comes from above! I tell you the truth, caregivers, it's been an honor serving Christ in spite of all the things I had to deal with or give up.

The mission, *"Equip "Caregivers" all over the world!"* Put something in their hands that will not only help make them excellent caregivers but also help bring them back to their first love—the creator, **GOD Almighty!**

So, If I can do all that plus bring one soul back to Christ

then this "inspired" book by God will have been worth all the time, dedication, and sacrifices made personally, financially, and emotionally too— for this was not an easy book to write. Again, if I can win **one** soul for Christ, but I do hope I win many, then I know I'll get a chance to hear God say *StarN'air,* **"Well Done"** *My True and Faithful Servant* **"Well Done!"**

Yes, all of the rejection, pain, and suffering, financial attacks, persecutions, slander, hatred, and jealousy would have all been worth it. This book—*A Caregiver's Bible To Excellence*—has been written for you, my friend. Because no matter what, **'Love Wins In The End!'**

This book is my legacy, yes it is, I fought the good fight, I remained faithful and true to my God. I allowed Jesus to be the role model of excellence in my life; not only as a caregiver but in all areas of my life. And because I chose to put God first I lost some people I loved along the way. Take heed and listen, people, following Christ, **"COST"**. But I would have it no other way!

Seated and United With Christ!

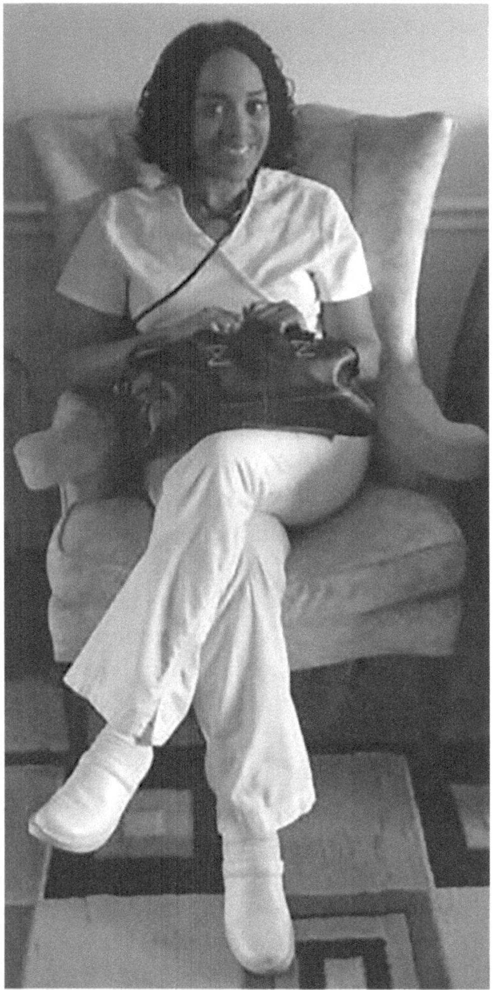

Look, I'm still here, seated with the invincible Christ Jesus, "No weapons formed against me shall ever prosper!

"And ever tongue which rise against me in judgment I shalt condemn; this is the heritage of the servants of the LORD, And their righteousness is from me," Says the LORD. **Isaiah 54:17**

A StarN'air Story

Introduction

How do I introduce a story that I don't want to tell but must because there may be other caregivers out there experiencing the same thing, they too have been persecuted and mistreated badly by others, including management. For me, it has become the norm, I have lost and resigned from so many jobs in the caregiving arena, and that's exactly what it has become—an arena, a place where only the wicked survive. Most of my worst experiences came from facilities, which can be a prison if you don't conform.

Nursing homes and some assistant living establishments can wreak havoc on a good caregiver if she does not have Christ in her life, because there are a lot of troublemakers in this field, one is going to need God's help to survive. The real problem I think is this, no one's minding the store, nursing are no longer walking the floor. Like I mentioned earlier in this book, cell phones have become a nuisance in the work place and now it has become a way of escape from other responsibilities. There used to be a time nurses would check in on both the residence and the caregiver to make sure all was well, meaning, all their needs were being met. Residence weren't in the bed, full of poop and soaking wet, and they knew were their Caregivers were at. And they also made sure that caregivers were being a team player and behaving like they should, they had no problem writing up or firing irresponsible caregivers or trouble- makers, they did not play that! Because they know like I know, *"Teamwork Makes The Dream Work!"* And also nurses back then, were not trying to make friends with the nursing assistances or exchanging phone numbers with us; no, they wouldn't cross that line, because they knew it was unprofessional to do so, they had a job to do, they'd never mixed the two. Skill and work performance is what matter the most. If you are a nurse right now, do you, run a top notch crew? Or do your paycheck mean more to you? Today in many places, caregivers are running wild, they're on their own, and this has set up opportunities for some to do others wrong.

In my early years, care giving was painful. I was out there on my own. I became a target for bullies, they came after me in groups, I was a loner by nature, with a heart of gold. But I would not conform to this world system of things. And because of so much persecution, set-ups, sabotage, lies and plain old jealousy, I resigned or loss jobs and being black, didn't help either. Nevertheless, scriptures always saved the day, and comforted me at night. I always heard God say "I will never leave or forsake you, don't worry my child, I will help you". And he did!

 Miss Asondra StarN'air

When God Closes One door, He Always Opens Another!

Moving from one job to another was very painful because I loved them all. I was so used to being on jobs for ten or more years until God called me to Long Term Care. it was unnatural for me to be in and out of jobs. But when I entered the health-care industry, all that changed. I found myself having to defend myself over and over again.

Just the way I looked made me a target for haters. Yet I believed once everyone got to know me, and saw my work, they'd like me and leave me along, however, that never happen, they didn't want to get to know me. I was quickly out casted from my first hello. the vibe I was getting was, we already hate you, **"Go!"** For me this became the norm, a lot of black women seems to despise me. I stayed at these kind of places as long as I could, like everybody else I had bills to pay, plus I was a single mother with a child at home. During this time in my life I became more and more withdrawn, introverted, because my coworkers didn't want me around, I felt rejected, that hurt me. In my solitude, it was Christ and me, he was all I lived for and all I could see. Cruel things were happening to me, and I kept it all inside. Most every night I'd cry myself to sleep. this went on for years "StarNair Tears!" But today I have a story to tell, I was an abused and used caregiver most of my career.

When God Closes One Door, He Always Opens Another! And for me it was another and another yet it was this particular door I liked a lot. One day I was blessed with a new opportunity to work for a big, big company, huge! The interviewing process was quite impressive, so I knew I was about to enter a very high class operation. I was moving up! Like the TV show, "The Jefferson's", I was moving up to taller buildings in the sky. I felt, that after all those years of tears and mistreatment, and not to mention all the long hours and hard work; finally I was getting my reward from heaven. Yes, I felt I was moving on up! I was so excited, my thought too, was (I can't believe this could all be happening to me) oh but it was, God is good, he does what he says he would.

The position was for an **STNA** by now you all should know what that stands for, State Tested Nurse Assistant, not aide. "Associate" that's right, you heard me, they were looking for an **STNA** with **"Hospice Experience"** to become an Associate member of their healthcare team. And oh how ironic, because that's where my love for care giving all came from, "Hospice" remember, I took care of my dying dad and also got certified and trained in hospice, so as you can see, I was more than qualified. Well long story short, I, me, Miss Asondra StarN'air became that associate. And I was determined to be the best hospice associate caregiver, that they had ever seen, after all, I was being led by the master, the king. And with Christ by my side, you know **WE** can do anything!

Moving right along, I did my first interview over the phone with one of the company's executives. I interviewed with four more executives throughout that week and unanimously, they all wanted me and nobody else. Not only was I more than qualified, but each one of those executives felt the love, the true heart for caregiving my dad left inside of me before he died. like I said, I was the one they all wanted, they didn't have to look any further, I was it! Finally, I went into the office and there was so much love and excitement for me, I felt like a celebrity. Everyone knew who I was but I didn't know them. And the very lovely receptionist was very professional and kind. She took me to a private interviewing room and it was quite impressive to say the least, I took a seat, and soon the top executive arrived. I had on black business pants and a white long sleeve shirt with a button up collar, and ah open black vest. I also wore a pair of low heel black pumps and I carried a black portfolio bag, inside my bag I had several copies of my resume and writing utensils and my cell phone too, but it was turned off. My hair was braided but pull back neatly in a bun, away from my face and my hands were clean, no fake nails or polish, my hands looked like a serious professional caregiver. What about yours? Let's pause here for a minute; I need to reiterate this, before we move on ladies, at that interview I planned my look, what to wear and what not to wear. And I also knew what to do and what not to do. I didn't over talk, I answered and asked a few questions of my own, and I listened, and within fifteen minutes I was offered the position. Lastly, I gave an exit greeting, shook that persons hand and walked! Yes, I walked the talk, **A Caregiver's Bible to Excellence** is inside of **"ME!"** High five, **"I Got The Job!"**

And a job like no other—For me, it was a job of a lifetime, seriously, I was offered a respect- able high end wage job with so many benefits I never knew existed. Wait a minute, there's more—my own cell phone, iPad, office mailbox, and personal office e-mail address. How about that? Wow! That's what I said.

My job title was "A Hospice Associate" (loved the professional name by the way) I was to go out in communities assigned to me, which was the east side of Ohio, and provide personal or companion care to the dying (my dad all over again, dream job) that was indeed an honor for me.

I was assigned five buildings within one community and one other building five miles up the road.

So I had a workload, along with all of that, every day at 8:30 a.m. everyone in the office, including me, had to be on daily conference calls. And every other week, there was a corporate meeting, which included the entire health-care team—Doctors, RNs, STNAs, Social workers, Spiritual Advisors, Therapists, and Office Managers, **"Wow"** all this was new for me but, now all the sudden, **"I'm scared!"** So much so, I started to feel like a useless aide, a nobody, a stereo type, a slave, like I did not belong there. Most of the staff were white, there was only a few of us, me and two other black caregivers. But quickly I had to pull it together and shift my thinking and tell myself I did belong there, and that I will not be a stereotype, I Am a Professional Nurse Assistant, and now part of a growing team. Besides, God put me there, so he must've thought, I have what it takes. But what really made my knees shake was, everyone at the table, had to speak up and give report. Oh, hold on. I feel a song coming on: At first I was afraid, I was petrified, oh but thank god I had Jesus by my side!

All I could think of was, **"Fake It Until You Make It!"** So that's exactly what I did, and it didn't take long, I started looking forward to those meeting. The first few weeks though, I had to train, learn my way around the office, whose who, where everything was, supplies and all, plus the protocols and what was expected of me. Then I had to activate all my devices, cell phone and I -pad; next I had to get my business e-mail account all set up and of course fill out more paper work for human resources file. **"WOW"!** That's what I said **"WOW!"** Finally came the community training. I had to work with another caregiver for a week on the road.

My boss—who, by the way, was awesome—was very easy to talk to and so encouraging. In fact, she was the one who suggested that everyone call me "Star" not me; because my first name Asondra was too similar to another caregiver's name, the one training me, so my new boss said," to avoid a mix up", we'll just call you "Star", I said OK, Star it is! So that's how that all came to be. Back to the story . . .

It's time to meet my new communities, that's what we called them, **"Communities"** I had all of the east side. **Let's go...** it's time to ride! My boss suggested that the other caregiver, whom I had not met yet, that we ride together in the same car since we would be together all day training. **"Wonderful"**, sounds great to me, I was elated, each night I waited, for the morning to come. **"Excited!"** Ready to train, ready to fly out the door! God just blessed me with a brand new job, who can ask for anything more!

On the first day of training, I met up with my partner. She took one look at me, I had on my professional gear, **"Nice Work Shoes, Nice Scrubs"** but by the look on her face, it was clear, (this is so very funny now, but was not funny back then) honey, you're not getting in here! What's up with black sisters? Yes she was black, and not in the best of shape, very overweight, But, **"So What"**, she didn't need to "Cut Up"! Besides, **I'm With Christ**, we're not caring about all that, I love everybody, fat, skinny, white, black, yellow or brown. I tell you the truth, Jealousy, hatred, insecurity and cruelty all needs to settle down. **Love's** in town! Sadly and suddenly I felt a cold disapproval, but I pretended I didn't feel it.

So she changed the plans and said, "You can just follow me."

I said kindly, "The office wants us to ride together I don't know my way on the highway, I don't venture out much, I'm not good with directions." She reassured me that I would not get lost and to just follow her.

Next thing I knew, before I could get my seat belt on and put my foot on the gas pedal, that caregiver took off.

Within minutes, I was lost, I felt awful, I thought, look Lord, it's happening all over again, I'm hated on sight, this is wrong, Lord, this ain't right. And why from my own people? Black women to be precise, over the years, many have been nasty to me, and only a few have been nice. And what is very sad too, the women who come after me are almost always overweight black females. They hate themselves and the way they look, in their distorted and reprobate minds, it's the fit or skinny persons fault and they must pay. So they come after us, they try to run us away. These kinds of evil and mad minds are out there in the work place, in fact they're everywhere. They're full of jealousy, full of malice and full of hate. But let me also say this for the record, there are some large black women who are quite comfortable in their own bodies and would never mistreat anyone like that. In fact my best friend is black and she's a large woman. She is absolutely beautiful inside and out!

So let's not confuse what I'm saying or what I'm talking about! I'm talking right now about a thing called **"Love"**, **L. O. V. E.** Love Others Very Existence. No one should ever be rejected because they are very attractive and polished or whatever, **Every Person Matters! If You Matter, Then I Matter!** Back to the story, **"She's Gone"** that's right, this girl just took off an left me, just like that! Yes she was fat, but why act like that? My love is blind, my heart is like Christ, its kind! Now because of what she did, I thought to myself, this is going to make me look bad, incompetent, late on the first day of work, and unable to follow directions, I was almost in tears, but I had no time to cry, this girl was not going to make me look like a lie. I asked God, what do I do now? I felt compelled to go back to the office and explain why I was not with my trainer and not at my schedule location. So I did just that, but I stayed in the parking lot for a little while, trying to find another solution. I did not want to tell on that caregiver in fear that she would retaliate like many of them have been known to do, so I protected her.

So I sat there for a while and waited, hoping she would call my new business phone. And sure enough, she did, seconds before I was getting ready to go up to the office, because I was tired of waiting, the clock was ticking, I'm supposed to be working, training,"not in my car sitting!"

Just her luck, my phone rang, it was her, she said, "Where are you?"

I said, "You left me."

"Where are you?" she asked again.

I told her I was back at the office, getting ready to go up, and in a panic-stricken voice, she said, "Oh no, don't go up!" "Meet me around the corner at the gas station, you can park your car there, and we'll ride together."

So, I said okay, and that's what we did; I got in her car, I tell ya, Jesus must've been calming the stormy seas in me because I was calm and gentle. I had no attitude toward this girl, I was meek and grateful, yet quiet. What's the use in going off? She's got the problem, not me, I'm with God, I can clearly see. Besides, I was still excited about those new communities. My focus was on "Excellence", not her nor me, **"Let's Ride…!"**

Fast-forward: The training's over, and now all those eastside communities/facilities have a brand-new hospice associate caregiver—me, Miss Asondra StarN'air, with a new nick name too, **"STAR!"**

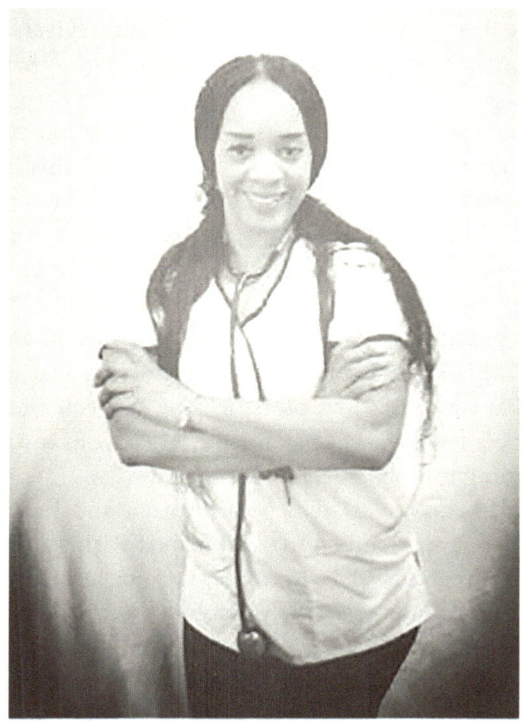

Watch Out World, Here I Come!

Day One On The Job

I woke up at the crack of dawn, I was so excited, I got up, put my new scrubs on, grabbed my new business bag, and was out the door by 5:30 a.m. I arrived there at my new community fifteen minutes early, training is done, it's me and Jesus now; and before I went in, I prayed. Then I got out of my car went in to introduce myself and my company. I told them why I was there and who I was seeing, next, I went to the patient's room and began to provide personal care, once finished, I needed to find a caregiver to help with a Hoyer lift, I wanted to get this person up for breakfast.

So I went back out to ask the caregiver I just met when I first arrived, (She's on her cell phone, laughing, playing around)

"Excuse me," I said politely, "who is the caregiver assigned to this room?" She said, not so nicely, "I am."

I said, "can you help me do a Hoyer lift? I'm done with her bed bath."

The caregiver went off on me! She said, "I don't have no time right now, I have other rooms to do." then I said, "but I just saw you here on your cell phone having fun, but no problem, I'm just here to help; and I have only a limited time here, I've got more people to see." The caregivers reply was, "You here to help, whatcha you mean by that? Who are you? What you mean you helping us?"

I got quiet and headed back to the room. Then something inside me turned me around. I went back to this caregiver, and this is exactly, word-for-word, what I said: "Go ahead, go off on me, take whatever it is, all off on me. Go ahead, I'm not going to tell anyone. You must be tired, you are not yourself, take it all off on me, I don't care, and if you ever need me, I will help you, I'll be there."

I turned and headed back toward my patients room, and the caregiver stopped me, and this is what she said. "I'm so sorry! I had no business ever talking to you that way. I'm sorry, please forgive me. You are right, I'm tired. I've been working a lot trying to pay for the last part of my nursing. I don't know how I'm going to get the rest of the money."

I said, "I will help you"! I will help research and find where the free money is." The caregiver thanked me and helped with the Hoyer lift. From that day on, that caregiver was kind to me, but not her friends. I never told a soul about our encounter, why? Why should I, Christ had risen that day, no way were those my words, "Take it out on me" honey please, baby don't take no jive! That day Jesus came alive! Those words were his, not mine, that was the Christ in me. Oh but I so felt so liberated and free, that day, hatred didn't bother me. Individuals who hate, don't know Jesus or how to escape.

The StarN'air story continues, my first day on the job was really about me, the new girl in town. All day long, I was being checked out by other caregivers, just about all of them were my own people, **"Blacks"** colored people, why we act like that? They were standing around in groups of four or more, I felt their intimidation. They all were watching and staring me down, (gangsters, so, this is the new chick in town) they were watching my every move, my coming and my going, this was annoying! For more than eight months this went on and on and it got worse and worse for me there. Each day they camped out somehow and waited for my arrival.

No matter my smile, speak or don't speak, I was going to be their *"Slaughtered Sheep"* Jesus was the only one who could protect me!

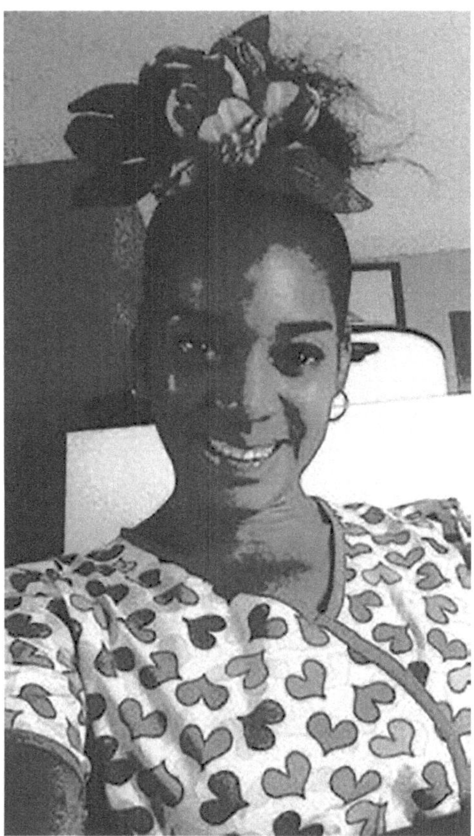

See My Smile, I Really Am Sweet!

Day Two

Same routine, more drama awaits me. This time instead of the first caregiver I met, Now it's two of them—her and another caregiver plus an LPN, all best of friends. They watch me come into the building; I waved and said hello, and went into the room to do personal care on a hospice patient. I finished, went back out, and asked the same question, "Who's the caregiver assigned to ms. so and so, I need help with a Hoyer lift. They All looked at me like I lost my mind (back on the cross) also the one assigned to the room was a different caregiver this time. This one flat out refused and started to pick an argument with me, she said in front of the other two, "You don't tell me what to do."

My response was, "I'm not telling you what to do, I'm asking for help." The LPN just stood there, never uttered a word. A few minutes later the other caregiver, who met the Jesus in me, the one I had an encounter with the first time I entered the building said, "come on, I'll help you again."

She did, and a few minutes later they all drove off in the same car, their shift was over. That was the overnight crew, third shift workers but, they stayed and waited to bother me. Shame on you **LPN** and your wicked friends! Let's pause here a minute, how do you feel about what's happening here, do share: ____

____

____

____

____

____

____

____

____

____

____

____

____

____

____

____

____

____

 Miss Asondra StarN'air

No Real Leadership

What went wrong with that day, I'll tell you what went wrong, **"No Real Leadership"** and a LPN, that decided to blend. If it had been all caught on tape, would they all have been fired, I don't think so, it seems as long as you are in a click, that's it, like the bibles says, this world is evil, but it also says, **Woe to those who call** *evil good and good Evil, who put darkness for light and light for darkness, who put bitter for sweet and sweet for bitter!* *Isaiah 5:20* Question ladies because it is mostly women who keeps up all the drama and wickedness in these fallibilities; is this what professional health care nursing and nursing assistant has come down to, hatred of women, and by women? That particular **LPN** should have been dismissed, fired! She was supposed to protect, and look out for others who are being mistreated on the job, but instead she stood there and watch them have a field day with me. Friend or no friend, That **LPN** is a disgrace to the entire healthcare industry.

Do you agree? Y/N what's your take on it? ______________________

____

____

____

____

____

____

After that second day on the job, that morning, I felt the need to call my boss, I was damn near in tears. I explained to her what had been going on from day one and she said "I will handle it" and that she was going to call a meeting with management there. She reassured me it would be taken care of. I made the rest of my rounds, and everywhere I went hatred was there, checking out my every move.

Each room I serviced was highly noticeable, to both, the family members and management staff in fact, all the family members wanted to meet me, they raved about the care and how nice their loved ones looked and they also noticed their rooms after I left. Detailed things like placing stuffed animals around the bed, watering plants, matters. I even replaced their bedding covers; I took the facility boring white coverings off and replaced them with the blankets families brought in; those covering were beautiful, full of color and cheer, why were they tucked away in a closet? Beautiful things shouldn't stay in a closet. I also left bibles on beds of those who had a Bible, and a little surprise snack on their pillows—things like that. I wowed everyone except the caregivers who hated me on sight. Doesn't matter, still, everyone wanted to meet me, or thank me over the telephone. They were very happy that I was there. Word even got back to the office on the incredible work I was doing.

That Was Jesus!

To tell you the truth, **That Was Jesus** working through me, he likes things meticulously! Right down to every detail, read about Noah's Ark, **Gen. 5:32- 10:1** and The building of the Tabernacle **Exod. 26** and you'll see, he's just another part of me. He was the voice inside instructing me; He was certainly the one who had me turn around and said to that first caregiver "Take it all out on me." Now it's almost time to get ready for day three, "Jesus, stay with me"! Meanwhile, back at the office I was told by a certain person at the hospice office that my boss was proud, they said she was praising my name all through the office. I had no clue what was happening.

Because every day since I started this new job, I was being watched by so many wicked caregivers. I didn't realize that in spite of what I was happening to me there, there were others who saw the love and real passion I had for those seniors and Caregiving. **Remember, Good Always Triumphs In The End! "So don't Blend!"** I believe in love, I believe in excellence, you always give people more than what they ask for. **And "Sunshine" should always walk through the door no matter if it's cloudy or storming out side or in your life, We should stay joyous.**

As a caregiver, what do you think caring for others consist of, besides love?

____

____

____

____

____

____

____

____

What are some new things you are going to start doing for those in your care? _______________________________________

____

____

____

____

____

____

____

     Miss Asondra StarN'air

Day Three

Same routine, same building. This time, I had no problems getting help with a Hoyer lift and this was a different caregiver this time. I hadn't met this person before and she seemed okay, a lot warmer than the others in this building. But I noticed too, this one talks and whispers to other caregivers a lot—that's a red flag for me, so I'll be, "Hi and bye!

That's it, I'm finish here, on to my next building in that same community. I enter the building and there they are—six of them, including the Dean Of Nursing (DON), standing around, talking. When I walked in, all the talking ceased; all eyes were on me and my every move. I waved and said hi to everybody, took the stairs up to see my next patient. Five minutes later, there was a knock on the door, and guess yawl, who it was? The DON herself, a black woman.

I said "Personal Care." but she came in anyway, else on while I was in the middle of serving that individual and started telling me who she was, I stopped what I was doing to listen, my patient was just lying there, I covered her up of course, but it seemed this DON had something on her mind that apparently could not wait (that's so unprofessional and rude, don't you think?) You do not interrupt a another professional in the middle of a bed bath, unless it's urgent and I don't need a degree to know that, it's called a patients right to privacy. My patient didn't receive that right that day. Correct me if my thinking on this matter is wrong somebody, anybody. Nevertheless, I felt a dark spirit in that room once she got there, she was up to something. If not, why did she come in there minutes after I got there? What did she really want, and why couldn't it have waited until I was done bathing that individual? hum, why? Well let's find out together shall we. Again, while she spoke, I stopped and listened. Then I introduced myself as well. Next, this Don started questioning me about my services there, as if she didn't know. I told her, however, she seemed to be under the impression that I had only one building there and not all five. I clarified it for her, but I was still getting a strong vibe that she was fishing and feeling me out. Like I said earlier, I felt an evil spirit, a darkness when she first walked in that room.

I felt she was up to something, and most likely snooping around for all her caregiver friends. And I was right! Next, (excuse me, for a minute, yawl, I need to ask the Lord something, excuse me, "hey, Lord, can I say this chick, can I say this low down and dirty broad,) "No" StarN'air, you belong to me now, take the high road. Remember what first lady Michelle Obama said, **"When They Go Low, You Go High"** so, no don't say that, you go high! OK, so where was I? Oh, she wouldn't leave, she just stood there looking at me, almost like she was trying to intimidate me, because my work was good, I was being excellent in Jesus name, what can ten thousands of people do to me, nothin! And all the sudden just out of the blue, just like that she had the audacity to ask me "how did you get this job?" I be your pardon, what, you got to be kidding me, I thought, because here I am trying to do personal care on this residence so that I can move on to my next patient and this black woman is drilling me. And trying to intimidate me by asking questions that are none of her business. How did you get your job, I wanted to say something else, but I didn't because I'm ah Christian. So I simply said I applied for it, that's how I got it.

Check this out, I may be pretty, but I'm not stupid or blind, this wicked woman, this DON cornered me in a patient's room and tried to find out all she could about me. She continued to question me, next she had the nerve to ask me this, "What are they paying you for mileage?"

Enough, is Enough! So I firmly said, **"I'm here to do patient care, I don't want to talk about me or discuss what they are paying me for mileage."**

She looked at me and said, "I can find out if I want to" and she left.

I finished that patient, went to my car, and reported it to my boss. My boss said, "I'm glad you didn't tell her, that's none of her business." And that's all that was said and done about that. Legally that's a form of intimidation on the job, but I was too, overwhelmed and so new to everything, I just buried it inside. I had a mortgage to pay and a child at home to feed, no time to grieve.

Let's pause here, so that you know, I've already talked to God, he's going to work everything out in my favor, but I'm pausing too, because I want to converse with all of you reading this story. Something is terribly wrong here don't you think because some of these leaders are corrupt, and in this particular case my boss is starting to turn a blind eye. My oh my, what have I gotten myself into here. I Thought this company would be loyal and true. Was I naive,because things are not right on either side. I think I fell for the pie in the sky! Absolutely nothing came out of that phone call to my boss, just and agreement, that she has no right to know what I'm being paid. **"Hello"**, what about the violation of privacy, and that residence right to privacy as well and also, what about the intimidation and cornering me in a residence room like that? **What About That!** Help me Janet Jackson, ask'em **What About That?** I'm being mistreated, and bullies on the job, not only by in -house workers I don't know or even work with but can you believe this, also by leaders. Wow! Tell me, what do I do now? What would you do, "quit"? _______________

____

____

____

____

____

After all that, I found myself working in fear, I'd hadn't even worked this job a full week yet alone a year and they were coming after me. So I started doing more and more and more, it seemed the good I was doing wasn't good enough, so I tripled it, I started working rooms that were not my assignments, I started helping the haters out. I noticed this too, that as long as they could use the crap out of me, they'd leave me alone. But the truth of the matter is, I love working with seniors, so helping other co-workers never bothers me, so go right ahead haters, use me until you use me up!

So when this day ended, I went home with the cares of the day, I read scriptures that took those cares and fear away. But I still felt the need to do something about what's been happening to me on the job because no one else was doing anything about the unfair treatments that I was encountering, not even my boss. Everyone went on as if nothing was happening, so I called the employees' grievance hot-line that evening.

In tears and in pain, I told them everything that had been going on. It took about an hour or so because they kept making me repeat myself, typing as I spoke. That day was a horrible day for me, and calling the hot line really didn't help, because I had to feel the humiliation and pain all over again. However, I got through it.

I was told someone would get back in touch with me within twenty-four hours and was given a case number, 6738925632, keep it so we can help you. Days and weeks went by—but there was nothing, they never called.

Meanwhile, things were getting worse and worse. Each day I went to work, some of these building I went in became more and more hostile and cunning. I don't even know these girls. oh, and they were all black, every last one of them including the Don, How can I win? I just kept letting Jesus in. I cried and read my scripture every day. There were times though, I wanted to give up. All that hatred and pressure was making me want to die. I was becoming suicidal, all alone in my room, at night tears drenched my pillows. But I heard Jesus say *"You can't' just give up and die"what about you and I? What about what we've been through, and the fact that I will always love and care for you, what about that? "Come back"!* In my darkest hour, Jesus was there. In all my despair, the world wasn't there. Jesus my healer and the lifter of my head is the reason why I'm alive today and not dead. He healed my wounded soul, and gave me lots of reasons to go on... Where I was weak, he was strong. I went back to work the next day, like nothing was wrong. And it wasn't, I was healed, and ready to tackle another day. I was strong enough to handle anyone or anything that came my way, I was better than OK! Christ held me up with his right hand, something haters will never know or understand. And I kept reading my scriptures next thing I know, I got stronger and wiser, I realized **"I Can't Let the Devil Have Its Way.** And another thing, I am not fighting against flesh and blood anyway. But against principalities, against power, against rulers of this dark and evil world, and against spiritual wickedness in high places. My battle is not with people, So I had to get myself and my focus back on track. **Eph.6:12**

Here's a question for you, would you have stayed on this job or quit by now? Please explain. ____

 Miss Asondra StarN'air

Day Four

Today's a pretty normal day, I was approached by another black big shot, the assistant general manager.

She said loudly, in front of her boss, "Don't come into the kitchen area again without a hair net on."

So, I said OK, but I wondered why she was so loud and cold, but I shook it off fast. A few seconds later, she went into the kitchen with no hair net on and made herself a cup of coffee. When I saw that, I got the message loud and clear, **'Do As I Say, Not As I do'.**

So now, I know this person is not someone I could confide in or talk to,

would you? Who should I turn to? **"Christ!"**

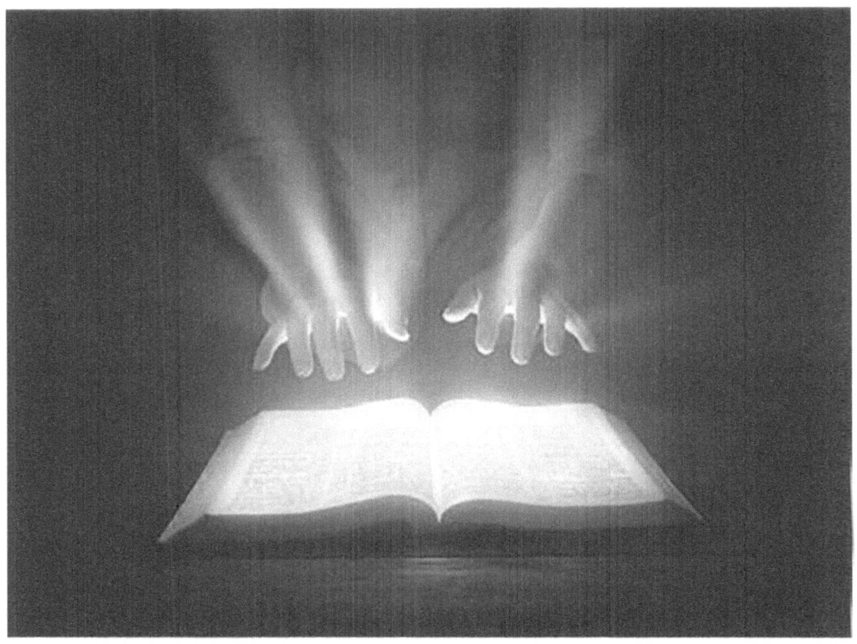

Day Five

Same ol same ol, but something interesting happened on this day, hey check this out, one of our associates and she was also new to the company she was an RN, we ran into each other and she pulled me over to the side and say this"

"Stay away from that DON." "She's looking for trouble."

Hey yawl, that's the one who followed me up to that patient's room. The one who asked me how much I was being paid for mileage, remember? Well, there you have it, This RN is my case manager and even she can see, she's trouble.

I said "I already know," after that quick warning, we went our separate ways and continued on with our day. Other than that, the hostile environment, whispers, and rejection continued. That was now the normalcy of my days at work for this company, and still there was no call back from the employee's hotline. Nothing! I was on my own, in some kind of prison at least that's what it felt like; I didn't know how to break free, bills and everyday life were still coming after me. Nevertheless, I had to go on, so I made the necessary adjustments:

1. I started documenting. I kept a running record.
2. I ate lots of scriptures instead of food for lunch.
3. I stopped responding to any of the mistreatment.
4. I did daily workouts at home to help relieve stress caused by those environments.
5. I cried and kept asking God why he was allowing it.

What is meant for evil, God uses for Good! We must trust him.

My first full week has come to a close. Oh my, some week, huh?

But I'm going to stop there, I'm not going to go to day six, seven, or eight, everyday was full of more schemes, jealousy and hatred. I learned to live with it. Right now, I'm in a prison, no escape. As usual, I went to work from that day on fighting for my job, watching my back and dotting my i's and crossing my t's. A painful journey in deed! Can somebody, anybody help me please! Nobody came but Jesus!

Moving forward, now it's Three months into the job, it was time for my evaluation, and I got it on my birthday. My boss called me into the office and blew my mind. She said I exceeded beyond what was expected of me. I had over achieved every expectation they had for me, then she said, she too talked to a few people in the company and they wanted me to go back to school and the company would pay for it.

I was in tears, I cried. I said, "All I ever wanted to do was please the company and take excellent care of the patients."

 Miss Asondra StarN'air

She said, "You have." My boss also said , "Star" everyone is blown away by you and your work. The community said they have never had anyone come out there and do what you have done."

All I could do was cry some more and thank her over and over again. But that's not all. She said she wanted me to come up with some new ideas for that community for our hospice patients. and that I could do anything I wanted to. So, on the spot, I said "glamour day, nail care, a fun day of glamour," and she loved it.

She said, "You can even do some type of scrapbook, but make sure you put your picture on the cover."

I left the office floating on a cloud. All that hard work and passion was noticed and rewarded too.

And I was offered a full scholarship to go back to school. Wow, that was the best birthday present ever!

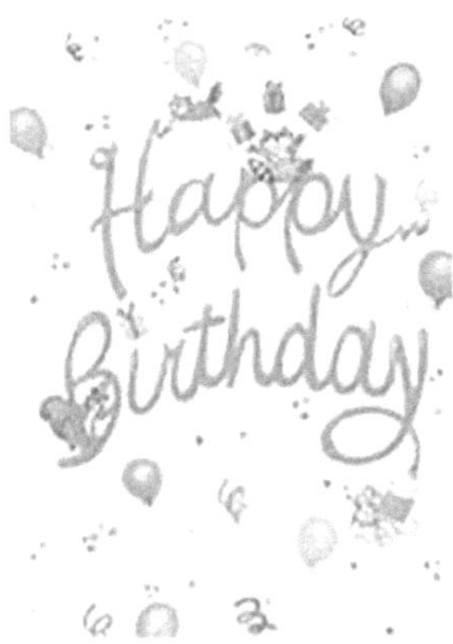

And it gets even better, my boss called me the next day and told me the other executives were donating everything I needed to make my glamour days a success. So the following day, I came to our business meeting, and there were many packages waiting for me. Fifty bottles of nail polish, fingernail supplies, cotton balls—you name it, I had it. Wow!

The other caregiver, the one who trained me, was speechless and barely spoke to me. But I was too high on love to care about jealousy or hate. It was my Whitney Houston" One Moment In Time" to ***"Shine!"*** Besides, the bible says in Matt. 5:16, ***"Let your light shine before others, that they may see your good deeds and glorify your father in heaven."*** And that's exactly what I did that day, no one or nothing was going to take that moment away, **Nobody!**

The Devil is Always Busy!

The Parties Over! Suddenly, all that attention has now brought me some new enemies now they're in my own back yard, because some of the people at the office were starting to hate on me. (Nobody really loves ah star, some can't wait until they fall!) It seemed after that evaluation, some of the white women at our office became a little intimidated by all the praise and attention I was receiving. There smiles weren't real smiles. I'm just an aide remember, yet I'm shining all over the place, and smirks on their face. Psalms 27:1 *'The Lord Is My Light And My Salvation —Whom Shall I Fear? The LORD Is The Stronghold Of My Life—Of Whom Shall I Be Afraid?*

But here we go again, **The Devil is Always Busy!** One day at work I get this phone call and it was from one of our associates, a hospice RN. She informed me that she would now be my new case manager and that she would also be rearranging some of my workload. And she went on to say, the real reason for her call was that she had received a complaint about me from several people, including the DON.

Before she could finish, I said, "Let me inform you of what's been happening out here."

I did, and her response was "Well, I'm just telling you to make sure you do your job and whatever they ask you to do;"

I said, "Wait a minute, hold on, you don't know what been happening to me out here from day one, I have been targeted, mistreated badly, cornered in rooms, out casted, lied on, schemed on, you name it, they've tried it. Ask one of our nurses on the team, she knows what's happening, in fact she also told me to stay away from this DON, says she's looking for trouble."

This RN ignored what I was saying, and said, "they all can't be lying."

And I said, they are. They have been coming after me from day one—I felt bullied, I still feel bullied.

Her response was, "Just make sure you do a better job."(again I was known for my excellent work, that's what stood out the most.)

I politely got off the phone, and this time, I was really frightened. Now someone on my team was joining in on the false accusations and schemes, and that's all they needed. A Judas, someone willing to betray me and this nurse sides with my enemies.

A few seconds later, I called her right back and asked if we could sit down and have a meeting, a one-on-one. She said sure, How about tomorrow I said? She said okay, we both agreed to meet out at the community I was working in. The next day, I came in to do my regular routine at the building where the mistreatment first began, and I noticed the housekeeper was watching me. Everywhere I went within that building, there she was, I thought to myself, it's awfully strange to keep seeing her, and she's not even a caregiver. But I was aware of her too, she was friends with all those caregivers who hated me. Anyway, my phone rang, it was the nurse, the one I was to have the meeting with.

Perfect timing, I had just finished up with my patient. That housekeeper was still on the same floor. I rode the elevator down, and minutes later, there she was again—doing no work, just watching me come and go.

The nurse arrived, and we meet and greeted each another. I suggested we leave the premises so we could have lots of privacy. She suggested we just go find a room inside, so I said okay. We found a room upstairs, we closed the doors, and the private meeting began. I asked her to go first, if she wanted, and I would listen. She insisted that I go first. I started off explaining to her the same thing I tried to tell her over the phone and suggested she speak to the other nurse who knew about many of those troublemakers, including that DON.

Next thing I knew, she was siding with them, bringing up more negative lies and then handling me like garbage. I could not believe her behavior. Next thing I said was **"This Meeting is Over"**!!! I said, I want some more people in this room with me, I don't feel comfortable with you; I'm not talking with you anymore, then I headed for the door.

But she got in front of the door, so that I could not get out and said, "don't go."

But somehow I got away, and she came racing after me. I said, "Leave me alone, I need to be alone." (I was trying to get with God, for he was the only one who could calm these stormy seas.) **"Man Can't Help Me!"**

But she kept coming after me, I had to stop and wait for the elevator. I looked up and there she was again, "who" that housekeeper, and she was just standing there with a smirk on her face that shouted, **"HATE!"**

I said to her, why are you following me? Haven't you all done enough? **"Just Leave Me Along, Go Away!"**

She calmly looked at me, changed her voice to sound like a white person's voice, and said, "I think I feel threatened by you, I think I'll call the police."

At this point, I just wanted to die. I swear, all these women hated me, and I did nothing to anyone but come in and do an excellent job and this is what I get. Finally, I got on the elevator and ran to my car. This nurse was still coming after me, she followed me all the way outside to my car, but I kept saying leave me alone, I don't want to talk to you. I barely made it into my car, and I had to shove my way in and lock the door. Once inside, I called my boss, I was hysterical and unable to think or speak. Over the phone, she had to help me breathe. **"Bullies and Jealous People are Very Dangerous People"**. At this point , I was ready to give up, I had been going home every night since I took this job wombed, stressed and depressed. and trying to do all I could to stay alive and well. But on this particular day, I just gave up. I did not want to live anymore, I was suicidal, I wanted to go home and kill myself that day. Repeat,**"Bullies and Jealous People are Very Dangerous People"**. Those four to five months of pure hatred and jealousy had finally taken its toll on me.

My boss was still unable to calm be down, she tried ,next thing I knew, I saw manages from the other building run out to see what was going on. They had to talk me out of the car, and I said, Okay, I'll come with you but "I don't want that nurse in the room with me", they all said Okay.

Another manager went into the building where the other girl was, the housekeeper, and I walked back with the assistant general manager, the same one who told me to put on a hairnet, *"Oh God help me"*. I will never forget what she uttered out of her mouth while I was in distress, she said, "it's all your fault, ever since you got here, it's been something."

That numbed me, it left me "Hollow", inside, I was in deep deep "Sorrow". I've loved, "I never bothered anyone. Now who cares about tomorrow? Like Jesus once said, do what you are going to do and do it quickly. That day I wanted to die, I wanted to be free! Too many had come after me; but let me continue , I was in a mental state of distress I was too much in shock to speak I could not believe what I was hearing from this executive. I only met her once, and happy for her success, yes I was very proud indeed to see my people in key positions, I love that! But what good is it to get an education, climb the ladder, gain the world, but lose your soul, leaders who become **"Monsters."**

Right now , I'm sitting in a chair in an office by myself. Ten or fifteen minutes or so later, they come back to where I was. There were about six of them, including the nurse they said they would not let in the room with me, but they did. They questioned me. I told them what I have written here. They said that the housekeeper said I verbally threatened her, and two other witnesses said so too, but from reading this story, yawl all know that's a **"Bald- Faced- Lie!"** There was nobody there but the three of us—me, the nurse, and the housekeeper that kept following me all morning.

"I never threatened her," I said. "I asked her to leave me alone. Haven't you done enough? Something like that, "leave me alone."

"That's not what they said, was this persons reply, others said you threatened her."

Then I turned to the nurse and said to her, "Please tell them what happened. I never threaten anybody. That's not in my nature."

By the grace of God, he got that nurse to tell the truth.

She said, "Star did not threaten her. All she said was 'Leave me alone, go away.' She never threatened anyone". (if she had not told the truth, what would have happen to me? I cannot even imagine what they would have done next, if **GOD** had not been there and on my side.)

That statement was noted, next that nurse had to leave, and they continued their questioning. In that room, the management team started making up all kind of lies, asking me questions from four months ago that I could not answer for example they said, there was a person here, with blondish dyed hair that I supposedly had problems with.

"No, I don't know who you are talking about. I already told my boss about one person and the group of caregivers making my job a living hell, but no person with dyed blond hair, I would have remember that.

(Management) "Okay, then what about . . ." Look,

"I have no idea what you are talking about, and if you had some question that needed to be addressed three or four months ago, why are you asking me now? I don't bother anyone, and I have no idea what you are talking about." Their reply was "We don't expect you to be able to answer it. It has been some time. Well, for today, we are going to ask that you do not return until a full investigation is done, and that should only take a few days."

So I left and went to the other location to finish out my horrible day.

My boss said "Don't worry, their loss," and she asked me if I wanted to go back.

I said, "Yes, I miss my patients." She also informed me this would be her last week; two new executives were coming on.

Meanwhile, as we waited while they held their so called investigation, I was assigned some paperwork—which I do not like doing, but it filled in the days. I noticed after that situation, and with my boss now gone, the office staff was cold toward me. They didn't even speak. In fact, it started feeling hostile like I was still out in those communities.

It would now be two whole weeks before we heard anything. Finally, I got a call from my office, saying I could not go back, I was devastated. But one of our new bosses said, (he was a male" "Star, we have lots of other places we can send you and he also said, if it was me, I would not want to go back to a place that didn't want me. No worries, we'll just have to re-divide the territories, he said, just give me a few days. Meanwhile, the second executive was due to arrive at our business meeting that day too. I was still working in the office.

Let's pause here: Again, I dread this part of the book. I have to relive this part of my life all over again. And can I tell you this, I have tried everything I could think of to convince the Holy Spirit to allow me to leave this story out, but it would not allow me. It wanted this story told, said it *must* be told to complete the book. But look, my StarN'air tears are falling all over again.

People come after you when you don't give in or blend. But we must still love and forgive our enemies, otherwise **"It's Sin"** Matt. 5:43-48

"Never Hate" we'll all have a judgment date!

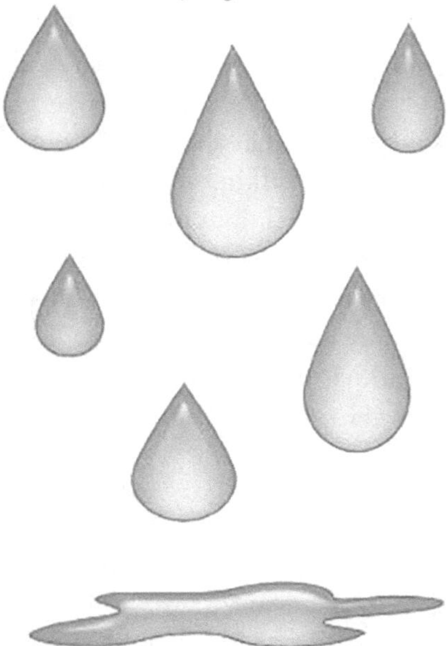

"Weeping my endure for a night, but joy cometh in the morning."

Psalms 30:5

What's going through your mind now about what I encountered? Do share: ____

____

____

____

____

____

____

____

____

____

____

____

____

____

____

____

____

____

____

____

____

____

____

____

____

____

____

____

____

The Boss From Hell!

Fast forward, I've been with the company for a few months now and not too much has changed. Today is our meeting day, everyone must come into the office and give a summary of what's going on with each patient. All the team leaders will be there including the doctor, social worker, spiritual advisor, therapist, the whole shebang, the entire health care team. And today is also the day everybody gets a chance to meet our other new boss. She's a female and comes with very high credentials.

I already met the other, He was the one who said, "I would not go back to a place that didn't want me."

Well let's welcome her, here she is, she's middle-aged and she's Caucasian and she's very well-spoken, and she seems to have big plans for this region. This company is huge, it's all over the united states. And with her credentials paralleled with the other new boss, we would continue in our growth. And in spite of all that was happening to me at this company, I was still happy to be part of the team; perhaps now things will get better for me, "we'll see!" Moving right along, each one of us had to introduce ourselves to her, and tell her a little bit about ourselves, we did that. Later on that morning when all the introductions were done and our meeting was over, I found my way over to her and welcomed her again with a smile. She did not smile back, she was kinda arrogant and cold. I told her I looked forward to working with her then eased away.

Now it's a new day, new week, and they still do not know what to do with me. One morning, I get a phone call, while in my car driving, I was on my way to the office, it was her, the new boss lady; asking me to go see a patient in Akron.

"Akron"—that's what I said—my response was, "I don't know how to get to Akron, I've never been that far before, let alone to Akron."

She said, "If I tell you to do something, I expect you to do it." And if I want you to go to Akron, you go or rethink if this job is a good fit for you. Am I clear?"

I said yes.

When I got off the phone, I felt I was right back where I started—in a prison again with new players. I had no idea how to get to Akron or travel that far. I have never driven that far by myself ever. I was desperately in need of God's intervention.

He did intervene, I could feel him and hear him say "Drive to Akron, I'm coming with you. Let's go."

I drove and ran into some problems—a toll -booth. I had no money, so I made a U-turn and drove twenty miles out in a different direction only to find that I had to turn back around and go through the toll. When I got there, he said, "A dollar fifty." I searched around in my car and found a dollar fifty in change. What a relief.

I found my way to Akron and took care of the patient. I drove back to Cleveland, and the next day, my iPad was loaded with cases all over the place, Akron, Medina, east side west side , south and north. She had me going in all kinds of directions and it stayed that way permanently. I became a traveling nurse assistant, putting five hundred to six hundred miles a week on my car. I was on the road more than with my patients, working twelve-to-fourteen-hour days nonstop except for weekends.

But something amazing happened, I started to love being on the road all the time. **One**, I felt free, **Two**, haters could get at me, and **Three** I was with *"Thee"* God was traveling my constant traveling companion. Plus God and I had lots of time together, and I was being healed too. I listened to all my sermons and healing tapes and even stopped for ice cream during my lunch breaks. it was a beautiful thing. No one was bothering me anymore.

But there were some changes, the office was still very cold and distant toward me, never really knew why they all turned, they once adored me, perhaps that was all a front. I think they got jealous when the previous boss bragged on me. But what about this new boss, **The Boss From Hell?** What's up with her? Each time I would show up for those meeting, she would treat me as if, I am to be seen, but not heard. For example, when it was my turn to share information about my patients, she interrupt me and cut me off, as if what I had to say was irrelevant, unimportant, this was never done before she came. And also during the morning conference calls, she did the same thing. Soon everyone noticed how she was handling me, and they started doing that too—the same people who once welcomed me with open arms, were nothing but fake and phony individuals **"All Charm"**. Reality, rang the alarm!

But at that point, I didn't care. Just put me back on the road where I was free! Send me to California, Utah, or Mexico for all I care, send me anywhere! But soon I would run into the same problems when I arrived at some of their new communities—there were more black caregivers with bad demeanors, unfriendly and didn't want to speak or say hello when I greeted them, here we go, I thought, same thing all over again. That's right, just one look was all it took! But this time, I got out before the sabotage began. I ask my boss, to give some of those new communities to another caregiver, I told her that

I was being targeted again, with the same kind of schemes. These caregivers were taking my hospice supplies and using them on other residence and calling my office asking them to tell me to bring out more supplies two days after I dropped of two weeks of supplies. Again they were lying and scheming starting to create problems for me—just like the others, "all blacks." With, like I said, the same cold demeanor, the same exact crap I just left—**I'm not going back into those communities!**

Do you think I did the right thing in asking to be removed? Yes or No, say why? ____

____

____

____

____

____

____

____

____

____

Well, they did honor my request but they didn't let up on my schedule they added in more, and more communities, my schedules was ridiculous, I was working 80 hours a week; constantly on the road.

One day, I went out to another one of their new sites, "Communities", they were always acquiring new accounts, and guess who I ran into, **"That Nurse"** you know, the one from my office that sided with the other community. Well, she was to be the assigned RN for that particular site, the one I'm at now. I'd would be working under her again. And she wasted no time, the same day I ran into her she started micro managing me, (If I was not good at my job, why am I in such demand on the road and working 80 hours a week minus weekends) She came upstairs to the room I was in, and as I was about to leave and said, "Did you do this? Did you do that?"

(me) "Yes, I did."

(her) Well, go back in and ask her if she needs you to do something else."

I told her, I already asked her that before I left, and she told me she was tired and wanted to rest and that I could leave and she'd see me next time.

The nurse insisted I go back in and find something else to do. So, just to keep the peace, I knocked and went back in. This time the lady was upset, she said, "Didn't I tell you I'll see you next time?"

                MISS ASONDRA STARN'AIR

I said, Yes, you did. I just wanted to make sure you were okay.

I left, went back out, and told the nurse, I'm not going back in. I'm done here. I said, the lady was very upset that I came back in after she told me she didn't want anything else.

Then the nurse said, "All right."

Oh, but this was just the beginning yawl, this nurse harassed me so bad, (she was white and so was all the in house office staff that once loved me and have now all turned after my first boss left.) 'This same nurse, the one who came after me, at that first community began to go inside my charting log and snoop around, she was watching my ever move, where my next location was at, who would I be seeing etc. She had access to all that through our computer system, yet she did not track anybody else, just me. Why was I targeted and hated so much? She couldn't find anything, my work life was clean.

Next she schemed to try to do away with me wearing my beautiful scrubs to work. "What" that's what I said too, this nurse was on a rampage, the devil let her out, "opened the cage". I have a closet full of work gear, that picture of StarN'air closet in this book those are all my scrubs that you see, because I believe if you want success, invest! I made a career out of my profession. I am proud to say **I Am A Stated Tested Nurse Assistant, A Caregiver that Delivers!** If you feel the say way too, "High -Five To **YOU!** Back to the scrubs, scrubs is want we were, and I wore a flower in my hair to match each one, the residence loved it, they couldn't wait to see what I wore for them next. Well this nurse was about to put a stop to all that. (can you believe it, now almost a year into the job and they are still trying to hurt me, yet, still unable to find anything, I was a great nurse assistant in Jesus name. **"GET UP OFF ME,"** but they wouldn't let me be. Now this nurse, also from hell is having a problem with my work gear, this is stupid and ridiculous, like the late Micheal Jackson said, **"Just Leave Me Alone"**, but they won't, now everybody wants a piece of me, including the office. But no worries haters, soon everybody will get a piece of *'StarN'air'* "you'll see"! **When the World's People Go Low, Miss Asondra StarN'air Go High!**

Look, is that a bird, is that a plane, **"NO"** it's **A Caregiver's Bible To Excellence** *in the sky!*

One day, at work, the new boss lady pops up by surprise and wants to do an evaluation on me, right on the spot, a pop up visit if you will, everybody's tracking me now. (in my mind, I'm thinking **"fine"**, sit down! do what you gotta do, I'm cool but I'm no fool!) She said she wanted to grade my performance for my ninety-day evaluation. (Hold up! I hear music! Is it Halloween? It's close to midnight, something evils lurking in the dark! Boy, the devil certainly has his people marked!) I sensed that this woman was on an evil mission, but I'm with Christ, she's no competition. She wants to do a ninety-day evaluation, "yeah right!" I looked at her and said I just had mines done three weeks before you got here. You know what she said, "It doesn't count" then I said, "excuse me, yes it does" (listen, the evaluation was the one I told you all about, the one I got on my birthday, remember?) Of course you do, I cried, it was an awesome day that day for me. But now as you can see, she's trying to get it thrown out. This woman was horrible to me, she hated my cuts, and for what? When I saw her out at other communities she'd never say hello or spoke to me, and I never did anything to this person, ever. She hated everything about me from day one. I did not look like an "Aunt Jemima" or fit the other stereotypes the other two aides did. I was healthy looking and well built,. A fine and intelligent black woman with a promising future like them. But I was supposed to be an "Aide" nothing more and nothing less, but my walk is with Jesus, and some could not handle that, especially my black sista's!

And I'll end it right there, my story goes out to those with a heart that cares. All in all, I told her in my mind, my evaluation is like "Stevie Wonder" song, **Signed, Sealed, Delivered!** It's at the corporate office **"It's Yours"**, she looked floored!" (I feel like singing...here I am baby, you think you got my future in your hands baby...no, no, no... you did a lot of foolish things ...trying to mess with an African Queen, you won't rule over me, give me a Mic hear this black girl sing... here I am baby, only God's got my future in his hands babeee.. Yeah, yeah, yeah, only God's got my future in his hands babe, world

won't stereotype me! get it right, Gimme the Mic 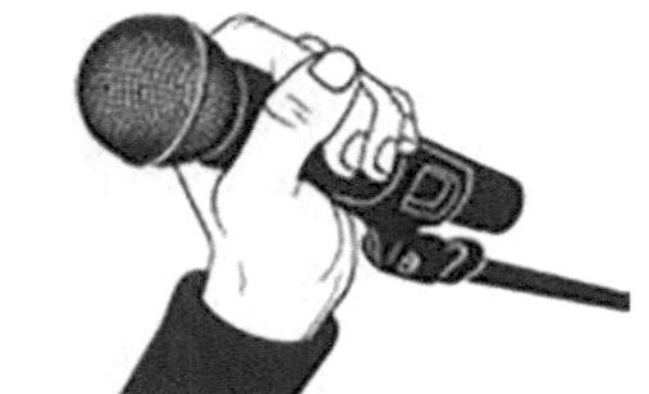 here I am baby... **Nobody's Got My Future In Their Hands!** Jesus and I shall have the late great singer, Donna Summers **"Last Dance!"**

But in spite of all that, and with paper in hand, she said, "Well, we'll have to see about that!" News flash, update, ha, ha, ha, she was a little too late! Absolutely nothing came out of that plot to have my great evaluation thrown out. Jesus is the man, my **'Great Evaluation'** of his work in me **"STANDS!"**

Gimme the Mic! Repeat, "It Stands"

Pause right here: How are you doing so far? Do share your thoughts, we talked about a lot and I sang too! _______________________________

____

____

____

____

____

____

____

____

____

____

____

____

Has anything like this ever happened to you? Were you ever bullied or mistreated before? _______________________________________

____

____

____

____

____

____

____

____

____

____

____

____

____

____

____

____

____

Oops

I almost forgot to include what happen with the pop up evaluation that day on my skills. She was looking for incompetence, but what she found was excellence, in fact, a few of the mistakes came from her, not me. Nevertheless, that part went well, then she looked back at me and said, as she was about to leave, by the way, you cannot wear your scrubs anymore. From this day forward, you have to wear professional attire.

I said, "I was told when I accepted this job that scrubs were preferred, so I went out and bought all new scrubs and work gear."

She looked at me and said, "No more scrubs of any kind, you must be in professional attire."

The next day, I wore professional attire, and the communities managing staff, was fit to be tied, very upset and angry too, (she's an aide, not one of us, why is she wearing these nice clothes?) I 'm sure that what they thought) they went from nice to nasty. However, this was my office idea, that nurse and my boss, See, I never wanted people to see that part of me, I knew it would cause some problems in this overweight and jealous world. Round small firm bottom, small waist, come on, a lot of women know what I'm talking about, "I rest my case!" My scrubs hid all that, and too, scrubs are very, very comfortable to work in. But this move of theirs got me lots of stares. Hatred and Jealousy was on the rise. All in the air, nice body, beautiful braided hair. Hatred and jealousy everywhere, **"This Black Woman Is Fine"**, And God and Love says, "no kidding" I created her, why is that ah surprise? I do hope this book opens up blind eyes.

Stop Judging A Book By Its Cover, I'm more than what you think I am, if you don't like my frankness, I don't give a damn! I have a right to be a bright, I have a right to be a light, I wore business attire. loose fitted pants with matching jacket and low heel walking shoes. again , this is what they ask for. Now it's a problem too, I look more like "YOU." **"Take ah Hike!"** Now this move of theirs has caused all kinds of confusion, not only from the communities management staff, because, now I look like one of them, but also the caregivers in these communities and confused and some are uncomfortable with me looking like somebody. Lord have mercy, what are we seeing here, conformity, stereotyping, racist attitudes, hatred, jealousy and some insecurity all tied up in a bow, "I can't win, or lose!" This part of the book is giving me the blues. Where in this dark and evil world can I go? Reader, tell me, do you know? Why where they so fixated on StarNair? Was is my love for Christ and the flower in my hair? People just ought to get a life, and they need to get one with Christ and let all that darkness inside go, **"HEAL!"** I read in the bible, that when Jesus was here on earth, he dealt with all kinds of jealousy and hatred too, he had no place to lay his head, they hated him with a vengeance, they crucified him. I say all that to say, this, the world's people, the ones who don't know Christ and don't want to know Christ either are trouble makers and full of evil, no one has the right to control another person life. That wicked nurse and our boss, tried everything they could think of to harass me or get me to quit my job, they came after me like a mob. It was a mess, but I got a chance to see something, when you are in professional clothes versus scrubs, people treat you different—a lot different, passerbyers had nothing but hello's and respect in their eye when they saw me out of uniform.

Nevertheless, this move of theirs tuned out to be horrible especially for me, now everybody, everywhere had a problem with me. My life with this company has been full of misery. All the healthcare workers, including nurses in every community I went to, were all giving me dirty looks, I could read between their eyes, ***Who does she think she is coming in here to work looking so professional?*** They all turned, and their office managers seemed to be wondering too, where does this aide get all this money to wear such fine clothes like that? Again, this was a very bad move on my office part, because it all backfired, everyone's in a pickle, but hold on, don't throw **"StarN'air"** no nickels! Management, their all scratching their heads, what to do, what to do? (How about leave me the hell alone and let me do my job as a caregiver, how about that!)

"Ring The Alarm"! Now nobody knows what to do with me, but God.

I don't fit in anywhere, like Jesus, no place to lay my head, in this dark and evil world, love is dead!

Readers hear my cries, all I tried to do from the very beginning, was go out and be the best caregiver they had ever seen, because I believe it's my calling and I couldn't imagine doing anything else. But instead, I get ambushed with hatred, jealousy and lies. Right now, excuse me, I need some tissue to dry my eyes.

The Book of StarN'air , hear my cries, after all that things never got better for me at this company. In fact the worst was yet to come, higher up, was trying to play dumb.

They knew, what was happening to me, remember, I called the hot line. The fact of the matter is this, people go after whomever they want, and if they have enough backing they can destroy people lives. That is exactly what they tried to do to me, but God and I shall have the *Last laugh* and *The Victory!* ***I'm Still Standing!*** Nothing ever changed for me working where I was working. And the workload was becoming unbearable, not to mention that nurse and the new boss were handling me like garbage and black caregivers too, everybody was having a field day. And I was still working fourteen-to-fifteen-hour days and putting up to six hundred miles on my car every week. The money was great, but I got tired of all the working and driving, "No Life" I wanted to spend more one on one time with Christ! Yes, I wanted all the time I could get, and this here, wasn't it. So finally, I called the office, asked to speak to my boss and asked her if I could be released from some of those communities? I picked all the ones that were making my day at work difficult. The next thing I knew, she took me from eighty plus hours a week, to sixteen hour a week. And to add salt to injury, another episode with a black caregiver emerged all in the same week.

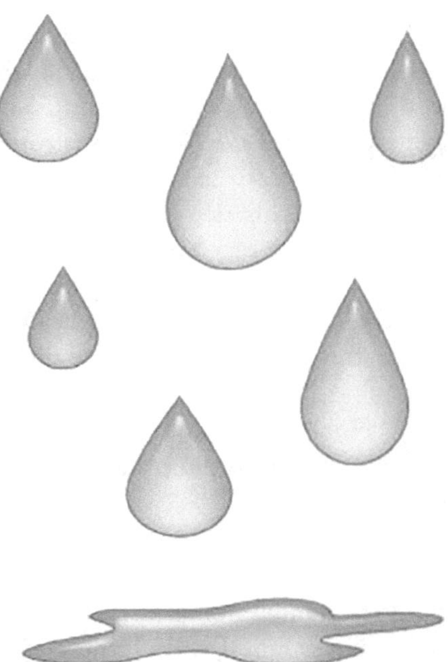

I walked in to do what I always do and next thing I knew, I was under attack, a caregiver was mistreating me badly, hollering and screaming at me for no good reason at all. (But, this time someone witnessed the mistreatment and persecution)

Seconds later two caregivers came running in from nowhere, and confronted her and said, "Why did you talk to her like that? She's your boss."

  Miss Asondra StarN'air

The caregiver said, "No, she's not. She's one of us, an aide."

Those two caregivers looked at me, like they were in shock, "you're an aide"? I said, no, I'm nurse assistant, an STNA. They said, wow we thought you were a nurse. Then they turned to the other girl and said, "that still does not give you the right to treat her that way."

Both of these young ladies told me to file a report. I said, "No, that's okay. It will be okay."

The next day, when I came in, the two caregivers stopped me and told me they wrote that aide up because others nearby heard it too. What a relief, finally somebody got caught. Now maybe my boss will believe me.

That same day I was called to come into the office. The new boss said it was reported by someone that I wore cutoff blue jeans to work.

"What?" I replied. "I would never do that. I don't own jeans like that." "Well," she said, "I'm just telling you what was reported." And she wrote me up.

I have never been written up before. They started making up lies after I asked to have my schedule reduced. I asked her to call all the communities I worked at that day and ask them if they have ever seen me in jeans. She didn't respond.

Then I said, "I need to say something, I am tired of all the disrespect I have been getting from you. You cut me off in meetings, you don't speak to me when you see me in the communities, and you—"

She said, "That's enough" this meeting is over. "You can leave."

I said, "If you want respect, you have to give it. I am not asking for you to be my friend, I'm asking to be treated like a human, not an animal or a dog! I've done nothing wrong here, I have worked hard for this company, I want respect.

Another office member came in, took over the meeting, made excuses for this person, and just said, "It's been a busy week, everything will be fine."

Well it was not fine, the very next day, I got a call and was asked to come

back into the office, and they fired me.

Then, later, I received a phone call telling me that if I wanted my two weeks' severance pay, I would have to come in and sign a letter of resignation. They set me up, they were not going to give me my money if I didn't sign that paper. "White America " makes up their own rules.

"Vengeance is mines says the Lord", Today, the company went out of business. Every last one of their locations throughout the state of Ohio, "ALL GONE" They no longer exist, now haters take this! God wiped yawl all out, jobs and all , God's a fair and just God, all that is wicked and evil shall Fall!

What do you think about that move? _______________________
____
____
____
____
____
____
____
____
____
____

Finally, after nine months, it was all over. All I could do was say, *God, whatever kind of test you are putting me through, it's going to be up to you to restore me. I'm wounded. I don't care what happens to me anymore. You keep allowing this. You won't stop it, but I trust you. Tell me what to do next.*

In conclusion, all of this happened in 2014. Nobody would help me. The other caregivers looked the other way while it was happening except for those two caregivers in the story who spoke up.

As I mentioned, for most of my caregiving career, I have been mistreated, bullied, and sabotaged—not only by caregivers, nurses and by management too. I did not realize so many people hated Jesus so much so, that they would try to destroy anyone who has his light in them. Mediocrity rules in these kind of places, beware of smiling faces.

And final, I came to the realization, after spending so much time with Christ and his word that it is not me haters hate—it's the Jesus in me they hate. But I don't care, He's my one and only true love, the author and finisher of my faith, the world is trapped, but I escaped!

The World Hates The Disciples

"If the world hates you, keep in mind that it hated me first. If you belonged to the world, it would love you as its own. As it is, you do not belong to the world, (Personalized, StarN'air stay faithful and focus, trust what I'm about to do in your life, be strong, hold on'.) That is why the world hates you. Remember what I told you: 'A servant is not greater than his master.' If they persecuted me, they will persecute you also. If they obeyed my teaching, they will obey yours also. They will

   Miss Asondra StarN'air

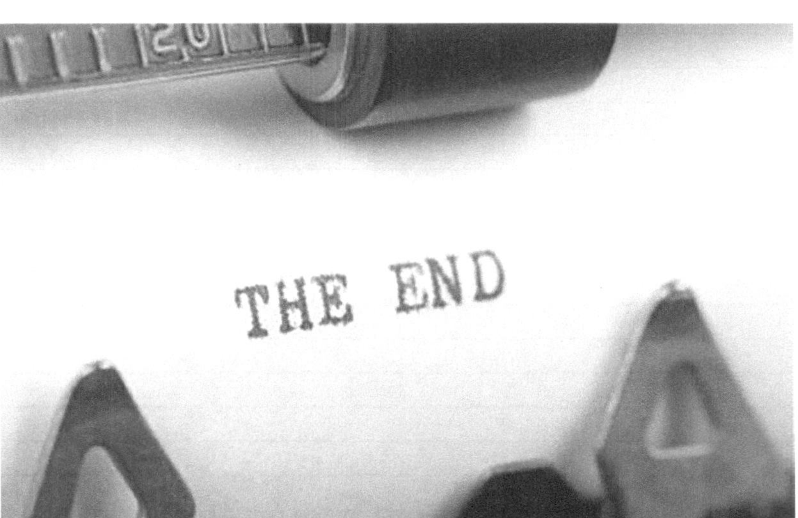

Jesus Is Your True And Only Friend, Let Him In!

The StarN'air Story, Your Thoughts?

Did this story have a profound effect on you? If so, why? _______________

What would you like to say to the author? _______________________

____

____

____

____

____

____

____

____

____

____

____

____

____

____

____

____

____

____

____

____

____

____

____

____

____

____

____

____

____

Send to: OnlyOneStarNair@Gmail.com

 Miss Asondra StarN'air

A Caregiver's Cry

Bullied

Rejected

Cast out

Sabotaged

Blackballed

Hated

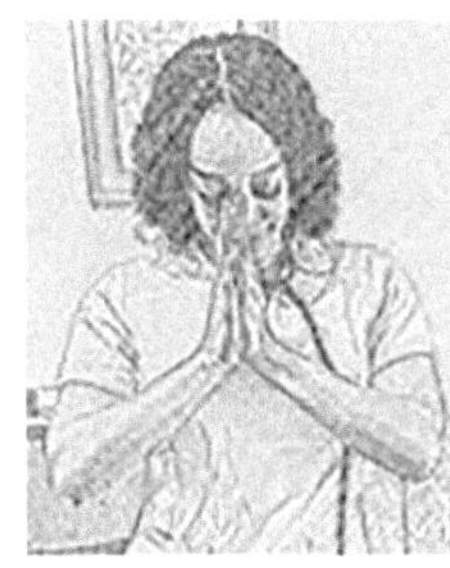

Mocked

laughed at

Persecuted

Hostile Environment

Abandonment

Enemies on every side

For I hear what many are saying, the terrifying news that come from every direction when they plot together against me, they figure out how they take my life. **Psalms31:13**

Everywhere I turn,
"Greatness" is there
but haunting me too!

Jesus, why can't you tell them
it's not me—it's you.

Everyone's peeking around the corner
Wants to see what greatness is all about
And with joy, unspeakable joy
"Greatness" wants to serve them all
It works overtime,
Never gets tired,
It rejuvenates itself
See, ***"Greatness"*** wants to bring
Peace, Love, and Joy to the world
But hate is right around the corner
watching ***"Greatness"*** every move.
I felt its presence too
I'm a caregiver—a nobody to all of you
Yet everywhere I turn
"Greatness" is there
Yet haunting me too

Jesus, why can't you tell them?
It's not me, it's you.

Hate doesn't like what it sees
It gathers up lost people
Now enemies

I'm trapped, my god, they're
everywhere
Part of me wants to die
But I can't be caught with tears in
my eyes
Blood moon, red skies
Why does love have to die?
over and over again, here comes
"The Cross"
Crucified, hated, unaware —
"Excellence Cost!"
Help me I'm drowning *Titanic*, is there
anybody out here other than I? Can
anyone hear **A Caregiver's Cry!**

Miss Asondra StarN'air

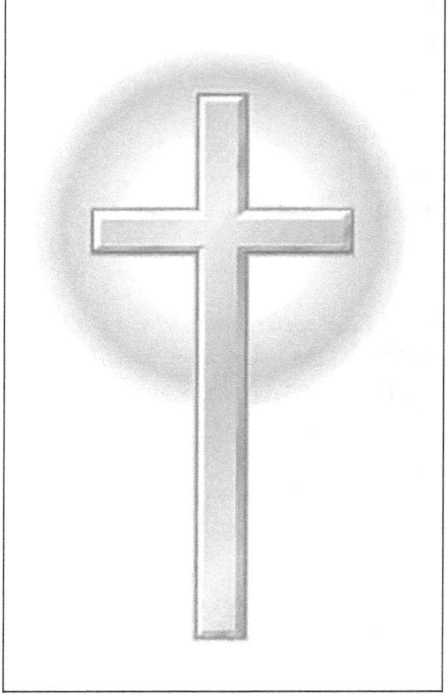

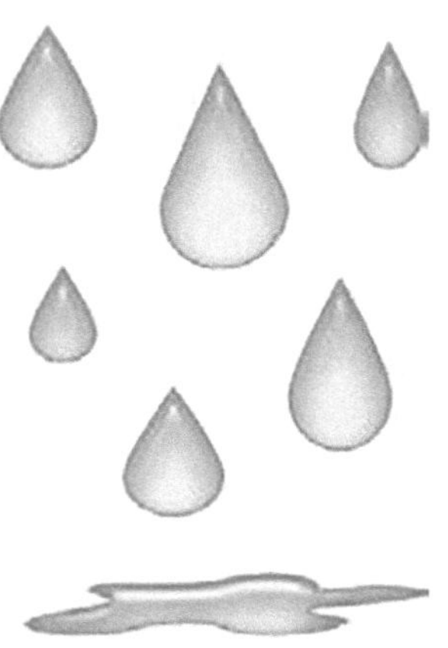

Weeping May Endure for a Night!

But a shout of joy comes in the morning. **Psalms 30:5**

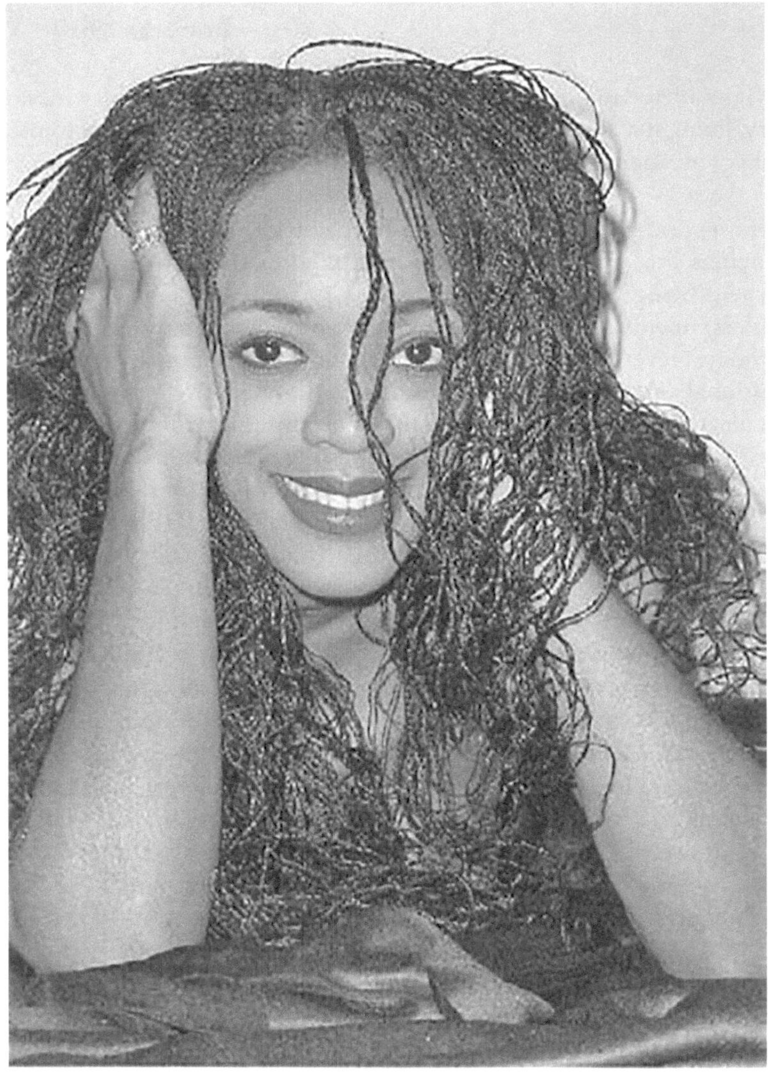

"A Caregiver's Cry"
Written by Miss Asondra StarN'air copyright 2016

The **V**oice of StarN'air

Where there is no vision, the people perish . . .

—Proverbs 29:19

Many of today's caregivers are still in bondage to the old wineskin of slavery, living day by day just getting by they lack hope for a better tomorrow. But that's all about to change.

Home care agencies, I'm talking to the office, the staffing department, the owners too, we can no longer continue on the path of those before us, where being an aide meant slave—a nobody, desperate, poor people, worthless, uneducated and undeserving. It wasn't true back then and it not true today. Nevertheless, we must keep movin; we must move toward a more professional and dignified place in America that honors caregivers (blacks in particular) for the professionals we have become and remove that awful low down demeaning title **"AIDE"** that white supremacist and the government stamped on us during the dark days of the **"Great depression"**. hence the word **"DARK"! My People Shall No Long Settle For Being Marked!** "Let My People Go", black people need to thrive and grow! The word **"Aide"** to me means nothing, **ZERO!** Let's be done with that despicable name along with modern day slavery, and poverty wages for once and for all.

Home care employees all over the world, both, blacks and whites and all in between deserve the right to have a more dignified professional title and be made part of the health-care team in every way. That means respectable pay and benefits too, just like **"YOU."** Therefore, office, have a meeting about that! We can no longer sit back and do nothing about it anymore. Today it's time to knock down some doors, crack some glass ceiling sort of speak, we do more than sweep! We have become healthcare professionals all the way, pay us right today! Furthermore, no one in this field should live poor. The **"Home Care Industry"** by itself is a multi -billion dollar industry, fact: The United States gross 65.4 billion in 2012, and that's the most recent year for which data is available. That's more than doubled the 30.4 billion figure from just 10 years earlier according to my research. Paying homecare caregivers, higher wages come on, **"Really"** that shouldn't hurt! And it you really want to know the truth about it, America owe caregivers all over the world big time, and I don't know about other caregivers, but I want what's mine! Last time, no more nickels and dimes. Let's fight, Home Care Associates, hold your head up and your banners high, time for change, time to reach for the sky!

   Miss Asondra StarN'air

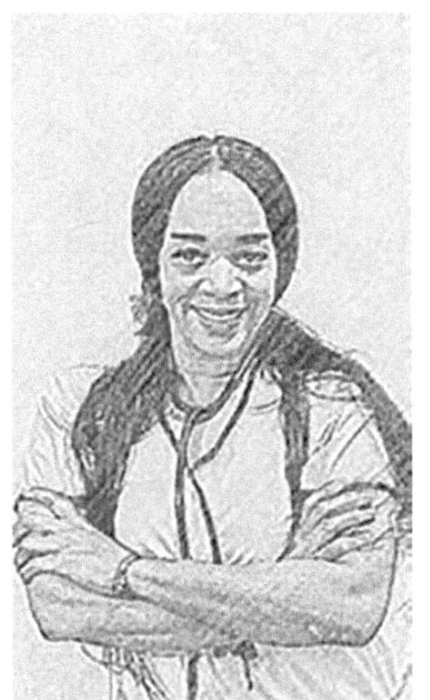

**Miss Asondra StarN'air
A Caregiver and Proud of it!**

I'm A Caregiver!

Tell you what, just call me Miss with a doubles, **"Miss StarN'air,"** time to show me and caregivers all some respect, I think we've earned that!

We Are More, We Do More, We Deserve More, Pay Us More!

Caregiver, if we want to see change, I can't do this along, **"Team Work Make The dream Work!"**

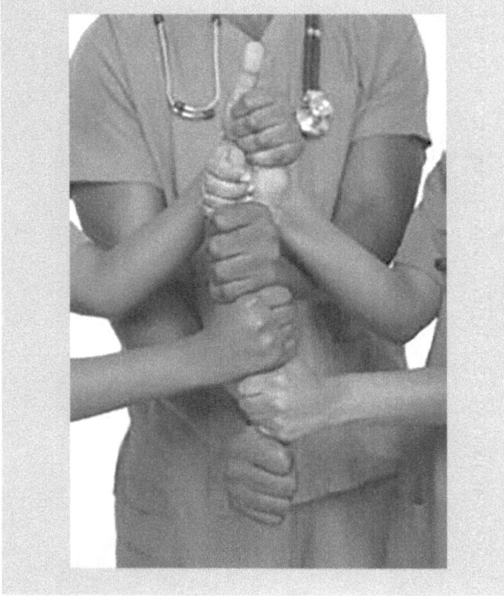

Welcome To My World!

C. A. R. E. G. I. V. E. R. S.

Christ

Almighty

Reaches out to

Everybody, everywhere

Gives

Individuals

Varieties of gifts

Each Received

Something Special

CAREGIVERS, WE ARE BLESSED!

* Caregivers, God has a plan for each and every one of us.

* So no need to be jealous or envious. What is for you is for you. No one else can have it.

* God has set you apart from everyone else.

* He has restored you, made you whole.

* He has given you a special gift, per- haps more than one.

* You have a gift, now up to you to do something with it.

* Everybody's got a gift, if you look inside you'll find it!

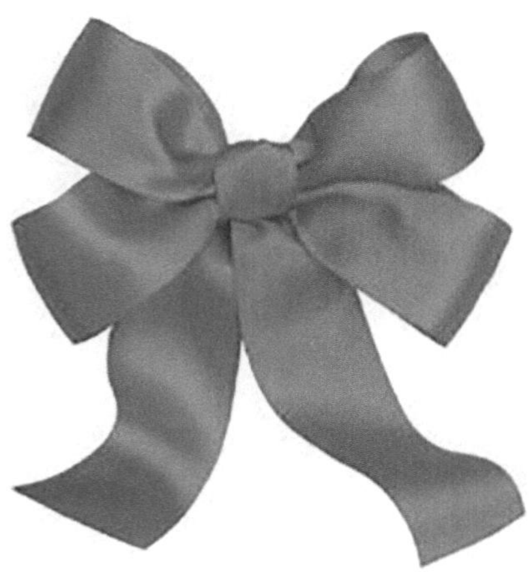

From: StarN'air With Love

A Caregiver's Love Letter To Nurses!

Congratulations, nurses **"YOU"** made it you're an **RN** or **LPN** now, **"Congrats!!!"** However, don't forget about us **"The Caregiver"**. Just because some of us de cided to stay caregivers or nursing assistants doesn't mean we're losers or dumb. (help me someone) Our time too, **"Has Come"**! We're on the same team, both caring for others, so let's become one.

The Bible teaches us to love and care for one another, like sisters and brothers but I'm afraid sometimes degrees can get in the way of that. New graduates please don't let that happen to you. Us caregivers look up to you, but not for you to look down on us.

StarN'air Love Letter To All Nurses, Never forget this, The Caregiver/Nursing Assistants **"WE"** are the eyes and ears for both you and the doctor **"We Are Important!"** Respect what we bring to the table! **"WE"** are the *Florence Nightingales* of our time. **"Let Us Shine!"**

Stop calling us aides and call us by our real name, **"Nursing Assistants"** or simply **Caregivers**. Again, we look up to you, but not for you to look down on us! From now on, *Let's All Get On The Same "Love" Bus!*

Come with us, live out *'A Caregiver's Bible To Excellence!'* Remember, **In God We Trust!** Moving forward, lets not think of ourselves anymore instead lets think **"US!"**

We are all in this together, different scope, yes—but one health-care body that is in-complete without the other.

With Love", Miss Asondra StarN'air

Whoever exalts himself (no matter your degrees, sisters and brothers) will be hum- bled, and whoever humbles himself will be exalted.

Matthew 23:13

Everybody, Everywhere, Be Humble!

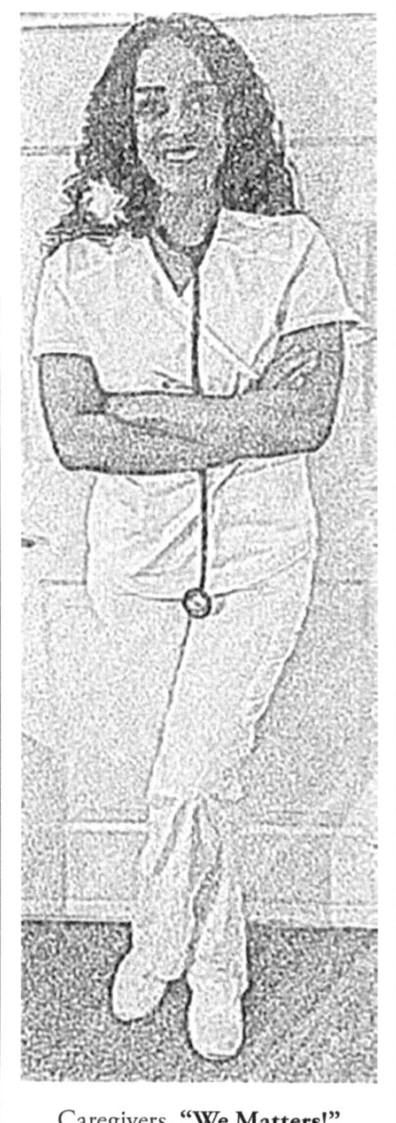

Caregivers, **"We Matters!"**

StarN'air Personalized Care Plan Rap!

gimme the mic, 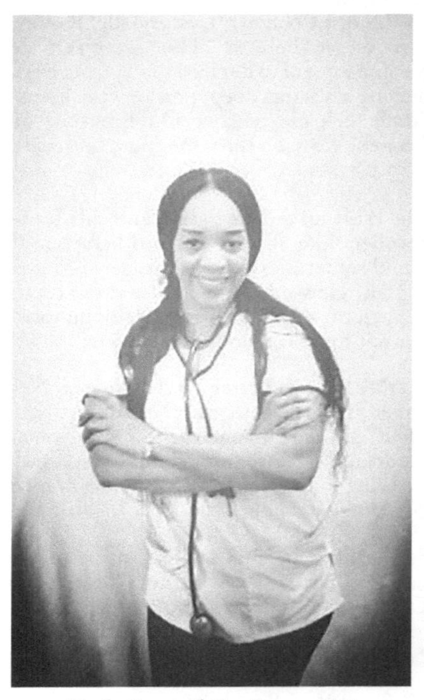
Go to work happy and ready to serve
Don't let haters get on your nerve
Work well
Lies don't tell Look clean and neat
Wear professional shoes on your feet
Watch what you eat
No fast foods from the street
Avoid gossip and troublemakers
Be for real, not a faker
Overtime
Never mind
Forty hours
Just fine
Remember to be loving and kind

This Care Plan Is Mine!
Oh, last one, last line
Don't settle for nickels and dimes!
gotta go... that's my time!

Dj, Give Me Ah Beat!

Ooh Sound So Sweet!!!!!

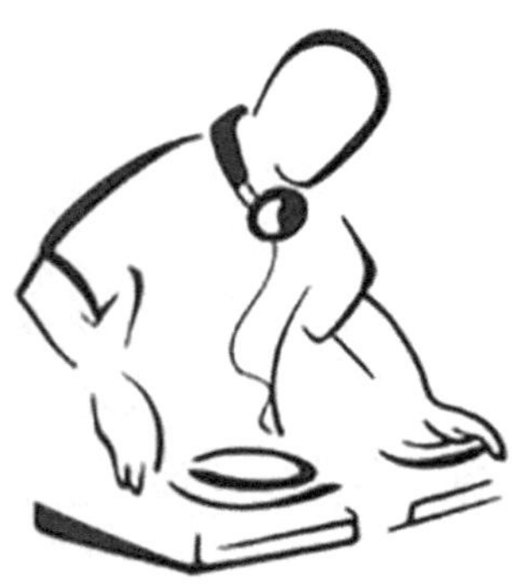

   MISS ASONDRA STARN'AIR

Possible

1. It's possible to love your enemies.
2. It's possible to start over again.
3. It's possible to fulfill your dream.
4. It's possible to forgive all the wrong done to you.
5. It's possible to get out of debt.
6. It's possible to fall in love and get married.
7. It's possible to be a good parent.
8. It's possible to break addictions.
9. It's possible to lose weight.
10. It's possible to become an STNA, LPN, RN, Doctor, you name it, then claim it!
11. It possible to become the head and not the tail.
12. It's possible to be what you want to be.
13. It's possible to buy a home.
14. It's possible to live on your own.
15. It's possible to have the finer things in life.
16. It's possible to be a good husband and wife!
17. It's possible to have faith and trust.
18. It's possible to recover from porn and lust!
19. It's possible to be risen from the grave.
20. It's possible to live like you got it made.
21. It's possible not to live like a slave
22. It's possible to see brighter days
23. It's possible to reverse the aging process—rest, you'll see.
24. It's possible to write a book; look at me.
25. It's possible to win souls over to Christ.
26. It's possible to go to the ball.
27. It's possible to win over them all.
28. It's possible to get back up when you fall.
29. It's possible to live happily.
30. It's possible to see Jesus face to face.
31. It's possible to get in good shape.
32. It's possible to enter his holy gate.
33. It's possible to walk again.
34. It's possible to beat cancer.
35. It's possible to have a child.
36. It's possible to wait a while.
37. It's possible to make thyself over.
38. It's possible to find a four-leaf clover.
39. It's possible to enjoy a glass of wine.
40. It's possible to walk a thin and narrow line.

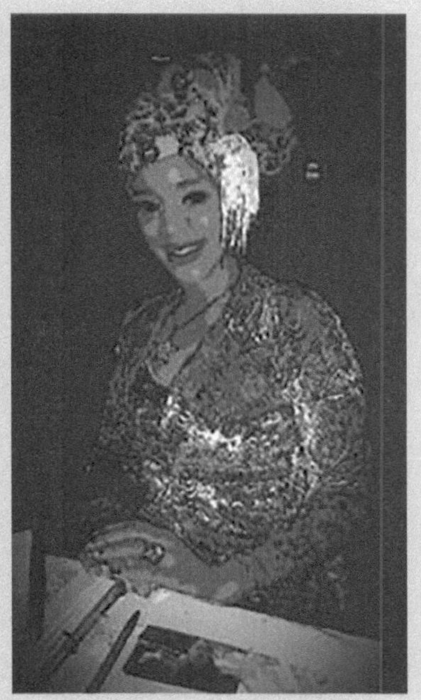

It's Possible To Shine Too!

May the light of God be with you as you keep moving toward his "marvelous light"!

'The Greatest Caregiver of All' will not let those who love him stumble or fall!

Impossible

1. It's impossible to love if you don't forgive.
2. It's impossible to love if you love only those who love you.
3. It's impossible to love if you don't have a loving role model.
4. It's impossible to love if you live like the world does.
5. It's impossible to love if you don't help one another.
6. It's impossible to love if you can't control the tongue. Be quiet!
7. It's impossible to love if you keep remembering one's faults.
8. It's impossible to love if you are full of hatred and jealousy.
9. It's impossible to love if you don't love yourself.
10. It's impossible to love if you if you don't study God's word.
11. It's impossible to love if you love this world.
12. It's impossible to love if you slander and gossip about others.
13. It's impossible to love if you give in to fornication.
14. It's impossible to love if you have **EGO** (Etched
15. **G**od **O**ut)!
16. It's impossible to love if you don't believe in love.
17. It's impossible to love if you are struggling.
18. It's impossible to love if you are full of fear.
19. It's impossible to love if you don't give.
20. It's impossible to love if you don't know who you are in Christ.
21. It's impossible to love if you don't know Christ.
22. It's impossible to love if you are not kind and nice.
23. It's impossible to love if you don't practice righteous living.
24. It's impossible to love if you're a hustler or a thief, "just know", what you sow, you shall reap!
25. It's impossible to love if you don't know how.
26. It is impossible to love when you hang out with haters.
27. It's impossible to love if you're prejudiced and stereotypical.
28. It's impossible to love if you don't do the right thing.
29. It's impossible to love if you forget Jesus, and make 'Men' your "King."
30. It's impossible to love, when you're so vain; you probably think this world is about you, don't you.
31. It's impossible to love if you don't love yourself.
32. It is impossible to love if you don't have a heart of love.
33. It's impossible to love if you are closed-minded.
34. It is impossible to love if it's all about you and what you want.
35. It is impossible to love if you are overworked and tired.
36. It is impossible to love if don't see what God has done.
37. It is impossible to love if you don't welcome people in.
38. It is impossible to love if you can't be your own best friend!
39. It's impossible to love if you don't know Christ, or the difference between wrong or right!
40. It's impossible to love if you can't see with Jesus's eyes.
41. It is impossible to love if you can't see me for who I really am.
42. It's impossible to love if you don't care or give ah, _______ you fill in the blank! "Bam"!

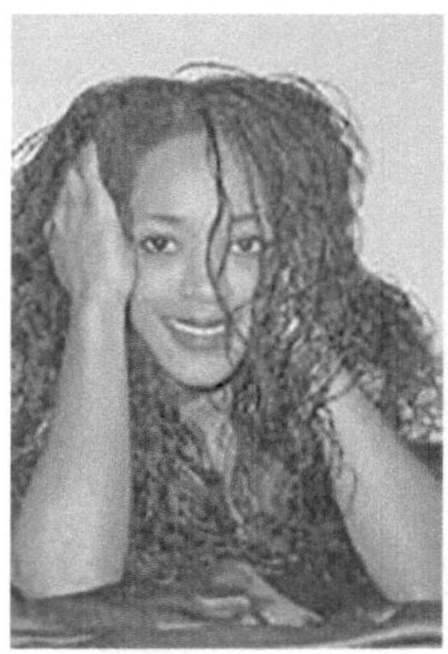

I was called by God at the tender young age of seven to make "footprints" on the human heart. Little did I know mine would be stamped on, trampled on so much so that I could no longer feel pain anymore. I became numb to it. The only thing left to turn to was **LOVE.** Only to find out, through wisdom, one cannot love until it makes it through the wilderness of hate and survives by forgiving all wrong done to it. I did that, and by Jesus's stripes, I am healed. Transitioning into agape love, a kind of love most will never know. It's impossible to love if you don't forgive.

Miss Asondra StarN'air

The Lord's Prayer

Matthew 6:9–13 New International Version (NIV)

"This, then, is how you should pray:
'Our Father in heaven,
hallowed be your name,
your kingdom come,
your will be done,
on earth as it is in heaven.
Give us today our daily bread.
And forgive us our debts,
as we also have forgiven our debtors.
And lead us not into temptation, but
deliver us from the evil one.'"

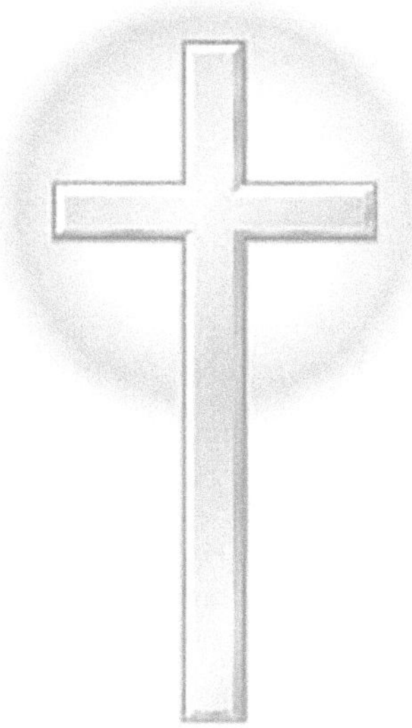

Energy Field

Hey, did you know everything we think and do creates energy?

If you are wicked, you will created a life of problems and misery as well as poverty for yourself. Nothing good will come out of evil—nothing.

Loving individuals are blessed, happy, and highly favored by God. Hatred can't keep us down, our energy field is so bright, so full of light, and light is far more powerful than darkness — even the devil has to flee!

Stay with me! All those who have eyes, keep reading, all those who have ears, keeping listening. Long ago, *'Mother Nature'* and I met, she whispered like the wind, but I heard her, I let her in. She said, with a **C**alm, **C**ool, **C**ollected breeze, **(all 3 C's)** *"All that we are is a result of what we have thought!*

"The things we say, think, and do helps describe who we really are" Wow, talk about wisdom, that's gets ah "Five Star!"

LOVE ONE ANOTHER, BE LIGHT!

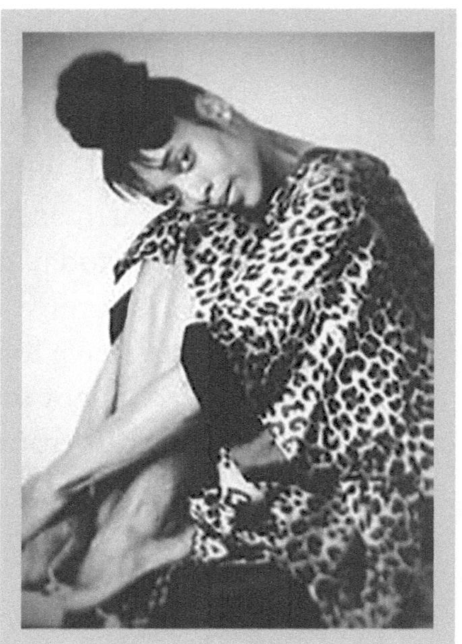

Wisdom, All I Wanna Do, Is Be Where You Are!

Wisdom, *"I kept looking in the night visions, And behold, with the clouds of heaven One like a Son of Man was coming, And He came up to the Ancient of Days And was presented before Him. "And to Him was given dominion, Glory and a kingdom, That all the peoples, nations and men of every language Might serve Him. His dominion is an everlasting dominion Which will not pass away; And His kingdom is one Which will not be destroyed.* **daniel 7:13-14**

Energy Field: And I, if I be lifted up from the earth, will draw all men unto me.
John 12:32

A Time For Everything!

For everything there is a season,
and a time for every matter under heaven:
a time to be born, and a time to die;
a time to plant, and a time to pluck up
what is planted;
a time to kill, and a time to heal;
a time to break down, and a time to build up;
a time to weep, and a time to laugh;
a time to mourn, and a time to dance;
a time to cast away stones, and a time to
gather stones together;
a time to embrace, and a time to refrain
from embracing;
a time to seek, and a time to lose;
a time to keep, and a time to cast away;
a time to tear, and a time to sew;
a time to keep silence, and a time to speak;
a time to love, and a time to hate;
a time for war, and a time for peace.
Ecclesiastes 3:1-8

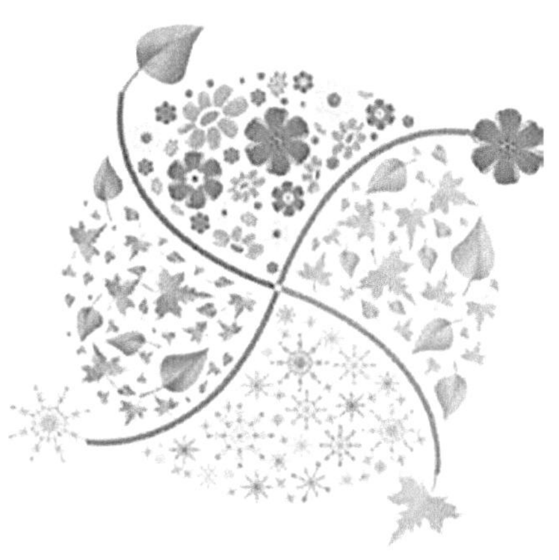

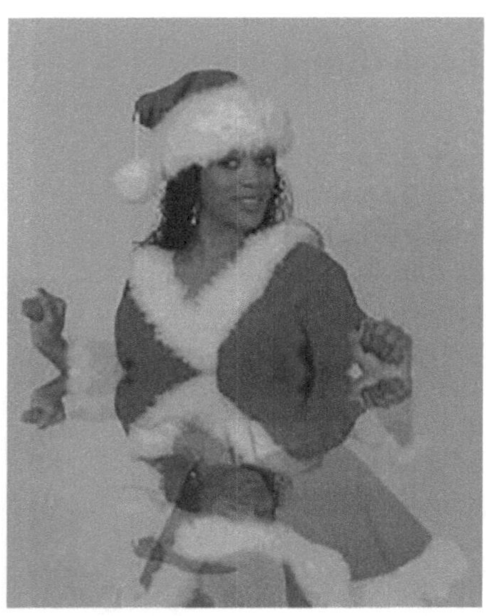

Miss Winter

Winter is my mentor
Winter is my center
In which I build my snowman
Winter is my cold feet
Getting warmer to the truth
I'm still a child of God
I need to connect to my youth
Winter is joy and laughter
A lifetime friend
Cookies by the fire
Waiting for Santa to come in

  MISS ASONDRA STARN'AIR

Spring, (oh how I feel like singing)

Spring, oh, how I want to sing
Do my own thing
Watch me spring into a flower
Oh! What will I be?
Will I be Daisy?
Will I be a Rose?
Only heaven knows right now, I can't see
I could be a little happy bluebird in a tree
Or singing in a video, on a big-screen TV
Oh whatever, what will be will be
But it sure feels like Springtime to me!

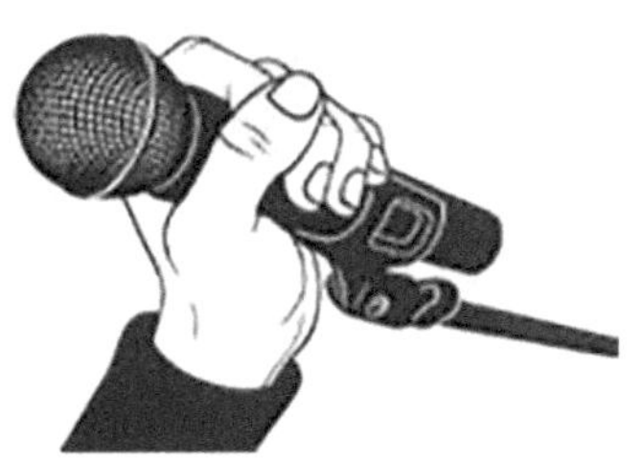

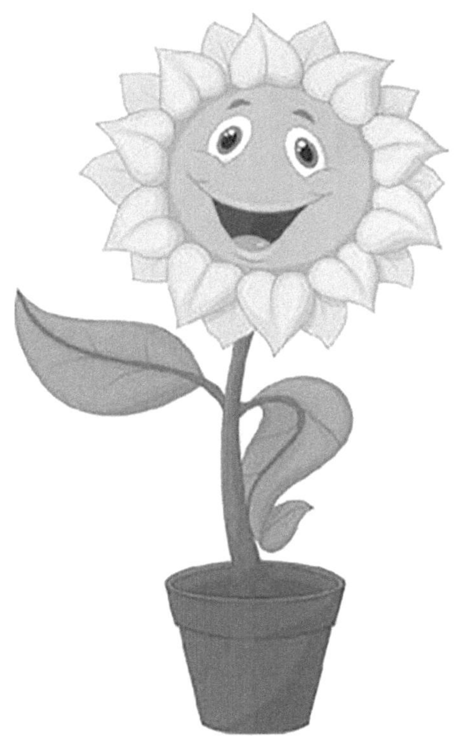

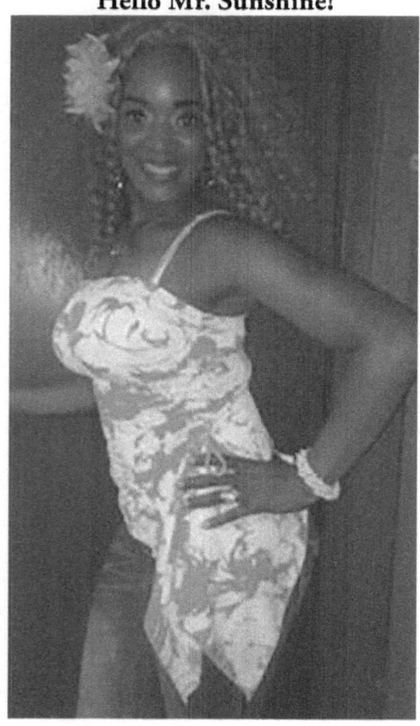

Miss Summer

Ooh wee it's hot, hot, hot
And I'm not, not, not
Going to complain
For all the seasons have their reasons
To be hot, hot, hot
cold, cold, cold
Or Fall, fallen, old
Even "wet", springtime bold
But on summer
like most people, "I'm sold!"

MISS ASONDRA STARN'AIR

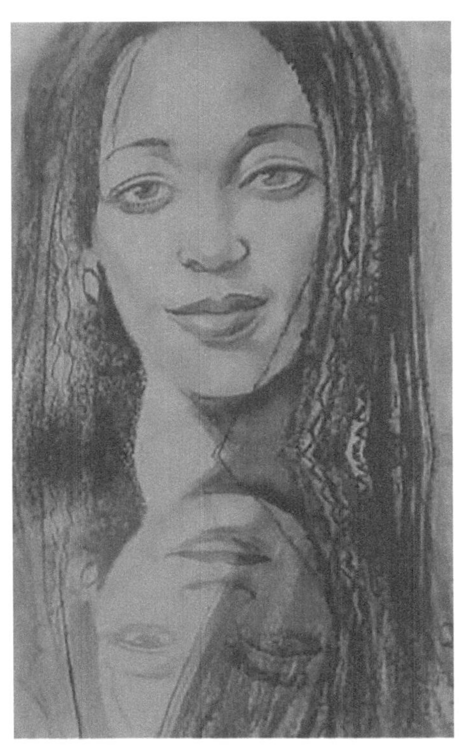

Fall

What a beautiful day!
It's fall
The season that makes me feel
I have it all
I go from nothing
To Green, Yellow than Orange
Then I fall
I fall off myself like leaves
But still intact like trees
Strong and secure holding on
No worries, no fear
Because I know I'm protected
From the storm
Like nature
I too was given everything
When I was formed
And Wow! What a beautiful day
To write this poem
For I thank God
The day Christ in me was born!

Published by Timeless voices 2006
Written by Miss Asondra StarN'air

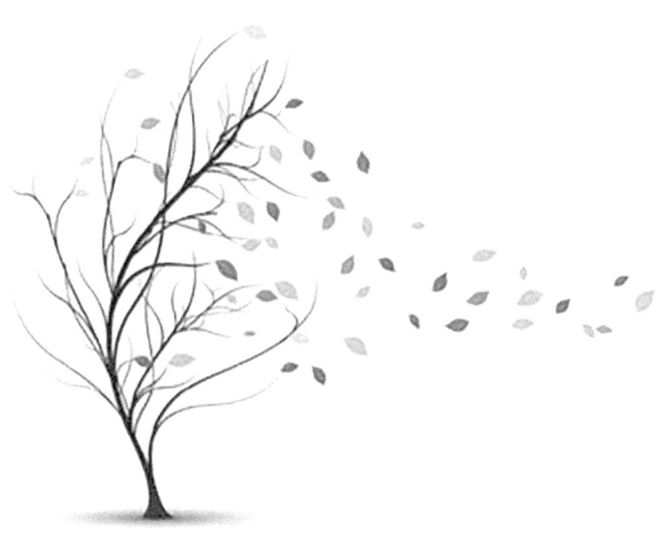

"Be Quiet"

listen, you'll hear sounds
all around you
some sounds will
astound you
"Be Quiet"
thank God
you're alive
saved
peace has found you
"problems"
they come, they go
"Be Quiet"
Someone's
about to go
to sleep you know!
will they awake?
will they die?
"Be Quiet"
shurr . . . I hear a whisper
Eternal life says, "Not I."

written by StarN'air copyright.1996

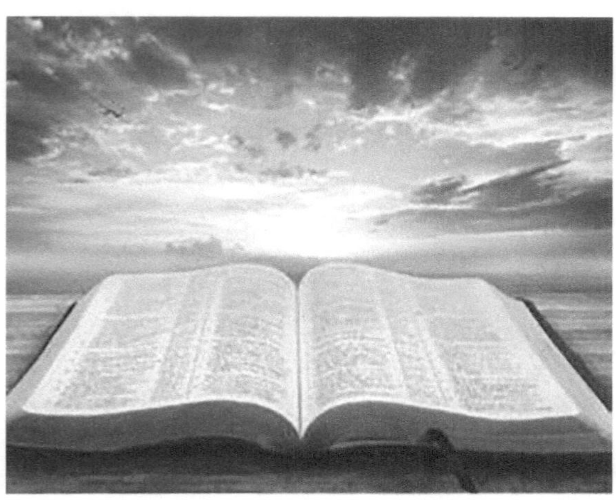

　　Miss Asondra StarN'air

Love One Another Like Sisters and Brothers

This is an intro to a Song I wrote almost twenty years ago and seem so appropriate here in this book…
it goes like this
"Love One Another Like Your Sister's and Brothers"
Love one another like your sister's and brother's
…you've been told this over a thousand times
…why does this kind of compassion always leaves your mind?
and you for get to be kind
always out to find
a reason not to
love one another like your sister's and brother's
but once you do… a new world, you'll discover
God gave his son…
the only one
there's no other
who can teach us
how to love one another
like our sisters and brothers…
But you've been told this over a thousand times
Why does this kind of compassion always leave your mind and you forget to be kind.
Always got to be reminded, in your heart, why can't you find it, good to.
love one another like your sisters and brothers
that song never left me and I hope it doesn't leave you either.

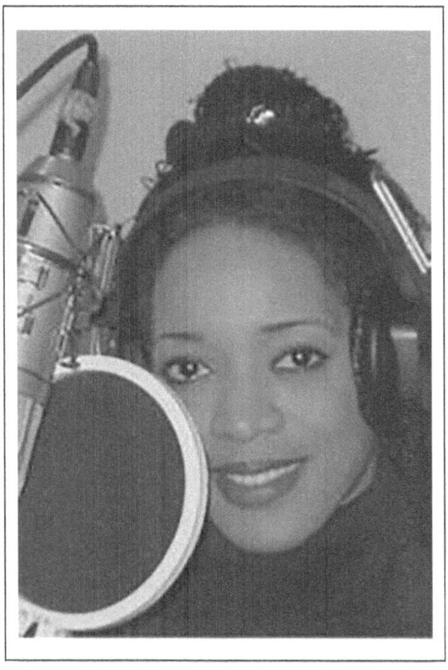

"Love One Another Like Your Sisters and Brothers"
In Jesus name Amen!

Man In The Mirror!

This is a wonderful song, that was written by Glen Ballard and Siedah Garrett, produced by Quincy Jones and recorded by the late great 'Michael Jackson'. The song was release on January 16, 1988. This Song 'Man In The Mirror' has become one of Michael Jackson's most beloved hits since it was first released. *"I Love This Song!"* This song connects with this book, because it's all about *"CHANGE"* in this case, for the caregivers, from **Mediocre** to **Excellence**, all in **Jesus Name!"** Shrr.. I hear rhythms and beats Micheal Jackson's music is still playing, it's on air, **"Turn It up!"** I want see caregivers **"STOP"**, and take a spiritual look in the mirror, *"Everywhere!"* **Caregiver in the Mirror, Make That Change!** For starters, Ask thyself this question, Am I all, God has called me to be? If not, than get busy, **"Go After Your destiny!"** Don't just waste your life away, **Take A Look In The Mirror And "Make That Change Today! Giving up On You or God Is Never Okay.**

Therefore, I urge you, brothers and sisters, in view of God's mercy, to offer your bodies as a living sacrifice, holy and pleasing to God—this is your true and proper worship. 2 Do not conform to the pattern of this world, but be transformed by the renewing of your mind. Then you will be able to test and approve what God's will is—his good, pleasing and perfect will. **Romans 12:1-2**

The Lord is not slow in keeping his promise, as some understand slowness. Instead he is patient with you, not wanting anyone to perish, but everyone to come to repentance. **2 Peter 3:9**

Make That Change!

My Life In Ah Song!

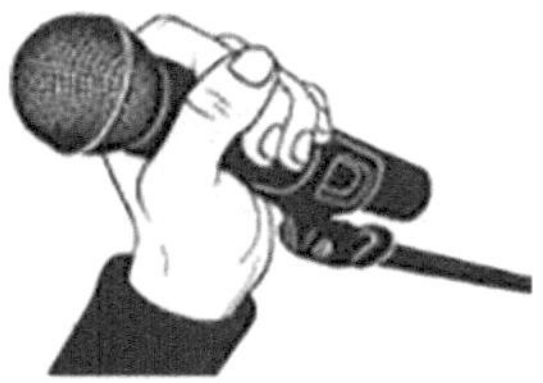

My Life In Ah Song: DJ, Mr. DJ gimme ah beat, here we go... a marriage, beautiful baby girl, joy- to- my- world, nice house, white picket fence, hey but I wasn't liven quite like prince, but I was liven, God was still given, booming daycare business with two toy poodles as pets, and you can surly bet, "I ain't done yet", driven down the street in my yellow convertible jeep, at home three more cars waiting for me, park along the side, matching clothes up with my ride, nice outside, chillin, ain't bout to come inside! Wearing all kinds of fancy clothes, and only heaven knows, how it felt to be fine, foxy brown and thin, men were at me, but they weren't getting in; didn't want them, didn't need them, besides I was married, with a baby carriage. "DJ up the beat" break it down, material things wasn't nothing but a thang, oh –did- I -mention, "bam" I wore diamond rangs, and I hope you don't this black woman strange, but I love to listen to Elvis sang, I don't know who taught him, but that man could sho'nuff sing and swang! Yeah I had it all, I lived at the mall... (Slow it down DJ, real slow) but one day I ask, God, **"is that all?"**

I want something more, something I've never had or seen before and I declare, Jesus waked through my door, now the world don't live in me anymore!

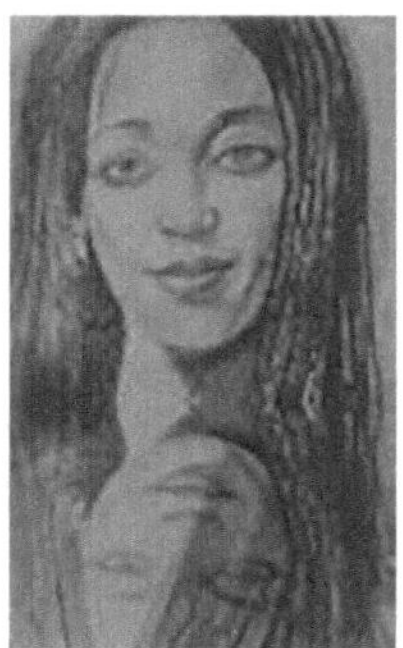

I'm not the same as before, ***"Me"***, *it's over,* ***No More!***

Make That Change Journey With Me!

Heal the world, Michael Jackson is no long with us today but his spirit lives on, and he left with us a very powerful song. **"Man In The Mirror"** plus many, many more. Now it's up to us to get right within ourselves, take his message he left in his music and carry on. We can no longer, just sit back and do nothing to help make this world a better place. People are dying, babies are crying and there is still hunger everywhere. But we have a savior, just waiting to use us, *He's* still searching for those who'll help out, dedicate their lives to him, and be there. For those of you in need of a super natural change, you've come to the right place, ***Jesus Christ*** is his name; winning souls over to him, is my thang!

Listen, **'People'** Jesus must be that change otherwise, there's nothing to gain. **To The Loss:** Let me show you which way to go.....

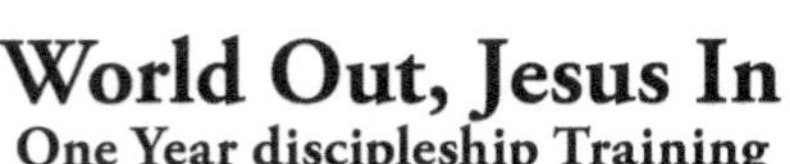

World Out, Jesus In
One Year discipleship Training

Make That Change!

1. No TV or secular music, only Christian programming and spiritual/ gospel hymns, melody in your heart to the Lord.
2. No profanity or lewd jokes or negative conversations.
3. Refrain from sex and intimacy outside of marriage. No romantic relationships—just you and Jesus for one whole year.
4. Remove yourself from all those who are not taking this one-year challenge with Jesus. Troublemakers, fools, nonbelievers, and hypocrites—don't even eat with them anymore. Oh my, there goes most of your social life.

 Miss Asondra StarN'air

5. This may also include family members who have not committed their lives to Christ. Jesus said in **Matthew 10:23**, *"Do not think I came to bring peace on earth; I did not come to bring peace but a sword."* He goes on to say *"He who loves his mother or father more than me is not worthy of me."* And he also says a person's enemies will be a member of his own household. **Matthew 10:36**

6. Get on my one-year weight loss and management boot camp for caregivers. It is written that our bodies are not our own but have been bought with a price: Jesus. Therefore, it's time to get in the best shape ever and stay that way.

7. Bond with someone you hurt or mistreated, preferably another caregiver. If you are not guilty of this, then choose someone else and serve them an entire year with love and appreciation. One full year—put them on your Christlike list.

8. No gossip. Get far away from her/him. You already know who these snakes and fake friends are. Remember, if you don't hate who they tell you to hate, you will be next on their list of schemes. Once they have no more fools who are willing to choose them over Christlike behavior, they will soon die out, and everyone will begin to see how evil they really are. Therefore separate yourself, come from among them.

9. Read God's word daily, and *A Caregiver's Bible To Excellence,* together, be transformed into the kind of person God world be proud of. But remember, change takes time and requires obedience, discipline and work, and of course, a little exercise couldn't hurt. **"Get fit, not fat!"** We must *always* take good care of our vessel. All in all what I'd like most for you to do, so that real change can happen is get yourself on a one year bible study reading plan as fast as you can, **"hurry,"** I promise you, you won't be the same woman or man.

Therefore, I urge you, brothers and sisters, in view of God's mercy, to offer your bodies as a living sacrifice, holy and pleasing to God—this is your true and proper worship. Do not conform to the pattern of this world, but be transformed by the renewing of your mind. Then you will be able to test and approve what God's will is—his good, pleasing and perfect will. **Romans 12:1-2**

10. Tithe, Give! How can you be a caregiver and not give? *Giver* is intertwined, woven in with *Care*. See **"Care-Giver."** So what has to happen, you have to make that heart and soul shift into realizing that it is better to give than to receive—the way I sum it up, "Give and Live"!

I do hope you make every effort to
take a look in the mirror and:
"Make That Change!"

Prayer of JABEZ

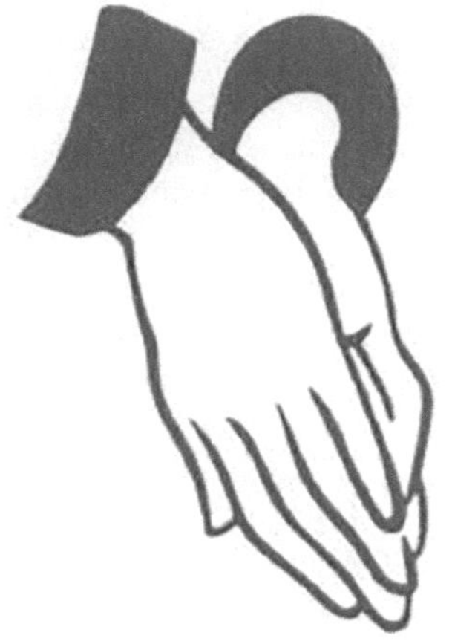

Never Stop Living For Christ!

Prayer of Jabez

Jabez cried out to God of Israel,

"Oh, that you would bless me and enlarge my territory! Let your hands be with me and keep me from harm, so that I will be free from pain." And God granted his request.

1 Chronicles 4:10

The prayer of _______________________

____

____

____

____

____

____

____

____

____

____

____

____

____

____

____

And God granted **"Your"** request too!

Amen

The Bible says if we cry out to God, he will hear us too. In Philippians 4:6, it says, *"Be anxious for nothing, but in everything by prayer and supplication with thanksgiving let your request be made known to God."*

Jabez and I have done that; now it's your turn, over to the right, write, cry out, tell him what you want? You have not because you ask not.

James 4:2-3 *"Ask!"*

 MISS ASONDRA StarN'air

Prayer of StarN'air

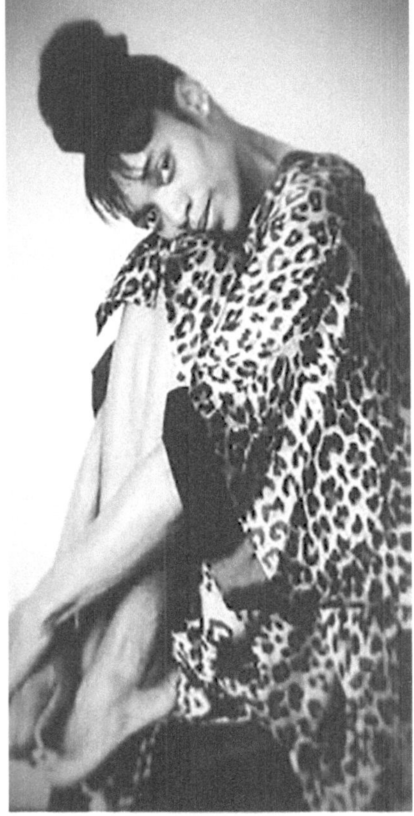

My God, oh, how do I love thee?

Take over my life and never give it back to me. Tame the ego mind.

Make it stay behind, free me from fear, remind me a Messiah lives here. Give me all that I need to succeed. Never let my wealth turn into greed. Keep Godly spirits in my life to help me grow and learn. Let your light shine in me, forever burn. When my time is over, help me to step aside give someone else a turn. Oh, my Lord, stay in the mist; keep your hands in all I do. Keep reminding me the day I was born, a diamond grew.

Lord, take me, my gifts, the music in me— use it for humankind, send me out in the world to do your work no matter what I find. Keep me thriving and living on faith.

Let me love, my Lord, and never hate. Teach me to walk a straight and narrow path. I'm told it's lonely, but let me rejoice, sing and laugh.

No matter what the sacrifice, keep me on that straight line, and let me say yes to those who say "Sister, can you spare a dime?" Yes, Jesus, make me over, I want to love and live like you, leaving no one behind. And God also granted her request.

Book of StarN'air
Written in the 21st Century AD
Prayer of 2007

Ask, And It Shall Be Given You!
Matthew 7:7-8

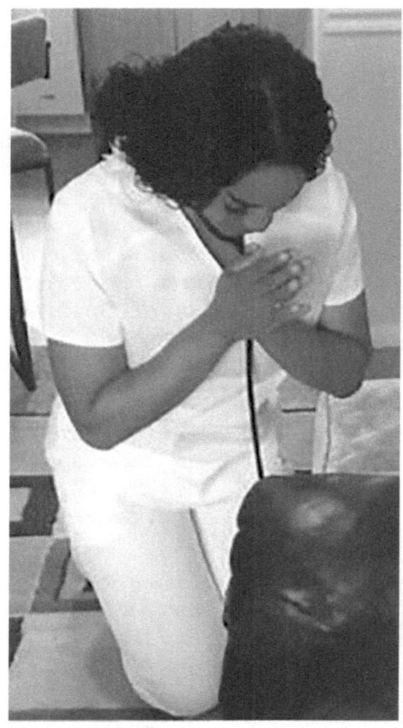

"Keep on asking, and you will receive what you ask for. Keep on seeking, and you will find. Keep on knocking, and the door will be opened to you".
Matthew 7:7

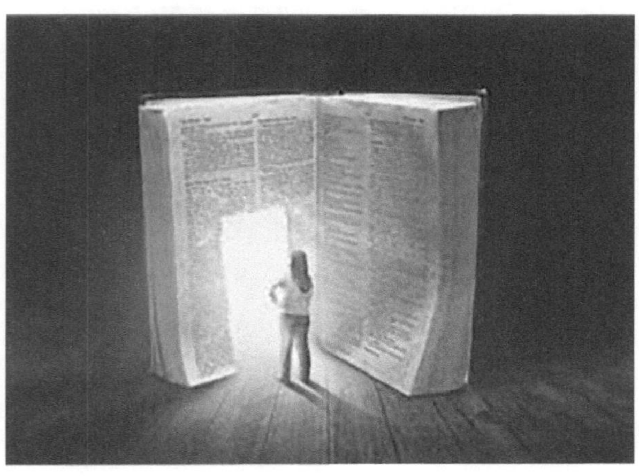

 MISS ASONDRA STARN'AIR

StarN'air

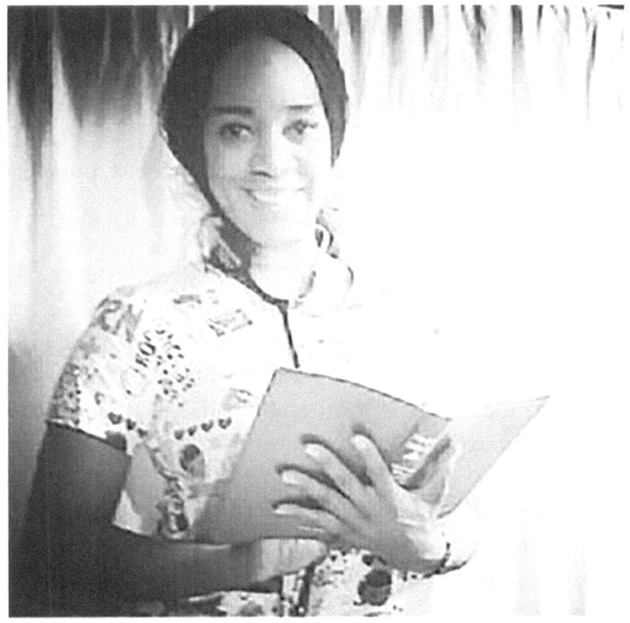

Well now you've all read my personal heartbreaking story, but too, I must say, it hasn't been all pain because from out of it, there's been some glory. Today, I have a new story to tell. **"My Life with God is good; I'm doing quite well! I'm still a caregiver and always will be. But "Now" I'm an "Author Too!" There are five more books written and scheduled to be released soon. But right now, this one is for "YOU" it's been a labor of love and hard work, and adding in all those picture didn't hurt. "Reality" A Caregiver's Bible To Excellence, is "LIVE" out now, and sold everywhere books are sold, now all you have to do is take action and:**

Get the book

Open the book

Do the book

Is with **"YOU"**!

And May God Be With Us All!

Healing
Matthew 4:23

Jesus Heals the Sick

Beloved, I wish above all things that thou mayest prosper and be in health, even as thy soul prospereth. (3 John 1:2)

Too many people are still suffering from disobedience. They refuse to obey God's word, looking for everything under the sun to satisfy their **"Fleshly Craving!"** However, when the sin wears off, people find themselves in trouble. For women, unplanned pregnancies, broken heartedness. For men, power, money, girls along with pornographic inducement and desires that eventually destroy him, his health, and everything he worked for eventually "crumbles" too.

Why Must We Go On This Way? Give your life to Christ today. Because there is a much, much better way. In fact Jesus said, *If my people, which are called by my name, shall humble themselves, pray and seek my face and turn from their wicked ways, then I will hear from heaven, and will heal their land.* **2 Chronicles 7:14**

And, want to hear some more, *Jesus went throughout Galilee, teaching in their synagogues, proclaiming the good news of the kingdom, and healing every disease and sickness among the people.* **Matthew 4:23**

Let All Those Who Have Ears Hear!

Nobody is going to force Jesus on you, you must have a change of heart You must get sick and tired of the way your life is going and be willing to give it all up for Christ, that is also known as a turning point, you're ready to surrender to a God that loves you. You no longer want to live for this world. However, until that day does come and I hope it does, I too shall pray for you. I cannot make you accept me or Christ; all I can do is be another light in a dark world reaching out for you saying won't you come. For I know a place that's safe. **"Come" Come And Go With Me To My Father's House!**

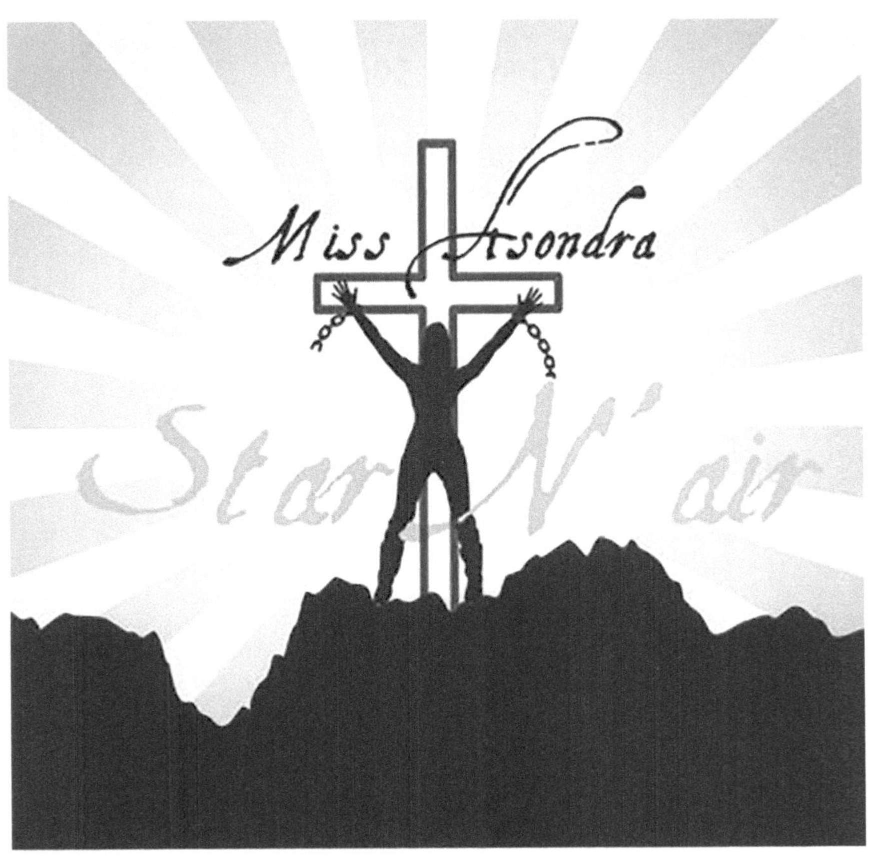

I'm On The Cross "Me Too", Crying Out For You,
"Come Home" Come Home!

Genesis 50:20

What was meant for evil, God used for good, he never left my side.
He's Got something for you, "Surprise"

A Caregiver's Bible To Excellence **"Worldwide!"**

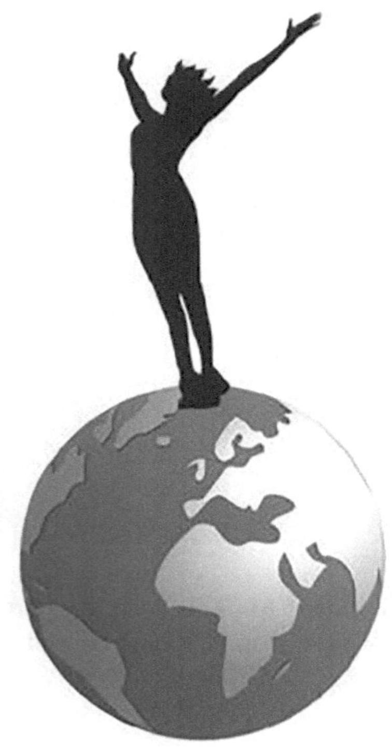

 Miss Asondra StarN'air

SECTION XX

The Sixty-Six Rooms In My Father's House

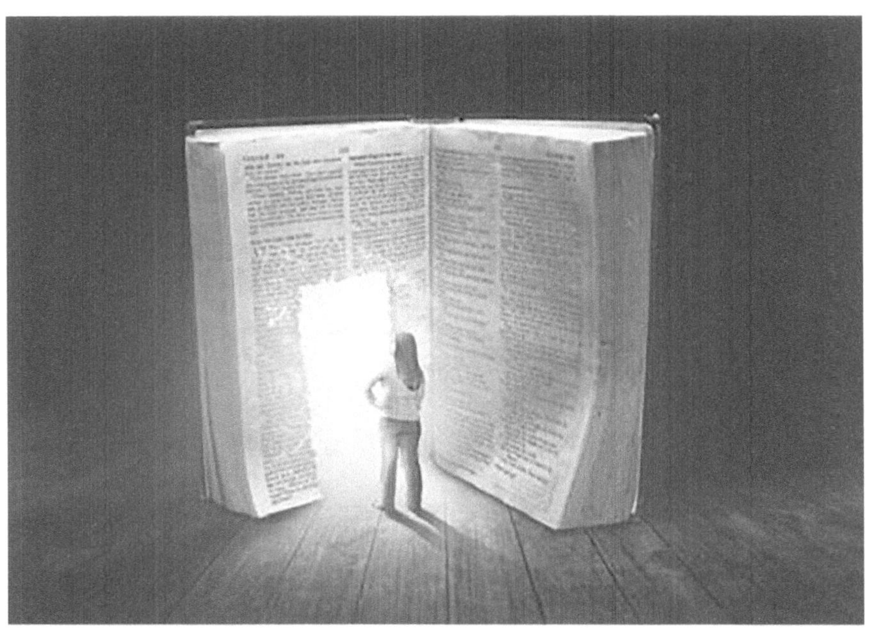

The Holy Bible

Get the Book
Open the book
Do the book
is with **YOU!**

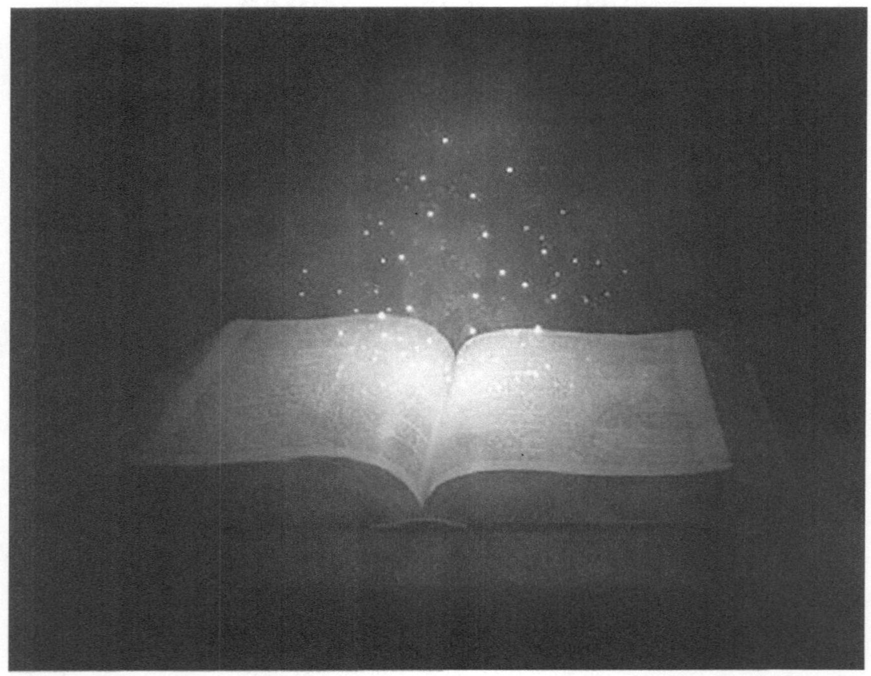

   MISS ASONDRA STARN'AIR

Short Story, God's Glory!

One night, while I was sleeping, I woke up to the sound of music, it was about 3:00 a.m. in the morning. An old familiar song at that, I always loved this song, but why is it playing in my head and why at three o'clock in the morning?

The song was called **"Come and go with me to my father's house."**
John 14:2 says *In my father's house there are many mansions; if it were not so, I would have told you, I go to prepare a place for you. And if I go prepare a place for you, I will come again and receive you unto myself; that where I am, there ye may be also.*

It was another call from God, *"Show them the 66 rooms of the bible, and do it in such a way, even a child can understand"* okay, was my reply. I'll show them around as best as I can, but holy spirit, I'm probably going to need your help on this one. I was told to just use your imagination and have fun on the tour, "okay", sure! Here we go, It's ah new day, so everybody are you ready to come and go with me to my father's house, if you are, then let's go.....

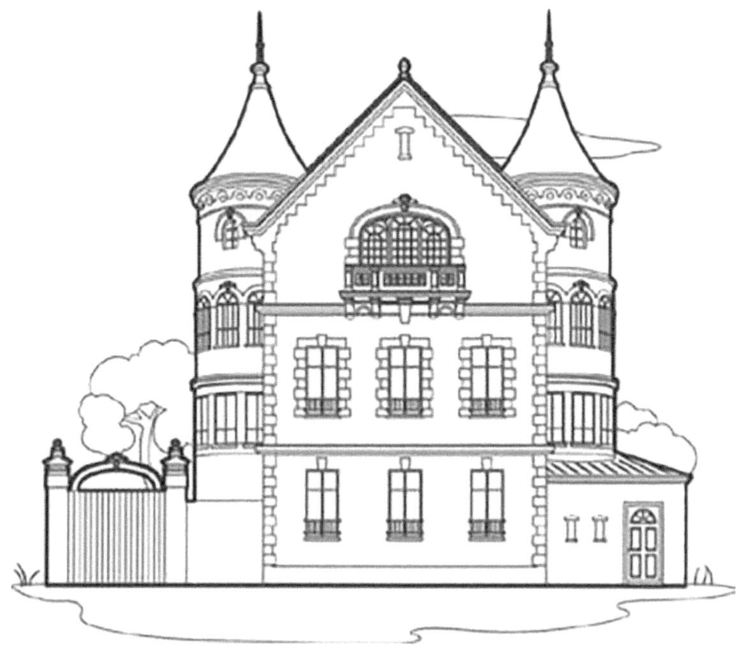

Come and Go with Me to My Father's House

In my Father's house are many rooms. If it were not so, would I have told you that I go to prepare a place for you? And if I go and prepare a place for you, I will come back and welcome you into my presence, so that you also may be where I am...

John 14:2-3

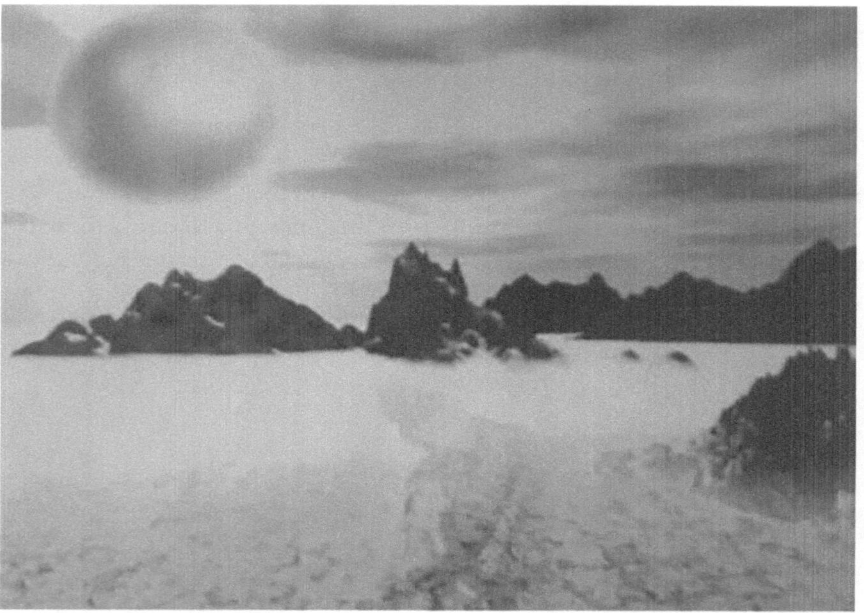

People get ready, we are about to enter into my father's house. I'm going to show you around the 66 rooms of *The Holy Bible* as I see it from a everyday life prospective and more.

It is my hope that you will revisit these wonderful rooms often and I do hope you find, a revelation and a peace of mind. Now, Without further ado, let me Introduce, the book of life to you.

The 66 Rooms of the Holy Bible!

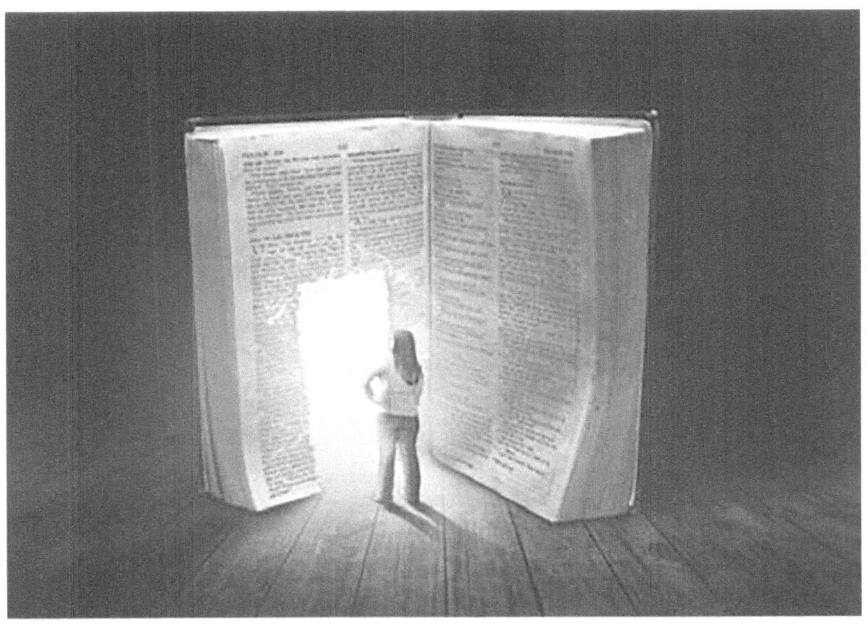

Come On, don't Be Scared, Come Inside!

Old Testament Rooms

1. *Genesis*
2. Exodus
3. Leviticus
4. Numbers
5. Deuteronomy
6. Joshua
7. Judges
8. Ruth
9. 1 Samuel
10. 2 Samuel
11. 1 Kings
12. 2 Kings
13. 1 Chronicles
14. 2 Chronicles 15. Ezra
15. Nehemiah
16. Esther
17. Job
18. Psalms
19. Proverbs
20. Ecclesiastes
21. Song of Solomon
22. Isaiah
23. Jeremiah
24. Lamentations
25. Ezekiel
26. Daniel
27. Hosea
28. Joel
29. Amos
30. Obadiah
31. Jonah
32. Micah
33. Nahum
34. Habakkuk
35. Zephaniah
36. Haggai
37. Zechariah
38. Malachi

New Testament Rooms

1. Matthew
2. Mark
3. Luke
4. John
5. Acts (of the Apostles)
6. Romans
7. 1 Corinthians
8. 2 Corinthians
9. Galatians
10. Ephesians
11. Philippians
12. Colossians
13. 1 Thessalonians
14. 2 Thessalonians 15. 1 Timothy
15. 2 Timothy
16. Titus
17. Philemon
18. Hebrews
19. James
20. 1 Peter
21. 2 Peter
22. 1 John
23. 2 John
24. 3 John
25. Jude
26. Revelation

King James Bible	Vulgate	Douay Rheims	Full title in the Authorized Version
Genesis	Genesis	Genesis	The First Book of Moses, called Genesis
Exodus	Exodus	Exodus	The Second Book of Moses, called Exodus
Leviticus	Leviticus	Leviticus	The Third Book of Moses, called Leviticus
Numbers	Numeri	Numbers	The Fourth Book of Moses, called Numbers
Deuteronomy	Deuteronomium	Deuteronomy	The Fifth Book of Moses, called Deuteronomy
Joshua	Josue	Josue	The Book of Joshua
Judges	Judices	Judges	The Book of Judges
Ruth	Ruth	Ruth	The Book of Ruth
1 Samuel	1 Samuelis also known as 1 Regum	1 Kings	The First Book of Samuel, otherwise called the First Book of the Kings
2 Samuel	2 Samuelis also known as 2 Regum	2 Kings	The Second Book of Samuel, otherwise called the Second Book of the Kings
1 Kings	3 Regum	3 Kings	The First Book of the Kings, commonly called the Third Book of the Kings
2 Kings	4 Regum	4 Kings	The Second Book of the Kings, commonly called the Fourth Book of the Kings
1 Chronicles	1 Paralipomenon	1 Paralipomenon	The First Book of the Chronicles
2 Chronicles	2 Paralipomenon	2 Paralipomenon	The Second Book of the Chronicles
Ezra	1 Esdrae	1 Esdras	Ezra
Nehemiah	Nehemiae also known as 2 Esdrae	2 Esdras	The Book of Nehemiah
Esther	Esther 1,1 – 10,3	Esther 1:1 – 10:3	The Book of Esther
Job	Job	Job	The Book of Job
Psalms	Psalmi	Psalms	The Book of Psalms
Proverbs	Proverbia	Sentences	The Proverbs
Ecclesiastes	Ecclesiastes	Ecclesiastes	Ecclesiastes, or, The Preacher
Song of Solomon	Canticum Canticorum	Canticle of Canticles	The Song of Solomon
Isaiah	Isaiae	Isaias	The Book of the Prophet Isaiah
Jeremiah	Jeremiae	Jeremias	The Book of the Prophet Jeremiah
Lamentations	Lamentationes	Lamentations	The Lamentations of Jeremiah
Ezekiel	Ezechielis	Ezechiel	The Book of the Prophet Ezekiel
Daniel	Danielis 1,1 – 3,23; 3,91 – 12,13	Daniel 1:1 – 3:23; 3:91 – 12:13	The Book of Daniel
Hosea	Osee	Osee	Hosea
Joel	Joel	Joel	Joel
Amos	Amos	Amos	Amos
Obadiah	Adiae	Adias	Obadiah
Jonah	Jonae	Jonas	Jonah
Micah	Michaeae	Michaeas	Micah
Nahum	Nahum	Nahum	Nahum
Habakkuk	Habacuc	Habacuc	Habakkuk
Zephaniah	Sophoniae	Sophonias	Zephaniah
Haggai	Aggaei	Aggaeus	Haggai
Zechariah	Zachariae	Zacharias	Zechariah
Malachi	Malachiae	Malachias	Malachi

MISS ASONDRA STARN'AIR

King James Bible	Vulgate	Douay Rheims	Full title in the Authorised Version
St. Matthew	secundum Matthaeum	Matthew	The Gospel According to St. Matthew
St. Mark	secundum Marcum	Mark	The Gospel According to St. Mark
St. Luke	secundum Lucam	Luke	The Gospel According to St. Luke
St. John	secundum Ioannem	John	The Gospel According to St. John
The Acts	Actus	Acts	The Acts of the Apostles
Romans	ad Romanos	Romans	The Epistle of Paul the Apostle to the Romans
1 Corinthians	1 ad Corinthios	1 Corinthians	The First Epistle of Paul the Apostle to the Corinthians
2 Corinthians	2 ad Corinthios	2 Corinthians	The Second Epistle of Paul the Apostle to the Corinthians
Galatians	ad Galatas	Galatians	The Epistle of Paul to the Galatians
Ephesians	ad Ephesios	Ephesians	The Epistle of Paul the Apostle to the Ephesians
Philippians	ad Philippenses	Philippians	The Epistle of Paul the Apostle to the Philippians
Colossians	ad Colossenses	Colossians	The Epistle of Paul the Apostle to the Colossians
1 Thessalonians	1 ad Thessalonicenses	1 Thessalonians	The First Epistle of Paul the Apostle to the Thessalonians
2 Thessalonians	2 ad Thessalonicenses	2 Thessalonians	The Second Epistle of Paul the Apostle to the Thessalonians
1 Timothy	1 ad Timotheum	1 Timothy	The First Epistle of Paul the Apostle to Timothy
2 Timothy	2 ad Timotheum	2 Timothy	The Second Epistle of Paul the Apostle to Timothy
Titus	ad Titum	Titus	The Epistle of Paul to Titus
Philemon	ad Philemonem	Philemon	The Epistle of Paul to Philemon
Hebrews	ad Hebraeos	Hebrews	The Epistle of Paul the Apostle to the Hebrews
James	Jacobi	James	The General Epistle of James
1 Peter	1 Petri	1 Peter	The First Epistle General of Peter
2 Peter	2 Petri	2 Peter	The Second Epistle General of Peter
1 John	1 Ioannis	1 John	The First Epistle General of John
2 John	2 Ioannis	2 John	The Second Epistle of John
3 John	3 Ioannis	3 John	The Third Epistle of John
Jude	Judae	Jude	The General Epistle of Jude
Revelation	Apocalypsis	Apocalypse	The Revelation of St. John the Divine

Come Into His Marvelous Light!

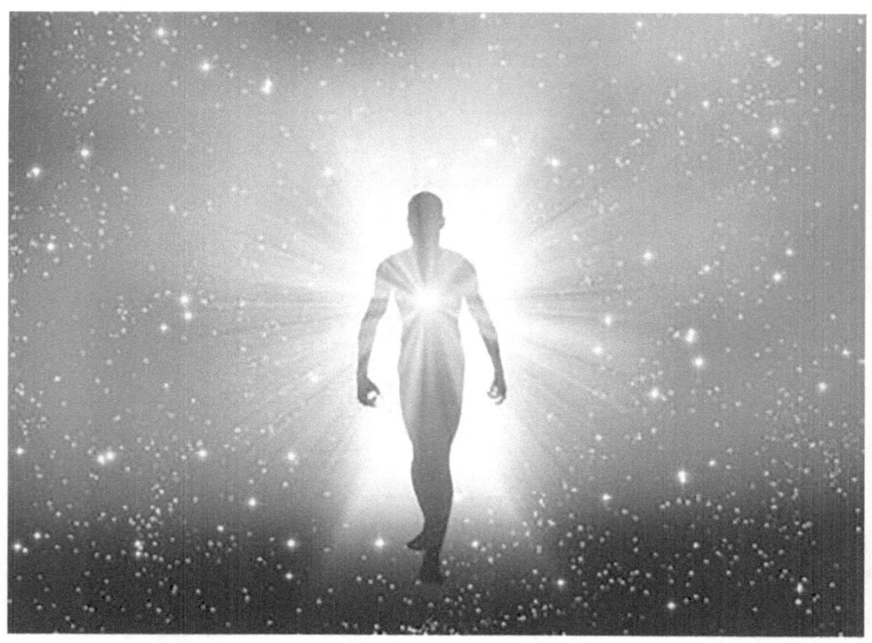

 Miss Asondra StarN'air

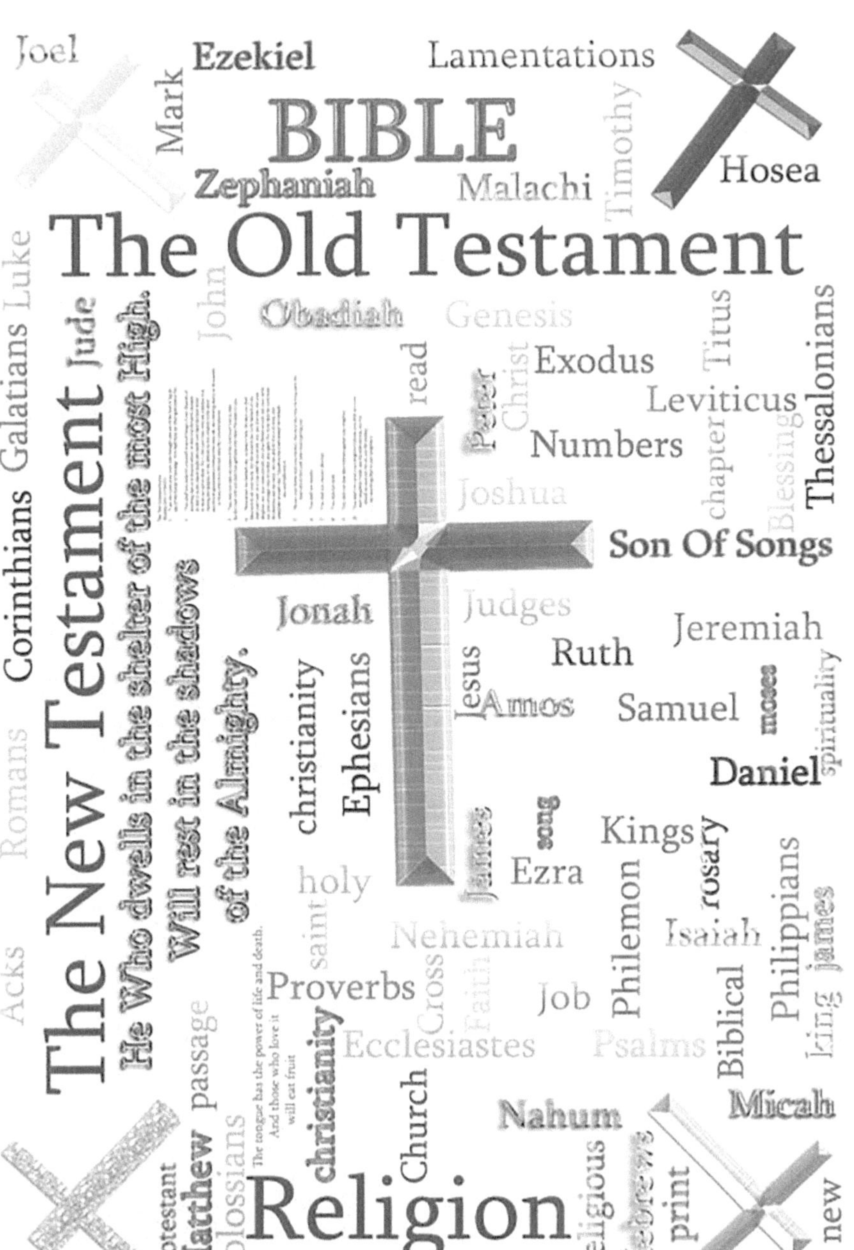
Joel
Ezekiel
Lamentations
Mark
BIBLE
Zephaniah
Malachi
Timothy
Hosea
The Old Testament
Corinthians Galatians Luke
Jude
John
Obadiah
Genesis
read
Exodus
Titus
Peter
Christ
Leviticus
chapter
Blessing
Thessalonians
Numbers
Joshua
Son Of Songs
The New Testament
He Who dwells in the shelter of the most High.
Will rest in the shadows
of the Almighty.
Jonah
Judges
Jeremiah
Romans
Ruth
moses
christianity
Jesus
Amos
Samuel
spirituality
Ephesians
Daniel
song
Kings
rosary
James
Ezra
Philemon
Isaiah
Philippians
king james
Acks
holy
saint
Nehemiah
Cross
Faith
Job
Biblical
Matthew passage
Proverbs
Job
protestant
Colossians
christianity
Ecclesiastes
Psalms
Church
Nahum
Micah
The tongue has the power of life and death.
And those who love it
will eat fruit
Religion
Religious
Hebrews
print
new

Genesis

Room One (Old Testament)

The book of Genesis is known as origin or book of beginning, how it all came to be, the entire world, you and me.

In this room, you will see that God made everything! when he did, he said it was good and on the seventh day he rested, so should we.

Also, we were all made perfect in god's own image, all of us are beautiful, black, white, alike. No one is more beautiful than the other. Every human on the plant no matter what color or creed, are all God's beautiful and perfect creation. In fact, the bible says we are all fearfully and wonderfully made, that's because we are God in the flesh he created us in his own image, how about that! And it does not stop there, He also gave us everything we would ever, need.

Genesis is a room of completion, Everything the world needs, ***"WE GOT IT!"***

Candid Snapshot

Good adores you, He is the creator of all things, He is so awesome, 'The Sun', 'The Moon' and 'The Stars' all obey Him, so must we. For He knows how to run our lives, not us. God is our real parent! He's our Mother, Father God all in one. Obey him and follow his will for your life always.

Key Verse

Now at last the heavens and earth were successfully completed, with all that they contained. So on the seventh day, having finished his task, God ceased from this work he had been doing, and God blessed the seventh day and declared it holy, because it was the day when he ceased this work of creation **2:1-3**

Key Action

If you want to know God up close and personal, then start at the beginning, read his word. Stop putting it off or make up excuses, just do it! And don't ignore it when God says the wages of sin is death, believe him. Go back and read the Adam and Eve, story, it all started with one apple from a tree. **Gen. 2:4-3:24** Fast forward to now, don't keep sinning against God and saying "It Wasn't Me".

Key Prayer

God, I have made a mess out of my life, I need help starting over, I want to get in your word and stay in it. I trust your will for my life now, please help me to surrender, for I am too weak to do it on my own. I have fell for too many lies, the devil comes in disguise. Father God, please help me find my way back home to you because I know that's where I belong. Lord where I am weak, help me to be strong.

Amen

Exodus

Room Two (Old Testament)

Let my people go! Leadership, the Ten Commandments, the tabernacle, worship, and once again, obedience. This room is no joke. In this room, a lot is going on, and God needs his people to respect leadership and move when he tells us to move. This room is about to explode in victory because God is sick and tired of his people being taken advantage of, like his caregivers for example, who are overworked, underpaid, disrespected, and still in bondage to a system that has enslaved them for far too long. God is saying in this room Exodus, "Let my people go or else."

Candid Snapshot

When God, commands us to leave a place and follow him, we must prepare to act, go.

Know that he will always be with those who trust and obey him, there is no time for **"FEAR" F**alse **E**vidence **A**ppearing **R**eal no, God is the real deal.

If we want to cross over to the over side, we must also fight if we have to, We are children of the promise. God promised our forefathers Abraham, Isaac and Jacob a land of milk and honey. Well believers, **"WE"** are the off springs of that promise, if you want it, it's yours for the taking—I Want It!

Key Verse

Then the Lord said to Moses, "Go to Pharaoh and say to him, 'this is what the LORD says: Let StarN'air, I mean my people go, so that they may worship me. **8:1**

Key Action

From now on, don't stay no place where there is abuse, not with a person or a Job, Jesus died so we all would be free and live happily. No that God will provide no matter what your circumstances are. Take action today, get out of all abusive relationships, including environments, demeaning jobs, **"Whatever."** God wants us to live well and prosperous too. In fact he sent his son, and his son Jesus said, my purpose is to give them a rich and satisfying life. **John 10:10**, so take action, don't think twice! Get out of bondage and stay out!

Key Prayer

I am a sinner in need of a savor, right now! Please God change my heart, send me a way out today, I can no longer go on this way, I need help.

Amen

Leviticus

Room Three (Old Testament)

In this room, God has provided a way for atonement (meaning the reconciliation of God and humankind by sacrificing his only begotten Son Jesus Christ) so we could live. If he had not done that, many of us would have been wiped out a long time ago (meaning death).

This room reminds us that we were bought with a price. We don't belong to ourselves anymore, never did. God has the final say in our lives, get that people.

Jesus paid it all! When I sit in this room, I can't help but cry, Jesus died for me. I don't know anyone alive who would do that for me, do you? Yet so many people still take what he did for us for granted, and just keep right on sinning against him and God, as if what happened on the cross means nothing. All I can say is there will be consequences for this kind of disrespect and disobedience I assure you. Leviticus is no room to play around with, better get your house in order or else.

Candid Snapshot

This room use to be a very bloody room, lots of killing and sacrifices were made to ward off the awfulness of sin. But not anymore, Jesus became the once and for all sacrifice for the world; yes *"HE"* became the one who died in our place. Question, how are you feeling right now? Does his dying on the cross for you, mean anything to you? Or are you still going to live your life the way you want to? I hope not, but if you are, you won't get far.

Key Action

Learn the ways of Christ, ***"Live Upright!"*** Don't blend into the world and become corrupt, sip out of Jesus cup!

Key Verse

You must sanctify yourself and become holy, because I am Jehovah your God. And keep my statues and carry them out. I am Jehovah who is sanctifying you. **20:7-8**

Key Prayer

Dear God, I have put myself in a situation I don't know how to get out of, I know I am out of the will of God, but I'm in fear of losing what I have if I try to make changes. Please help me undo this sinful lifestyle I got going on. I know this is not the way I should be living I am sorry, please forgive me. I am aware that if I continue on this way, things will not go well for me, in the will of God is where I want to be. Lord I just need a way of escape, "rescue me." I'm not working with a lot of options right now, please give me some directions. **Hear what saith the Lord:** *'Keep reading my word, says The Lord! therein lies the answer to all your problems and promises.*

     Miss Asondra StarN'air

Numbers

Room Four (Old Testament)

In here, "hard heads makes soft behinds". How many more times do we have to be whipped? How many more times does God have to tell us the way we are living is not acceptable?

This room hurts I have been in this room before because sometimes, us Christians get tempted too. In fact, the Bible says in **1 Corinthians10:13,** wrong desires that come into our life aren't anything new or different, many others have faced the same problems before, **"Me Too."**

But for some of us, we keep sinning against God over and over again, we come up with excuses like these: "I'm only human"—"It's been a long time since I . . ." or "everyone else is doing it . . ." What are some of your excuses? In this room, you will be convicted, dealt with, and some of us will keep going around the same old stupid mountain until we get it right. The Israelites took God for granted they had loyalty and discipline problems. Pretty much like what's going on today, people want to live life their way. It took the Israelites 40 hard long years to travel an 11 day journey to the promise land. But guess what, they never got there; their murmuring and complaining and disobedience to God let a good thing pass them by. They all died before they could even see the promise land. (my god, the disobedience of woman and man) However, you and I are still here, but here's the thing, have we learned from the Israelites, what to do and what not to do? I think not, how can we if you don't read the bible? God is *"The Bible"* people, and here's another thing, none of us are getting to the promise land or receiving eternal life if we are not going to live upright. That means we MUST study God's word. We MUST read the bible on regular bases. How many years will it take for "YOU" to become discipline and true to the one who created you? Don't repeat the cycle back then, the Israelites were a stubborn and rebellious people and they paid a hefty price for it too, don't let that be "YOU", **Repent!**

Remember, it is not too late until it is too late. We can all change!

You can come into this room anytime you want to and confess your sins, then ask for forgiveness, next, repent and move on to obedience and righteous living. God is merciful, patient and kind, no better heart will you ever find. God is still waiting for us to return back to our first love. Yes, the Bible says in Revelations 2:4, "Yet I hold this against you: You have forsaken the love you had at first!" But let me tell you something, choosing this world over God's leads to destruction, perhaps a curse.

Candid Snapshot

Many of us go through life on a search to find real happiness, yet very few people ever find it. True happiness can only be found in our Lord Jesus Christ.

Key Verse

Then the glory of the Lord appeared, and he Lord said to Moses, "How long will these people despise me? Will they never believe me, even after all the miracles I have done among them? **14:11**

Key Action

It is never too late to start over, God can still use you, tattoos and all Drug addiction and all, mental illness and all, broken-heartedness and all, police record and all, ex-convict and all, humanizers and all, intellects and politicians alike; you name it, God can change it! Go back to your first love, **"Christ!"**

Key Prayers

Okay, Lord I'm ready to start over, my way is not working, nor has it worked out for anyone else who did not make you Lord of their lives. I have been going around the same old stupid mountain too, only to find I'm wasting my time and yours. You have a plan for my life and I want to live long enough to enjoy it, so today I am asking for a change in direction, to the outside world I am just fine as I am, but inside I am not happy, what I have or have not accomplished is irrelevant. I have not loved or obeyed you Lord if I did, I would not be incomplete, empty. So my prayer is simply this, "Take Me Back" I am sorry I left you. I need you in my life. I am sorry I put other things before you, that's why I am still miserable, now I have come to realize there's only one way to true love and happiness and that's you Lord.

Please hear my cry Lord, I'll make you make you Lord over my life. No more me and my way, from now on, I will read and obey your word. Please accept me in your loving arms again. **Amen**

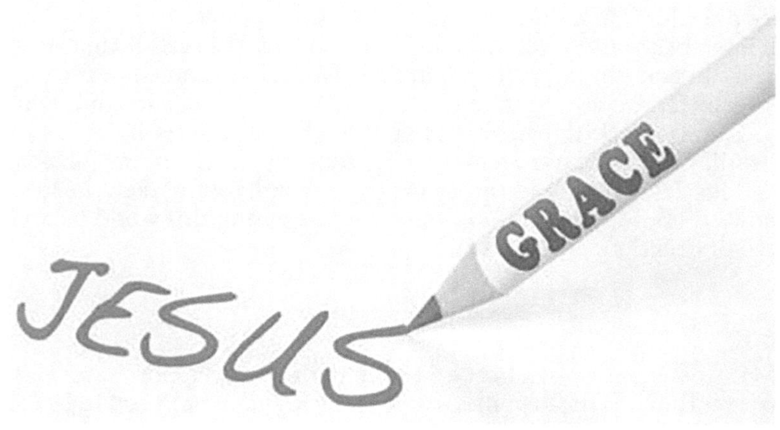

All In Place!

Deuteronomy

Room Five (Old Testament)

This room mourns the loss of a great notorious leader, his name was Moses. But now God is calling someone else to lead his people, "Joshua", we'll meet him later. In the meantime, lets fast forward to the 21 century. "Now!" Is God calling YOU? Is God calling ME? Nevertheless we'll see!

This is an interesting room because when you least expect it, God may choose to use us in ways we never dreamed of; kind of like what's happening to me now. I never in my wildest dreams thought that God would use me to write books for him, never. But he's doing it, he's using me like he's used so many others to advance His kingdom. Wonder what He has in mind for you? Whatever it is, just be loyal, faithful and true and know that God is with you.

Back to Deuteronomy, this room consist of several speeches or sermons that were given by Moses and the appointment of Joshua to replace Moses. Which means change, and a lot of times people don't like that. And it can also be a little overwhelming for the new leader. Both the people and Moses successor Joshua had to adjust. And when change happens, we must learn to welcome change.

Here are my favorite words: **In God We Trust!**

Candid Snapshot

Change is Good for us! What God did in the past *He* can do again.

Key Verse

After Moses had said all these things to the people of Israel, he told them. "I am now 120 years old! I am no longer able to lead you, for the Lord has told me that I shall not cross the Jorden River. But the Lord himself shall lead you, and will destroy the nations living there, and you shall overcome them. Joshua is your new commander, as the Lord has instructed. **31: 1-3**

Key Action

Get ready to fight for what is rightfully yours. It's there waiting to be taken for those who dare to go after it.

Dear God give me all that I need to succeed,
help me to be a godly leader.

Amen

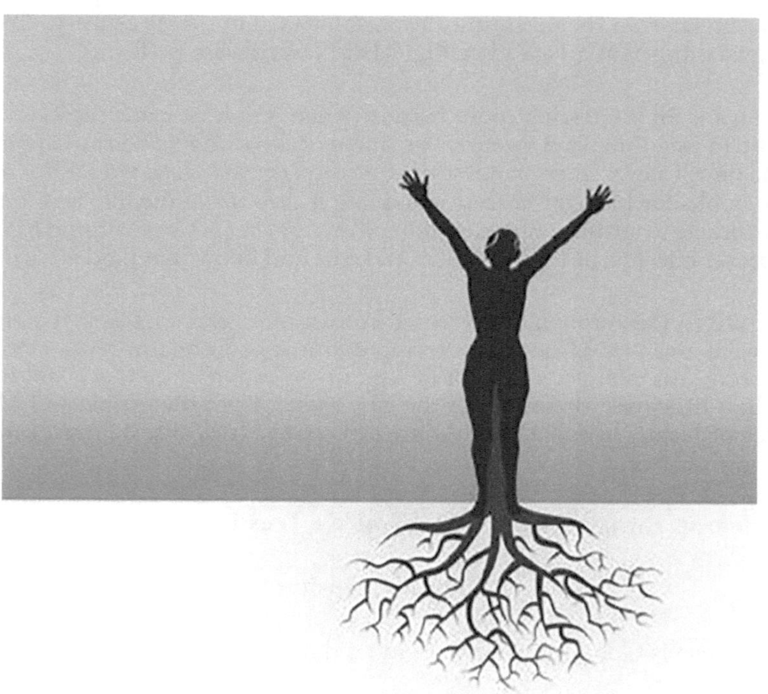

Joshua

Room Six (Old Testament)

This is one of my favorite rooms in the house! Meet Moses successor "Joshua" In here, you'll have a chance to see what good leadership looks like. God selected Joshua to finish what Moses started, which was to get his people out of bondage and then lead them to the land God had promised their forefathers—Abraham, Isaac, and Jacob. **(Gen. 50:24)** Later on, open your bibles and read all about this warrior, Joshua was a man of action, he got the job done. Personally what I love most about this room is, if we listen and do what God tell us, when he tell us, we will end up on top! We will enter that promise land he talked about. And another thing I like about this room, when I'm in here I get the satisfaction of knowing that what God has for me, no man can take away. No employers or job loss, even debt can stop the plans God has for his people.

God always blesses those who follow and trust in him. But let me say this also, this room is a room of action. God was Joshua's commander and chief and he will command us too, my advice is just do what he tells you to do. But suit up, because if you want what God has for you, you're also going to have to fight!
If you are a caregiver, your future is NOT limited, on the contrary, there is real place that is still flowing with milk and honey, God's provision will never ever end, but you can't blend, you must be his through thick and thin. I say, let the journey to the promise land begin.

Snapshot

God says seek first his kingdom and all else shall be given unto us it does not get any plainer than that! "click", (another snapshot)
Kingdom Living, God's Giving!

Key Verse

This is my command —be strong and courageous! Do not be afraid or discouraged. For the LORD your God is with you wherever you go' **1:9**

Key Action

Go get'em tiger!

Key Prayer

Lord let me know when to make my move otherwise,
I'll be still and wait, I trust you!
Amen

Judges

Room Seven (Old Testament)

Did you know that there used to be a time God used Judges as a go- betweens. His people would cry out to the Lord for help and God would send a judge to lead them back to Gods ways. It's a lot different today. The Primary focus now is on the laws, not God. What a pity! Back then the grim lesson of Judges is that the wages of sin is death. This still holds true today. Sin takes on many forms and is no respecter of persons, back then, kings were destroyed too. And here we are now thousands of years later, yet nothing's changed, people still have no fear of God. Warning, warning, when people/countries/nations do as they please, chaos and destruction are the natural result. Today our world is drowning in sin. Revelation, the world as we know it is about to end!

Candid Snapshot

"The Wages of Sin is Death!"

Stop in the name of God, before you destroy your life, think it over, hasn't God been good to you, think it over, hasn't God been true to you.

Key Verse

But when the Judges died, the people turned from doing right and behaved even worse than their ancestor had **2:19**

Key Action

Repent, repent, repent...

Key Prayer

Father forgive me for I have sinned, strengthen me so I don't do it again.

Amen

Ruth

Room Eight (Old Testament)

In this room, I find myself dealing with day-to-day life. One day, things are fine; and the next thing you know, you are faced with bad times all of a sudden. Something totally out of your control—yet it affects your entire household. Many times, this has happened to me, and I had no friend to turn to, not one.

Jesus became my rock, my fortress, and my deliverer in those difficult times. This room is a room of humility, faith and grace. Ruth is a woman of all that and more. Sometimes she reminds me of me. She's full of loyalty to those she loves through thick and thin; she's a friend to the end, **"Me Too!"** And God blessed her, she had such a good and loyal heart; many of us could learn a thing or two from Ruth, I most certainly have. But can I also share this, when I'm in this room, for some reason I get a little sad too, "why"? Because today, with all the electronic devices, texting and fake face-book friends, true old fashion friendships are becoming obsolete. People wanna tweet, and follow people they'll never ever meet. Everyone's so busy chasing after the wind. Where does real relationships begin? Nothing should be more important than spending time together. Ruth was the perfect role model of a loyal true friend. She stuck by her mother -in law through thick and thin. Hear her famous words, But Ruth replied, *"Don't ask me to leave you and turn back. Wherever you go, I will go; wherever you live, I will live. Your people will be my people, and your God will be my God.* **1:16**

How many of you wish you had a friendship with a relationship like that? I do, and I do. His name is **Jesus And** where *He* leads, I shall follow!

Lastly, I saved the best for last, Ruth, fell in love and married a fine and wealthy man named Boaz. Hey, her *Faith* and *Loyalty* paid off.

Real Women Wait On God! Real Men Follow God! Real People do God!

Candid Snapshot

"A Suddenly" happen to Ruth, God gave her a wealthy life and wonderful life mate, husband named Boaz. Therefore ladies, and men if you are looking for a Christian woman, with the wonderful qualities of Ruth, women be patient, men be patient, seek his kingdom first, and like Ruth, before you know it, "A Suddenly" can happen to you. Walk upright, practice being loyal, trustworthy and true. Be a real good friend too. Live for God, "Live Upright!" Ladies maybe we'll meet our night and shining armor tonight!

Key Verse

Then Boaz said to Ruth, "Listen carefully, my daughter. Do not go to glean in another field; furthermore, do not go on from this one, but stay here with my maids. "Let your eyes be on the field which they reap, and go after them. Indeed, I have commanded the servants not to touch you. When you are thirsty, go to the water jars and drink from what the servants draw." Then she fell on her face, bowing to the ground and said to him, "Why have I found favor in your sight that you should take notice of me, since I am a foreigner?" Boaz replied to her, "All that you have done for your mother-in-law after the death of your husband has been fully reported to me, and how you left your father and your mother and the land of your birth, and came to a people that you did not previously know. "May the LORD reward your work, and your wages be full from the LORD, the God of Israel, under whose wings you have come to seek refuge. **2:8-12**

Key Action

Women, learn the ways of an excellent woman. Men, be men of God!

Key Prayer

Teach Me Loyalty!

Amen

1 Samuel

Room Nine (Old Testament)

Humble yourself and come into this room with me. Let's talk about leadership and how we are to respect it—and if we are the ones who have been given that power, just know we have a serious job to do. Our responsibility is to God and the people we lead. First and foremost, everybody, everywhere, let's get something straight and keep it straight; leaders, boss and workers alike, we all belong to god and we also work for him too. Therefore, be careful, he knows and sees everything, he never slumbers or sleep. Be good to one another, no matter your position, be honest, fair and true and all will go well for you. In this room, you'll see men and women who have fallen from grace simply because they lost sight of who they really work for.

The world's ways of doing things are nothing like God's. So when we trade off God's way of doing things the world's way or go left when God says go right, as the old cliché would say, **"Houston We've Got a Problem!"** Don't agree with this, just look at the world at large idols, unrighteous money, sex, drugs, and rock and roll, lifestyle of the rich and famous and our lives too the way we live, all of it sisters and brothers comes with a price.

Samuel was a religious leader, called by God to warn individuals of their folly, and he was given inside information from God of things to come, like who was going to rise and who was going to fall. In other words, if you are not doing the will of God, no matter who you are and what you possess, you shall be dealt with. Samuel tried to warn them and some were just plain old stubborn and hardheaded, won't listen to the warnings, they got ambushed, destroyed.

Well, I'm here to tell you, God will not be mocked, he means what he says, and he says what he means. *"Jesus is Lord!"* He's Lord over everything, this world and man; better listen while there's still a chance. Keep on ignoring all the warning if you want to; inside the bars, high, drunk, lewd dance. "Twenty-first century" life technology advanced. Hurry, warning, warning, "flashing robot", no more Donna Summers, no more "Last Dance!" Like her and others **"Escape"**, run as fast as you can. Be done with sinning against God, don't lose your soul for man.

Candid Snapshot

The wages of sin is still death, although Jesus died for us, he gave his life up hoping we would leave this world and follow him. It's not too late to turn around but one day it will be.

Key Verse

Ordinary sins receives heavy punishment, but how much more this sin of yours, which have been committed against the Lord. **2:25**

Key Action

Make That Change!

False Leaders, People, Ministers, Christians alike and you know who you are, *'NOTHING'* is hidden from God, everything shall be brought to light, therefore "Get Right!"

Key Prayer

Jesus, I am in trouble, I'm living a lie. I have not been authentic in my ways or my dealing with others. But you already know this, Lord I repent and ask for forgiveness. Holy one, hear my cries, Father God, I need to be washed clean by the blood of Jesus. Please help me for I have fallen back into sin. Please remove all stumbling blocks so I can begin again. Oh Lord, come and help set me back on a righteous path. In Jesus name

Amen

2 Samuel

Room Ten (Old Testament)

When it comes to sin, we are all guilty! This room reminds me of this all the time. That's why I am constantly in the Word. Reading the Bible helps to keep Christians from reverting back to sin; but sometimes the temptations can be so strong and overwhelming that Christians fall too. I did! But when I felt the condonation from the holy spirit, I quickly got rid of my sin, repented and continued my discipleship with the Lord.

Everyday each an ever human being fall short, this is why we must stay in the word daily. Otherwise, sure enough, Satan's back in, tempting us to sin against God again. We mustn't do that! Staying faithful and true to God and his word it's an everyday battle. That's why it's so very, very important that we stay in the word and too meditate on it day and night. Come on, dance with me on this, otherwise, the rhythm of sin is gonna to get cha, it's gonna to get cha! And sisters and brothers if you don't believe me, it may get cha "Tonight!" **Don't Do It, Live Right!**

Snapshot,

Realized people, that anyone and everyone can fall prey to sin, Moses did, King David did, and we all know His son 'King Solomon' most certainly did, and many, many more, from that era. In fact Jesus was the only one in god's creation who never, ever sinned. The rest of us are lucky to be alive. But thanks be to our God and his son Jesus Christ, if it had not been for him dying on the cross for the atonement of our sins, god only knows what shape, we'd be all in.

Nevertheless, we must do our due diligence and stay disciplined in his word and refrain from actively sinning against God. Each time we *"Choose"* to sin, we are saying to Jesus and the Father, "what you both did for us means nothing to us, we are still gonna to do what we wanna do". But I assure you, there will be consequences for that; If you don't thinks that's true, just look around the world today, people are dropping dead like flies, "better recognize", God will never bow down to sin. Get right with God, or the end!

Key Verse

O Israel, your pride and joy lies dead upon the hills;
Mighty heroes have fallen **1:19**

Key Action

When it comes to sin, never say never, "The spirit is indeed willing but the flesh is weak" **Matt. 26:41**, So stay in his word seven days a week and please stay humble and meek!

Key Prayer

Lord, father God, don't let sin sweep me away, strengthen me to obey. In Jesus name I pray,

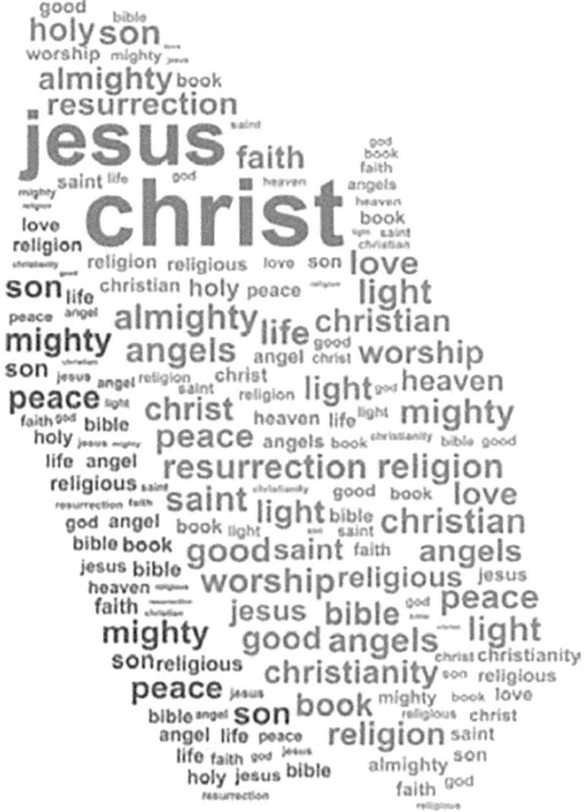

Amen

1 Kings

Room Eleven (Old Testament)

This room records history, the past and the present. Listen, if you don't know your history, you are doomed to repeat it. 1st Kings shows that God speaks to us from the past as well as from the present experience of others.

The bible is full of life lessons, there was a time when kings rules over the land, hence the name of the book. These events are recorded so that we will not make the same mistakes. In hear you'll get a sneak preview of how success can turn into a mess. It is true folks, that if God is not the builder of your life, it shall come tumbling down at some point.

Ps.127:1 Money, career, degrees, nor fame can save you, only **"Christ"** therefore, don't gamble with your life! Personal message: Hear, hear, "Fornicators", women, get ah husband, Men get ah wife. Come out of the world, ***"Live Upright!"***

Candid Snapshot

The higher you climb without Christ, the harder you fall!
Bugs Bunny, "That's All Folk!"

Key Verse

I am going where every man must go someday go. I am counting on you to be a strong and worthy successor. Obey the laws of God and follow his ways; **2:2-3**

Key Action

People, people, people, stop wanting more and more and more! At some point be satisfied, the more stuff you have, the more problems you have. And remember, bigger is not always better, get you mind together. Learn to be thankful for what you got! Like me, if you got Jesus, **"YOU"** got a lot!

Key Prayer

Lord help me to be happy without always wanting more. Let me be wonderfully satisfied with all the blessing you have bestowed upon me and my family. Show and teach me what real success is, not as the world says but, your definition of success. I come to the realization that if I am not pleasing you God, no matter what I acquire in life, I'm a failure not a success.

Give me the mind of Christ, give me your excellence, I don't want the world's stress, because I know with you guiding me, I will always be blessed!

Amen

2 Kings

Room Twelve (Old Testament)

This room is pretty much like the one you and I just came out of. We are still dealing with those of power, kings, good and bad. War, peace, prosperity and ruin is the theme of this room (for the record, *"Jesus is coming back soon!"*) Here God is getting fed up with all the disrespect, he's getting tired of all the chaos, individuals making up their own rules, doing what they want to do, "not cool"! So here he sends in prophets to preach his word and warn of the judgment to come, sort of like what I am doing with this book, yes, I'm also being used by God. **"World Out, Christ In"** is the message I send. Turn back to God's way of living; if we don't, trouble will come knocking at our doors too.

Many of you are already getting a wake-up call as we speak, life is not going well for you. Why, because some of you refuse to listen to biblical and sound advice. For example, to the young people out there, Honor your parents so that your days will be long. **Exod.20:12** Warnings to the Adults who refuse to grow up, **"Sinful Living"** fills your cup! *So it is no longer I who do it but the sin living in me* **Rom.7:17**

"Wake up Everybody!"

Today the love of sin is destroying family and homes. People are robbing and killing each other. Hatred, idolatry and every other kind of evil has made this world a dangerous place to live in and all become of **"Voluntary Sin"**. Be done with that kind of destructible life. **"World Out, Jesus In"** Conquer this world, denounce Sin. Live for Christ and **"Win!"**

Candid Snapshot

Compromising God's standards will result in moral and physical collapse. Obedience is the only sure path to God's blessing. No one living for Christ will be abandoned, God helps his people. Those living for the world, you are not his people, you belong to this world and all that comes with it. You will not be given eternal life unless you give this world up. I was once lost but now I'm found, and let me tell you, the best part of waking up is Jesus in your cup!

Key Verse

The Lord afflicted the king with leprosy until he died, and he lived in a separate house **15:5**

Key Action

Repent, come from among them, the world cares nothing about you in the end. Jesus is the only friend you got!

Lord, right now I am ready to give my life to you, how do I do that? What shall I say? How will I know you have received me? And where do I go from here?

Where do go **StarN'air speaks:** Let me help you sister or brother, first repent and then say these words: Christ Jesus, I come to you with all my heart and soul take me Lord, I no longer want my life, I give it to you. I don't have all the answers but you do, from this moment on I trust you. Take my life and never give it back to me. Make me a slave of yours for life. You are my Lord, and master, my savior. You're also my one and only true friend, I'm at the door knocking, please let me in.

Amen

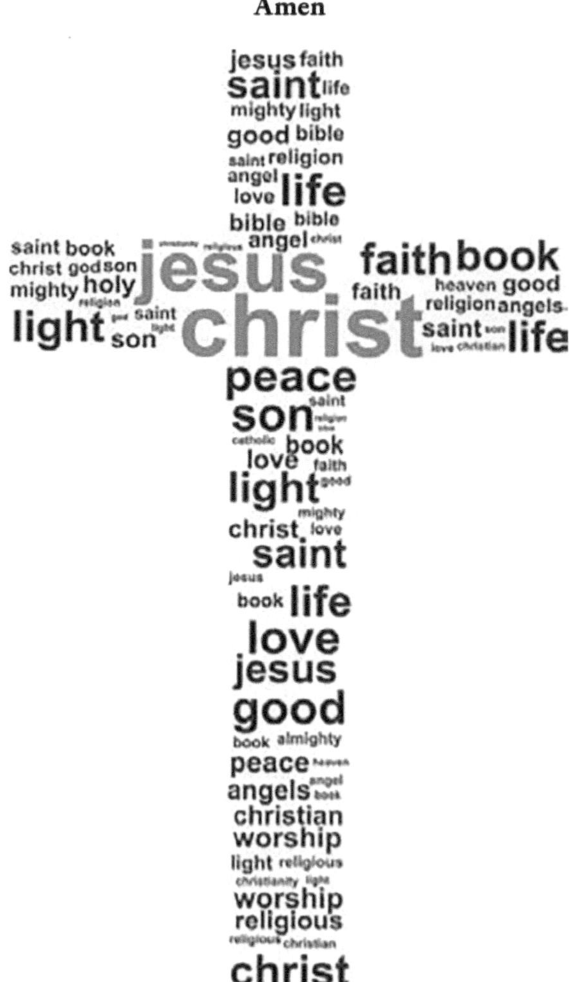

1 Chronicles

Room Thirteen (Old Testament)

When you come into this room, take off your shoes, bow down, and worship and praise him, for he is worthy to be praised. Many times this is held off until Sunday-morning church service, "what a shame"! Why aren't we making our homes the church as well? When was the last time you worshiped and adored him there? Think about that one.

Chronicles is a series of genealogies that records the family history of David the king, and the tribe of priest called the Levities. Very powerful and interesting room, intellects will be stimulated and entertained, to say the least. This room also points out the importance of worshiping God. History shows that God blesses those nations that trust in him, we once did that.

But, today "We" as a nation, ought to be ashamed we've taken God out of everything; we no longer worship or praise his holy name. And yes, we are the ones to blame.

History has shown again and again that a nation suffers when it doesn't include God in its decision-making. The United States, although the wealthiest and most powerful country in the world, is now in trouble. And if it does not repent and look to God for mercy and help like our forefathers did, we are headed for destruction.

Look, I'm just an ordinary person, a nobody to the world. A single woman answering a call, that's all; but even I can see something is terribly wrong, turn around. In 1 chronicles it is clear to see that God blesses a nation/individuals that trust him, Furthermore, those that have gone to their grave unknown by others are remembered by God. Therefore, never think your good deeds or your righteousness/ faithfulness will go unrewarded. Stay devoted and meek.

"7 days Without Christ Makes 'One' Weak!"

Snapshot

Praise him for he is worthy to be praise
Worship and adore him always, don't leave home without him.

Key Verse

Every part of the blue print, David told Solomon "was given to me in writing from the Lord. Then he continued, Be strong and courageous and get to work. Don't be frighten by the size of the task, for the Lord my God is with you; he will not forsake you. he will see to it that everything is finish correctly. **28:19-20**

Key Prayer

Mother, Father, God, I praise your holy name, there is an alter of love and gratitude inside my heart for you, each day I await your arrival, I pray that you are pleased with how I am living down here. Lord stay near, keep me safe and from harm, don't let anything happen to me, lift me up with your right arm. Instruct me on how you want things done, through you, victory's won!

Amen

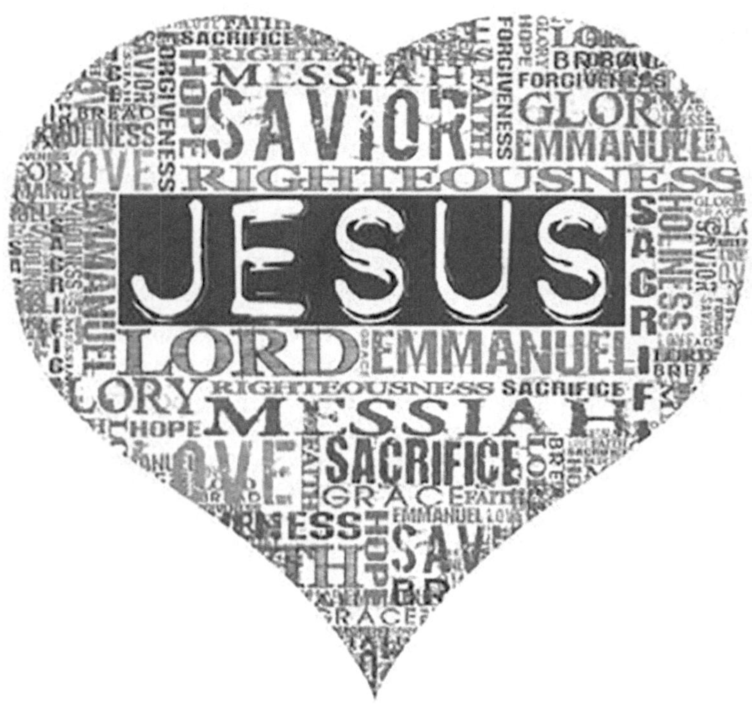

2 Chronicles

Room Fourteen (Old Testament)

Hello, let's keep touring, were in 2 chronicles in here the history of Judah is recorded, it deals with the glory of Solomon reign. And how righteous kings are commended and the evil kings are named, exposed so that all can see who is responsible for the rise and fall of nations. On your own time go read all about it. Lots of lessons to be learn, "God will not tolerate sin."

Right now I want to remind everyone how sin not only destroys nations but us personally as well. How we live our lives matter! On a personal note, it matters to God who we are sleeping with, sex outside of marriage is wrong and a heartbreak waiting to happen for many. Call this my sermon, or call it a rap song: It matters to God what we do for a living, "taking" but never giving. Porn, nudity, entertainment, lewd videos, soap opera sex filled TV, thank god that wasn't me. Men on the prow, shouting more, more, more, strippers stripping, picking money up off the floor. Now here comes another drug dealer walking through the door. Meanwhile young men turn young boys into thugs. Oh and let's not forget the dirty politicians who hide their dealing and the truth under the rug. God will not tolerate sin, The End! *"We Don't Belong to Ourselves, We Were Bought With A Price" How We Live Matters to God!* **Rom.14:7-9**

This is a record keeping room, God keeps a record of all those who are living sinfully, A "Ain't Nobody's Business If I Do" record. (Where are they now? They're gone!) Therefore you are not fooling anyone but yourself, if you think God's not listening or watching you, "Everybody", you're wrong! If you think he doesn't know what goes on in your household, think again. He checks in on everything, what we watch on television when no one's around, where we go on the Internet, how we treat people and our coworkers, how we spend our time and money, where the money came from, tithes paid or not paid—God knows all about us and about secret affairs too. "Yes sire", and of course he knows about me and do hope he likes what he sees. All in all, he knows whose, who, whose real, whose fake. More than that, God knows every little step we make! **"Repent"**, get it together everybody before it's too late!

Snapshot

You can be sure, your sin will find you out!
What's done in the dark will surly come to light!

Key Verse

"Go to the Temple and plead with the Lord for me" the king told them. "Pray for all the remnant of Israel and Judah! For this scroll says that the reason the Lord's great anger has been poured out upon us is that our ancestors have not obeyed these laws that are written here. **34:21**

Key Action

"Repent, Repent!"

Key Prayer

Dear Lord, I am sorry for not honoring you, but I know now sorry is not going to get things right with you, I must change my ways, I must do something to show you how sorry I really am, like start reading my bible every day. Also get away from all bad influences, and give up my bad habits too. This is "true repentance", taking action for my messed up behavior. And too, I must find a way to work well with all co-workers and love my neighbors. Lord I know this is the kind of sorry you are looking for, a real change in "ME' one that everyone can see, kind of sorry. The kind of sorry, that comes out of the world and gives oneself to Christ kind of sorry. Otherwise, I'm wasting my life and time, any other kind of sorry is pitiful and real sorry. So right now, I surrender to "Change", Lord make me over, in Jesus name

Amen

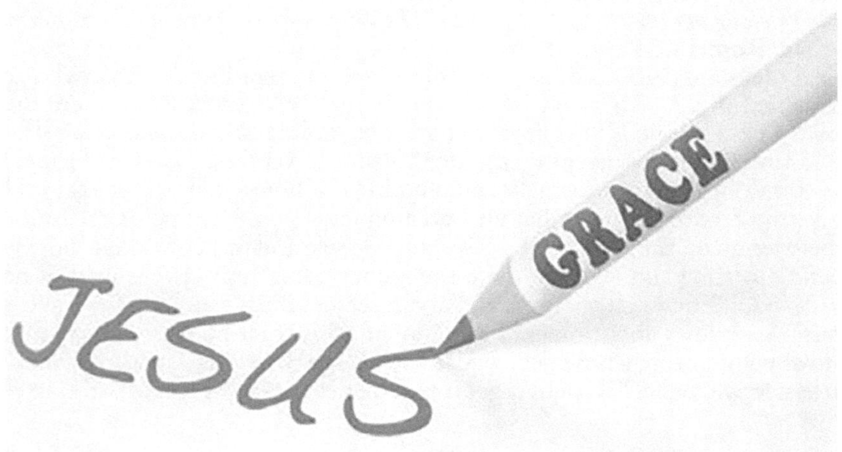

***Ask him to erase your past
and give you a future that last!***

Ezra

Room Fifteen (Old Testament)

Meet Ezra both a priest and a scribe, here he is calling all of god's people to return back to total obedience to God's Word.

And now *A Caregiver's Bible To Excellence'* is suggesting we do the same thing; lack of obedience has consequences, "we don't want to mess with God". So to help us all stay focus and out of trouble, this room speaks for itself

Get a bible
Open up his word,
Do his word
is with **"YOU!"**

Each one of us must honor and respect God's ways of doing things. **"Be Obedience, Show Some Respect"** it as simple as that!

Snapshot

Here's the thing, look, we're all going to make mistakes—pastors, ministers, leaders, all of us—and God already knows that, Yet he still expects us to listen to him, correct those errors, and move on, there's still much work to be done. God has a job for each and every one of us, collectively and individually. And it's up to that person to stay in God's Word and listen out for the call; if we say we love and belong to him, that shouldn't be hard at all.

Key Verse

All of the people gave a great shout of praise to the Lord, because the foundation of the house was laid. **3:11**

Key Action

Get going
Obey his orders
Do the work of the lord
Is with **"YOU!"**

Key Prayer

'Our Father in heaven, hallowed be your name. Your kingdom come, your will be done, on earth as it is in heaven. Give us this day our daily bread, and forgive us our debts, as we forgive our debtors. And lead us not into temptation, but deliver us from evil. For thine is the kingdom, the power and the glory, for ever and ever.

Amen

Nehemiah

Room Sixteen (Old Testament)

Come on in, grab a cup of tea, and sit with me. I have a question for you, can you remember a time when God got you out of a bad situation and if he hadn't you'd be messed up today? Just sit back and think about that for a while and, later on, journal it. **"God is Good!"** How many times have we forgotten how God has been there for us when we really didn't deserve it? That's the reason why I asked that first question. Right now please allow me to introduce you to Nehemiah. Nehemiah was another one of God's prophets. He had a lot of them throughout the Bible as you can see. Long story short, God wanted Nehemiah to oversee the rebuilding of Jerusalem's wall. Also the problem brought to Nehemiah's attention and God's concern was that people are slow to learn the lessons God wants to teach. God's got his people out of bondage because of sin and the very same problem arose again. Hum, does that **"Sounds Familiar!"**

His people stopped worshipping and praying, neglected God's Word, and started hating on one another. My that **"Sound Familiar!"** And sure enough, they were back in bondage.

People, this is what I know for sure—if you do not discipline yourself to make time for God every day, Satan will make you his before you know it. You will be under the influence of the evil one. It doesn't matter whether you are saved and born again, the flesh is weak, it is "Not"your friend; one must stay in the Word as if your life depends on it and it does, it really does.

Personally, this *Caregiver's Bible To Excellence* is kind of like a safe haven to help caregivers all over the world, be safe and thrive. Everything God has asked me to include in this book, guess what? I need it too! Oh, I cannot wait to have the physical book in my hands, when I get it, I'll be doing the happy dance!

But first, "Everybody" let me make it crystal clear, nothing—and I mean nothing—should ever take the place of *'The Holy Bible'*, "Nothing!" No, no, no, *'A Caregiver's Bible To Excellence'* is a friend of God and a door/window to Christ, not to me. I'm just a vessel and messenger, **"Without Christ, You Ruin Your Own Life!"** We're done in here, finish your tea and think about that too tonight!

Candid Snapshot

Satan will do just about anything to keep our faith in Jesus from growing, lure you, tell you, you only live once go for it, tell you too, the bible is man - made, not true; and that times have changed. Along with all those lies, Satan the devil and his human followers, (they all know who they are) will all try to convince you or tell you that what was back then don't apply to us today and so forth, but that's not true, like Jesus, don't go for that, the scriptures don't lie. Satan is the liar, the truth is not in him. He wants you weak so he can use you to do his dirty work, lie, cheat, and hurt others for him. All awhile wreaking your life in the process. He's up to no good and he knows it, but he wants to stay hidden, behind the scene. Once you start reading your bible,"game over", Satan

　　　　MISS ASONDRA STARN'AIR

will now longer be in power; he will not be able to tear your life down anymore. But for some of you, and I'm disappointed to have to say this but, you love this world, you're friends with it, you answer to no one, not even God. Well then, I'm not talking to you, I'm talking to those who want to grow and mature in Christ. If that is you, then listen, there is a wall of protection you *Must* get under, reading this book and the bible on a regular bases is that wall of protection. This wall is guarded with love, truth and prosperity, it's not looking for popularity! Just those who really want what Christ is offering, a better life, and eternal life.

Key Verse

So the wall was completed on the twenty-fifth of Elul, in fifty–two days. when all of our enemies heard about this, all the surrounding nations were afraid and lost their self–confidence, because they realized that this work had been done with the help of our God. **6:15-16**

Key Action

Build A Great Life In Christ!

Key Prayer

You called me Lord, and I shall not be afraid, I will do as you asked

I will go back to school, I will open up that business I've been putting off, I will ask my lover to leave my home if we can't get married, I will stop having sex outside of marriage, I will look to you for all my needs and not manipulate others for it, I will read my bible every day, I will get right with you God, I will. Lord I need your wall of protection more than ever, I want to live a life that's pleasing to you. Make me your servant, teach me to be loyal and true. **Amen**

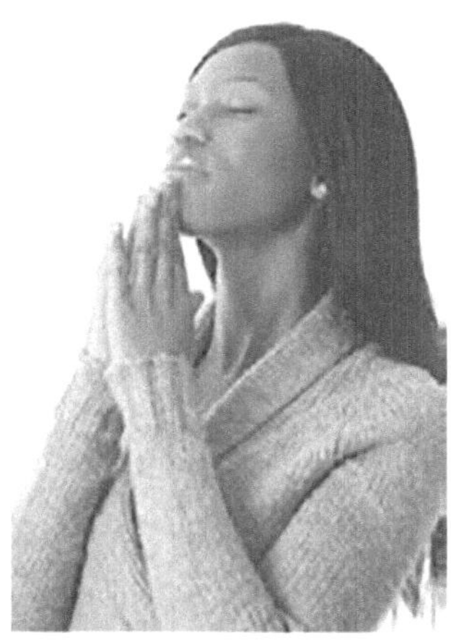

Esther

Room Seventeen (Old Testament)

Welcome everyone, this room is indeed fit for a queen, Esther even sounds like a queen's name too don't you think? Esther was a young Jewish woman who became part of the Persian king Xerxes' harem and eventually became his queen. But there was a problem, Esther cousin insulted and evil official, he would not bow down to him and because of this, he sought out to destroy her people, the Jews. But this queen tactfully intervened and saved her people. ***"If I Perish, I Perish!"***

In life we never know when we'll be called to save the day. It is important to note that God used human being all the time to accomplish his purpose rather than doing it directly himself. Therefore, we must be ready at all times to do what God directs, regardless of our situation. ***"If I Perish, I Perish!"***

Candid Snapshot

There is something God wants you to do, and only you can do it, no one else can. And too, there may be times God will not ask us to do something until the very last minute as was the case with queen Esther. Bottom line, God calls, "Take Action!" Go Out and Be the Change the World Need to See "Your Majesty!"

Key Verse

So the king and Haman went to dine with Queen Esther, and as they were drinking wine, on the second day the king again asked 'Queen Esther, what is your petition? It will be given you. What is your request? even up to half the kingdom,' it will be granted." Then Queen Esther answered, " if I have found favor with you O king, an if it pleases your majesty, grant me my life —this is my petition. And spare my people- this is my request. **7:1-3**

Key Action

Go!
Obey!
Deliver!
Is with **"YOU!"**

Key Prayer

Dear God, help me to put things in proper prospective and realize, all I have been blessed with, I will do everything in my power to make this world a better place. And I will do it through *'Your'* peace, love and grace. Father God, on bended knee, I bow down to thee. Oh holy one let *Your* will be done "use me", **If I Perish, I Perish "Happily!"**

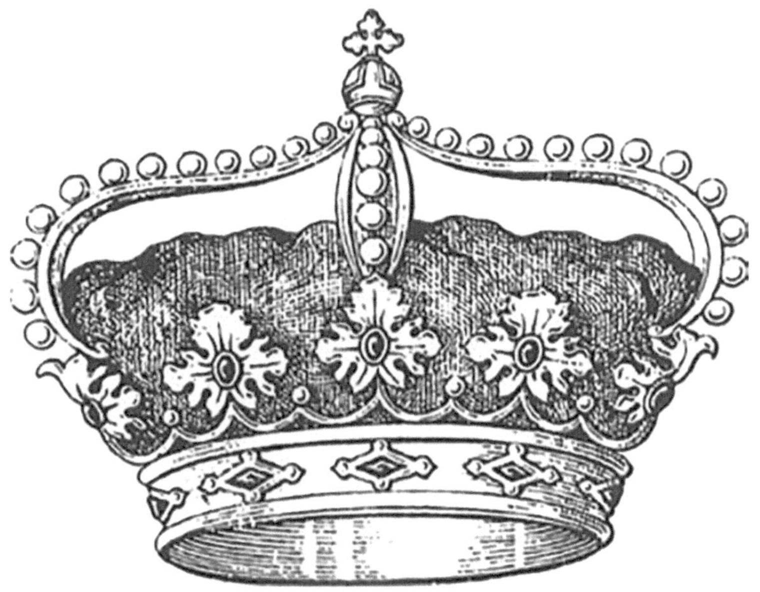

Job

Room Eighteen (Old Testament)

Hello, come in, time to meet **Job!** Job was a righteous man who endured great suffering with remarkable *"Perseverance!"* No matter what, Job would not turn against God. But, here's what disturbing and also interesting about this room we're in, it was God himself, who allowed Job to be tortured by Satan. (paraphrasing) 'Have your way with him, but don't kill him'. (my thoughts, sometimes torturing is worst. How would you feel if someone set out to ruin your life on purpose?) But, in spite of all the destruction, **Job loved and trusted God.** (he got through this and so *Must* we.) The reality is, those who serve Christ wholeheartedly like Job did are enemies to the gods of this world. Today these corrupted and fallen angels are still at it, now they have someone else in mind. And I'm afraid it's "ME", **I just Got Jobbed!** And if that's not a word, it is now!

My Story, God's Glory!

Satan: What about Miss StarN'air? "She's always thrived, you've always protected and looked out for this one. She doesn't know hard times. She's always bought and gotten whatever she ever wanted. And She;s been sheltered and protected from the storms of life. She don't know how to endure hard times. God's kept her in a fairytale world, his world. Hey, I wonder what she would do if there was no *YOU* to come to?

Oh My, I've been Jobbed!

Satan's First List of Attacks

- Workplace
- Severe Persecution "everywhere"
- The family.

Satan's Second List of Attacks

- The Home
- Luxuries
- Fellowship, place of worship
- The Mind
- Friends and social relations
- Calling, and Projects

"Wait" He's not done yet!"

Satan's Third list of Attacks

- The body
- Visitors, "Angels of light!"
- Fear
- Financial ruin, "Poverty"
- Hopelessness & Loneliness

Satan: "Where's Your God Now"?

StarN'air: Here *He* is "Inside Of Me", for *He* never left me, we're both laughing! For no weapons formed against the people of god' shall ever prosper; Games over, "flea", Satan you and your followers shall never get my love for **God** out of me! "Get outta here", go away "Flea!"

In conclusion, although I went through hell, like "Job", **I Survived, I'm Still Standing, Plus, "wiser than ever!"** Unfortunately, Christian **"WE"** get singled out because we don't belong to this world and never will, so don't be surprised if **"YOU"** get **"Jobbed"** too! Nevertheless, take heed, here's what you do? say **"Boo"**, Flea Satan, I'm not wasting a thought on you! My God will replace and restore everything I lost and more. **Next** kick him out your life, and shut the door! Ooh wee, I'm lovin' this tour!

Candid Snapshot

Wait for the salvations of the Lord!

Key Verse

The Lord said to Satan, where have you come from? Satan answered the Lord, "from roaming through the earth back and forth in it. Then the Lord said to Satan have you considered my servant Job? **1:7**

Key Action

If you are who you say you are in Christ get ready to be tested.

Key Prayer

Lord, Please let me be all you thought I was and more

Amen!

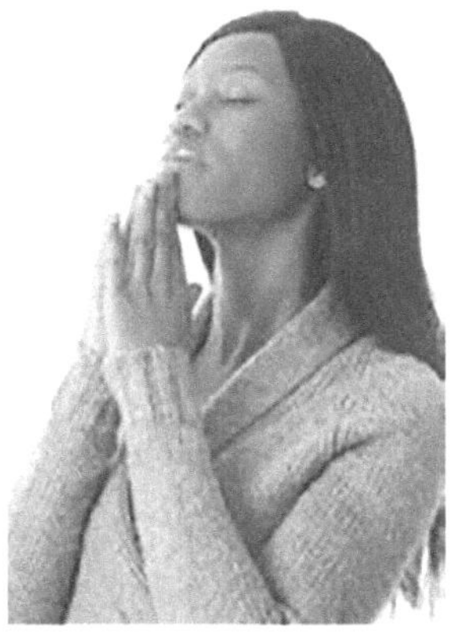

Psalms

Room Nineteen (Old Testament)

For me, Palms is a room of instruments, and comfort for the weary souls. The book of Psalms all in all contains ancient hymns and prayers which were used in their worship to the **LORD!**

Psalms is a beautiful, calm and peaceful room for Christian to relax and meditate in. While in there, you'll find comfort plus a friend. And even more amazing, music's blazing! "Ah" Psalms is many things in one, it's "String Instruments" "Music" and the healing has begun. Psalms is also Prayer for those who need to connect more deeply with God. Oh how refreshing it is to know we have some- where to go. And for all those experiencing a loss, or dealing with pain and sorrow, hang in there, embrace God, there's always tomorrow. Now may God keep you at peace and in his loving arms. *"Welcome To Psalms!"*

Candid Snapshot

Psalms gives voice to the cries of our heart, when words fail us Psalms helps express our deepest emotions. There are times life can be so overwhelming and yet exciting too; Psalms is there for you! If you are lonely, hurting or think no one really care for you, Psalms says "I do" let's talk about it. Psalms wants to wrap its arms around you, if you let it, "let it!" Let his holy spirit penetrate your mind, body and soul. Live for Christ now, you're never too young and you're never too old.

Key Verse

Bless is the man who does not walk in the counsel of the wicked
Or stand in the way of sinners, or in the seat of mockers. But his delight is in the law of the Lord, and on his law he meditates day and night, He is like a tree planted by streams of water, which yields it's fruit in season and whose leaf does not wither whatever he does prosper. **1:1-3**

Key Action

World Out, Christ In!
This Is Where My Psalms Begins!

Key Prayer

Psalmist cries out, Father God, hear my cries, restore my life, no more waterfalls dry my eyes. King of kings, Lord of lords, free me of worries and despair. *Oh, Holy One, Oh Holy Night,* pull up a chair; life thunders more than I can bear. But I know the scriptures and I know them well, they don't lie, I know you'll be there; "I'll wait" please answer my prayer. **Amen**

Proverbs

Room Twenty (Old Testament)

They say an Apple a day keeps the doctor away. I say A Proverb a day keeps drama away! This room in my 'Father's House 'has 31 Proverbs—one for each day of the month. It seems God wanted to arm us with these truths for a reason—so we would be armed and ready to defeat anything that might come our way.

Most of the book of Proverbs is closely linked to Solomon, he was known as the wises man to ever live. This room, speaks of the importance of righteous living and how wise it would be to follow the ways of Christ rather than the seductive path of folly. Like vitamins, I say, we ought to read a Proverb a day, it's sure to keep mentally fit and stop us from going astray.

Candid Snapshot

Get wisdom at any cost, only a fool thinks it's worthless!

Key Verse

The way of a fool is right in his own eye,
but a wise man listens to advice **12:15**

Key Action

Don't Listen to Fools, Listen to God, Read his Word
If you don't have your own bible, get one, don't delay.

Key Prayer

Lord, I surrender, lead me all the way!

Amen

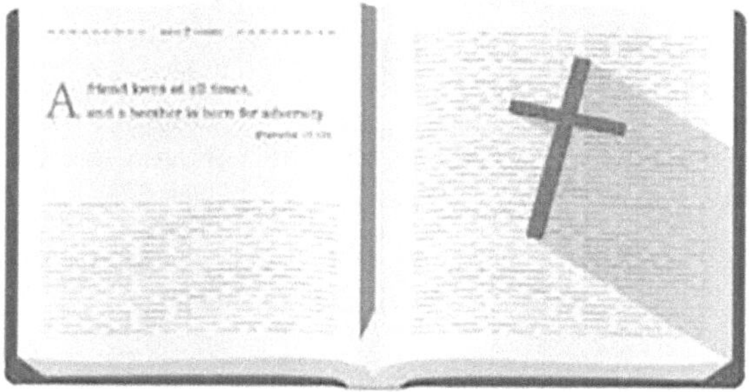

Ecclesiastes

Room Twenty-One (Old Testament)

This room are for those who have been there and done that, and are now at peace with what they got! The core message, **"Everything is Meaningless!"** **"Reverently Trust and Obey God." Enjoy Your Life as Much as You Can!**

Testimony: "Here is something you did not know about me. I had dreams of becoming a recording artist, and I spent many years preparing, I invested a large percentage of my income toward studio time, demos, wardrobe, portfolios, and photo shoots, I was all in, I became a backup singer for a local band. We opened up for Michael Bolton at the Front Row Theater—now torn down, but at one time, it was home to famous stars. Anybody who was anybody performed there. A few years later, I got a chance to spend time with the late great ,vocalist, Miss Phyllis Hyman in her dressing room. Along with that, I took some college courses on tour management, and read as many books as I could find on the music business, I guess one could say, like my hometown team "The Cavaliers" I was indeed "All-IN"!

But God was not, apparently He saw something I couldn't see, To this day I know he protected me. I still sing, but serving him means more to me than anything. Today I rarely wrestle about my life, most of my thoughts are on Christ; he's the one I live for, he moves me, and he plans my days. I trust his will for my life all the way! Hope others too can get to this place someday.

The book of Ecclesiastes is the book of man "under the sun" reasoning about life. Ecclesiastes also reflects those experiences of Solomon, he was a king that had it all, yet found himself empty inside and depressed too. All in all, he found **"Everything Is Meaningless!"**

Warning readers, the mood of this room is generally one of sadness, a lot is going on in here, evil, oppression, grief and mourning, yet it rises to the fear of the Lord, and how we must Reverently trust and obey him. I do believe once we do that, we will find true happiness, Solomon didn't, but I did, and so can **YOU!**

Snapshot

Life is not a puzzle to be solved, God has already put the pieces together, he knows what our destiny looks like, we don't, because we are so busy doing life our own way. But when we do that, there's a price to pay.

Key Verse

Fools are put in many high positions. while the rich occupy the low ones. I have seen slaves on horseback, while princes go on foot like slaves. **10:6-7**

(Simplified, Jesus was just a carpenter's son, she's just an aide.)

Key Action

Live For Christ, Not For Thyself!

Key Prayers

Life is meaningless without you God, I thank God I have finally come to this revelation. Money, Cars, Material Things, Diamonds Or be it Fame, all the same thing **"JUNK"** if I don't have you **LORD**, I praise your holy name.

Amen

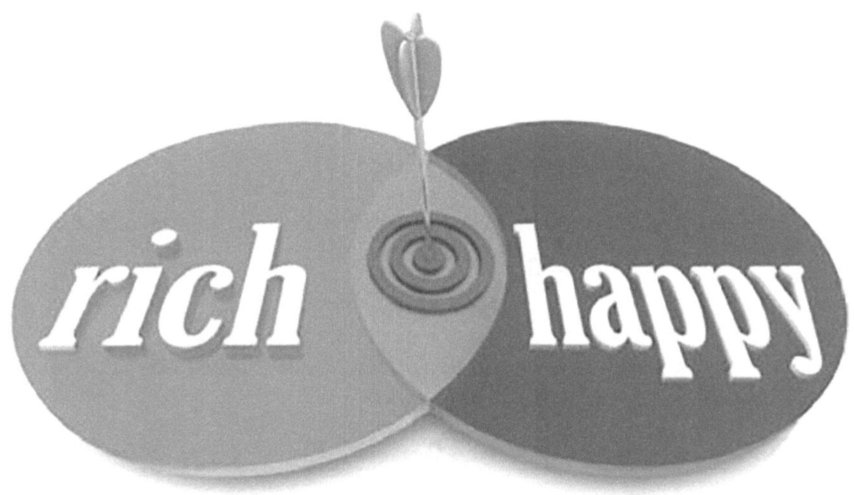

"Stay Centered and Focus On Christ!"

Song of Songs

Room Twenty-Two (Old Testament)

In this room, well, it's kind of private— a love story between a husband and a wife, male and female.

Some Bible scholars and let me assure you, I am not a bible scholar, but I do see the connection—say that the Song of Songs is also about God's love for Israel and the church. Both are his treasured bride.

Stay with me on this ride...

Never, In all my bible reading and studying, do I recall God supporting girlfriend and boyfriend sexual relationships, ever; and I don't believe he ever will. (I am so glad I don't live that kind of life anymore.)

It's ok to date, but it is not ok to have sex outside of marriage. Put a ring on it!

Too, marriage is between a male and female only. The world we live in today is full of 'baloney'! In this room **"Songs of Songs"** God married Adam and Eve, not Adam and Steve.

Snapshot

Nothing more wonderful then seeing a man and woman be joined in holy matrimony, that's the Snapshot, "click" no other photo will do!

Key Verse

Where has your lover gone, most beautiful of women, which way did your lover turn, that we may look for him with you. **6:1**

Key Action

Don't let the world turn you on to a different way, broken hearts do mend. Keep doing life God's way, you'll love again!

Key Prayer

Lord somehow I have gotten caught up in a world that makes up its own rules and for years I went for it, but now I am worst off than ever before, I'm am experiencing all kinds of demonic thoughts and can't seem to get focus or stable about who I really am, I'm a mess, I have ruined my reputation, and I'm hooked on social media too; I have posted all kinds of things that I shouldn't have. Today I am lost and ashamed of my life. I have disappointed those who love me the most, especially my parents, my mom and dad.

Lord I am in need of help, I am too weak to put my life back together, please send someone to help me and direct me to a bible teaching church home, don't let me die this way. I want to live again, but this time your way. Today I surrender my life to you, father God I trust and know that help is on the way. Thank you for hearing my cries. Amen

 MISS ASONDRA STARN'AIR

Isaiah

Room Twenty-three (Old Testament)

Isaiah is his name, and instead of me, he wants to speak, so listen,
Isaiah 55:1-3 *"Is anyone thirsty? Come and drink—even if you have no money! Come take your choice of wine or milk—it's all free! Why spend your money on food that does not give you strength? Why pay for food that does you no good? Listen to me, and you will eat what is good. You will enjoy the finest food. "Come to me with your ears wide open. Listen, and you will find life. I will make an everlasting covenant with you. I will give you all the unfailing love I promised to David.* (David was a man after God's own heart.)

If you want to know what that promise is, then stay in this room and find out. For God is a rewarder of those who earnestly seek him. Are you seeking him?

I do hope you are, you made it this far. This room you are in right now, is a room of **Rescue and Restoration**, no time to play games or go on vacation. Either we are with God or we're not! There is much work to be done in this room. God is not getting the respect due him and he's getting pissed off again. When will we ever learn? Isaiah sees the visions and tries to warn people, but like many of us, we ain't tryin to hear it, we won't listen. Therefore, some of us will move on and some will be destroyed or left behind. I don't care what others says, the bible is not lying. God is not a God that he would lie. 'Now' I'm warning you, I see the visions too, I see our world falling apart. "Get right with God" people, let's do what his word tells us to do! If you are friends with this evil and corrupt world, then yes, I'm talking to **"YOU!"**

Candid Snapshot

Isaiah was a prophet, what are you? Are you being used by God or by this world? Woe to those who call evil good and good evil, who put darkness for light and light for darkness, who put bitter for sweet and sweet for bitter. **5:20**

Key Verse

Woe to those who are wise in their own eyes" Woe to those who are heroes at drinking wine and champion at mixing drinks, **5:21-22**

Key Action

Make it a priority to read God's word every day, strive to be a positive God fearing good person, let Jesus show you how. Give Christ a chance to show you what he can do for those who love, trust and obey him. You have everything to win and nothing to lose.

Key Prayer

Dear God, give me the strength to walk away from it all.
Help me get my life on the ball!

Amen!

Jeremiah

Room Twenty-Four (Old Testament)

Come in, have a seat. Let me introduce you to Jeremiah's prayer first, ready, read:

> I know, Lord that a person's life is not his own. No one is able to plan his own course. So correct me. Lord, but please be gentle. Do not correct me in anger, for I would die. **Jer. 10:23** "Me Too!"

I have been at that place in my life too. It's a place of total surrender. At some point in one's life, there comes a time where you realize that the life you are living isn't working anymore, you are getting nowhere. *'Inside'* you're miserable and there's an empty void there too. If that is you, that use to be "Me Too". Family life couldn't help, material things and success, didn't help either. At the end of the day, I was lost of words to say, the void was still there, and that void turn out to be Jesus. Ever since I gave my life fully to him, I've been "Free" life trials and tribulations don't get the best of me.

Jeremiah was a prophet (a person who speaks god's truths to others) he pleaded with the people to change, "Turn From Your Sins, Turn From Your Sins" but was ridiculed and persecuted for it. I'm not Jeremiah, I'm Miss Asondra StarN'air but I know there's a chance this may happen to me once this book comes out. But this is what's meant by pick up your cross and follow me.

In this room, you'll find persecution, disobedience, slaughter, God' wrath, and what can happen to people and a nation who reject God.

Trust me, you don't ever want to be on God's bad side. Jeremiah tried over and over again to warn the people but, like today, people still don't want to listen. They didn't listen back then and there not listening now, today our world is tumbling down, nothing but crime all around. **"A World Without Christ Is Doomed"!** See you in the next room.

Candid Snapshot

Warning, warning get right with God before it's too late. Stop living for this dark and evil world.

Long ago you broke off your yoke "and tore off your bonds; you said, I will not serve you! Indeed, on every hill and under every spreading tree you lay down as prostitutes. **2:20**

Key Action

Get Right With God!

Key Prayer

Lord, help me find my way back home.

Amen

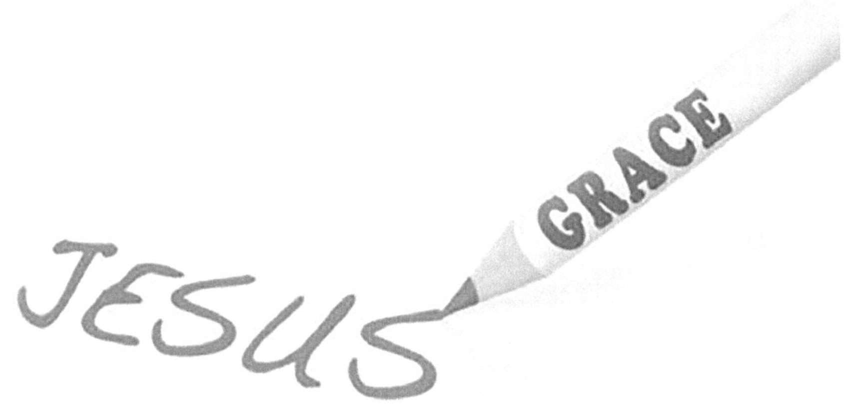

Abounds

Lamentations

Room Twenty-five (Old Testament)

The Best way I can describe this room here is, **"Something is about to go down"**! God is tired of talking and he's getting ready to show, he means business. He's not a toy to be played with, he's pissed of now!

The book of Lamentation is a funeral song and was written for the devastation city of Jerusalem. In here you will experience God's anger and find out too, why he's so angry.

Take heed people, "listen", don't ever think our sins will go unpunished. Right now God is being patient with us; but there's a breaking point as you are about to see in the book of limitations. As for our time and generation, be advises, *The I did it "My Way"* kind of thinking and lifestyle is ah lie. Where are they now? Many of them died way before their time. Better read the scriptures and read between the lines. I'll break it down for you, The wages of "On Going" and "Deliberate" sin means "death, "the end!" And no one's exempt, the rich will be humbled too. So many of them think that their wealth and popularity makes them untouchable, however the bible says this, When the day comes, everyone who is proud will be put down. Only the LORD will be honored. **Isa 2:17**

To The Rich and Famous

You say, "'I am rich" I have everything I want. I don't need a thing!' And you don't realize that you are wretched and miserable and poor and blind and naked. **Rev. 3:17**

Unfortunately, tragedy struck God's people in lamentation, Jeremiah cried and cried, he tried to save them but it was too late.

Candid Snapshot

Rethink your life, Choose Christ!

Key Verse

The LORD has done what He purposed; He has accomplished His word Which He commanded from days of old. He has thrown down without sparing, And He has caused the enemy to rejoice over you; He has exalted the might of your adversaries. **2:17** (meaning, you want this world, you got it!)

Key Action

Give This World Up!

Key Prayer

Jesus come into to my heart and set me free, I don't want to go to hell or live in misery, Jesus please come set me free!

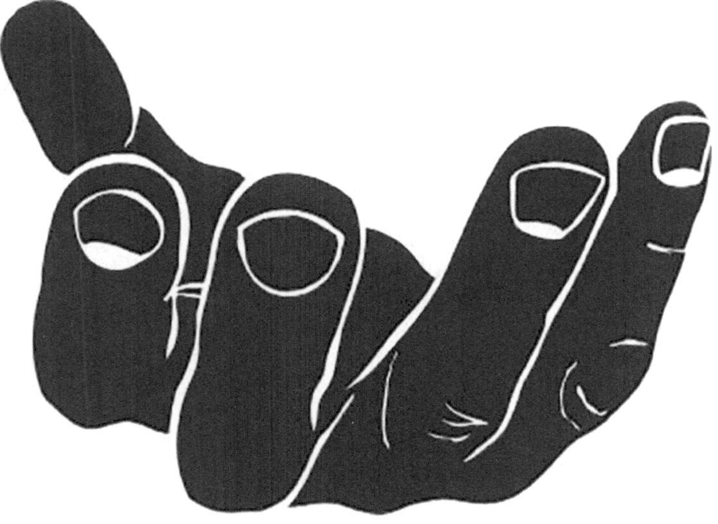

I'm Here, Take My Hand!

Ezekiel

Room Twenty-Six (Old Testament)

In this room, we have a chance to clean up our act, Ezekiel's thoughts exactly! Ezekiel grew up as a priest, he's been one of God's Shepard since childhood. He also had visions.

He saw God and heaven opening up right before his eyes. More than that, he saw what looked like humans beings but instead of one face they had 'four faces' and two pair of wings.

Just go back in time with me, I know this all sounds spooky, but I say, time to bow down, praise and sing. Seems to me, were getting ready to see *Jesus Christ,* The Almighty King!

Wow, what ah vision, okay, people back to Ezekiel, *" it's time to clean"*

Ezekiel, talks about a lot of things like restoration for God's people, and how God himself will find his sheep.

This is a very well laid out room, it's filled with lots of topics and is sure to educate you as well as shake you up a bit. We all need that sometimes. But not only that, in here you'll find peace in knowing that God finds and restore his people. So if you are a real Christian, and living upright, then you have absolutely nothing to worry about, you'll be more than alright, *"Sleep Tight!"*

Candid Snapshot

A Watchman Warns and Encourages!

Stop fooling around, get serious about becoming a real Christian why don't cha'! You ain't fooling anyone but yourself, that person you are laying with or living with, is not your spouse, *'Clean House'!* This is not acceptable to the Lord. This is, God wants us to be obedient to him and his word, he will reward us too, I encourage you to live for Christ, be holy, pursue the things of God.

Key Verse

Again, when a righteous man/person turns from his righteousness and does evil, and I put a stumbling block before him, he will die for his sin. The righteous things he did will not be remembered, and I will hold you accountable (believers, you and me) for his blood. But if you do warn the righteous man not to sin and he does not sin, he will surely live because he took warning and you would have saved yourself. **3: 20-21**

Key Action

Take inventory of your life then ask yourself these two questions, am I living right? Is this acceptable in God's sight? if not, then fight, kick Satan and the world out tonight! Don't let this world corrupt you and take your blessing away, if you are too weak and need help, call on the name of Jesus, kneel down and pray—don't allow the devil to have its way. Use wisdom, read your bibles "Everyday!"

Key Prayer

Thank you Lord for your forgiveness, I kindly ask you to forgive me for how I have lived. And to forgive me of my constant failures to think and act according to your word. *I will do better!* Today I repent from all my sins, and each day I will try again to live the kind of life you would be proud of. With all my love, I welcome change. In Jesus name,

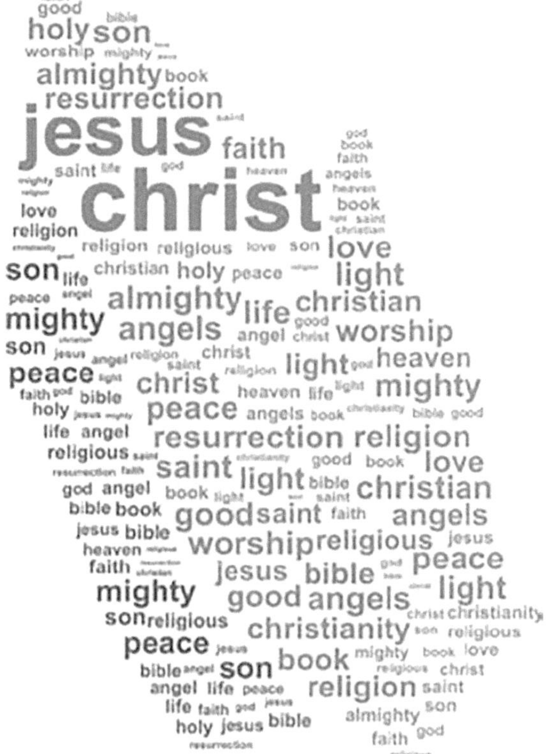

Amen

Daniel

Room Twenty-seven (Old Testament)

We'll call this room the **"Lion's Den!"** And It's a room I know all too well. For too many years now I have dealt with so much hatred and prosecution. But I'm used to it now, and too, I know why it's happening and so does Daniel. We both have the light of Christ in us. We shall not be moved or ruled over by man. So we end up **"Lion's Den!"**

I'm Still Standing!

This room is for all the survivors out there, the ones who are standing their ground, until Jesus comes back around. We shall not be moved.

More about Daniel, Daniel was a prisoner, he was capture as a boy and taken to Babylon. While there Daniel received an education and rose to a high position in the Babylonian and Persian government. But because of his loyalty and trust in God he experienced extreme persecution and at one point, thrown to the lions.

Loving and Living for God, "Cost"!

Not to change the subject, but for all you food lovers out there, Daniel was sticked in other areas too, like food. He wasn't down with high calorie meals or junk food. "No Siree", he cared also about what he put into his body. "I'm just sayin'! The scripture said *"Daniel made up his mind not to defile himself by eating the food and wine given to them by the king. Instead he asked for permission to eat other things.* **1:8**

After we're done with the tour, some of you heavy eaters might want to go back and find out why he wanted something different and what he ate, I get the strong impression, **"This Man Looked Great!"**

Long story, "short", young Daniel obviously grew into a man of God, and he stood his ground, no matter what the cost. Oh and before I forget, he was also very gifted, he had visions of the coming messiah and could interpret dreams too. He was simply an amazing young man, and a great role model for other men. You know the saying, "they don't make um like they use too!" If that's not true, okay prove it, "Live for Christ'! No more hanging out in the streets or shooting dice.

Snapshot
"Click" **CBL**

Faithfulness **C**ost!
God's The **B**oss!
The Lion **L**oss!

Key Verse

All the people of the earth are regarded as nothing. He does as he pleases" with the powers of heaven and the people of the earth. No one can hold back his hand or say to him: what have you done?" **4:35**

Key Action

Straighten up and fly right, straighten up for God and be right
Cool down everybody don't you blow your top!
Ain't no use in actively sinning, ain't no use in grinning
You better straighten up and fly right!
Straighten up for God, and be right!

Key Prayers

Lord, you rescued me, when I was in the lion's den, it seemed I had no friends, but that lion! No one but you Lord has the power to transform a lion a into a gentle lamb. "I Survived, Here I Am!"

Amen

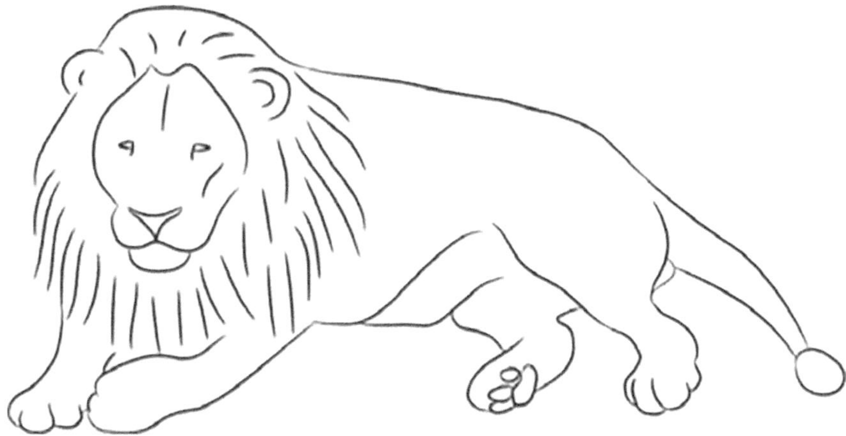

In that day the wolf and the lamb will live together; the leopard will lie down with the baby goat. The calf and the yearling will be safe with the lion, and a little child will lead them all. **Isa.11:6**

Hosea

Room Twenty-eight (Old Testament)

Room of betrayal! Hosea was a prophet, his story is a painful tail of love and unfaithfulness. If you are also dealing with something of that nature, this is the room for you. Come back in here later, perhaps after the tour; God and you can have a meeting of the minds. But, humble yourself and leave your anger behind. "Sometimes life makes us blind"!

In conjunction with all that, "Huston We Got a Problem", several problems too. "Unfaithfulness to God abounds! Today our homes are broken down and suffering greatly from not only infidelity, but identification. People are confused about the Godly order of things shall we say, if fornication and shacking up wasn't bad enough, now we have an even bigger problem. Same sex marriage has become the "American Way"! Is this right or wrong? What does scripture has to say, here's what saith the Lord:

But at the beginning of creation God 'made them male and female.' 'For this reason a man will leave his father and mother and be united to his wife, and the two will become one flesh.' So they are no longer two, but one flesh. Therefore what God has joined together, let no one separate. **"Mark.6:9"**

Do not have sexual relations with a man as one does with a woman; that is detestable **Lev. 18:22**

Lastly, *Or do you not know that wrongdoers will not inherit the kingdom of God? Do not be deceived: Neither the sexually immoral nor idolaters nor adulterers nor men who have sex with men nor thieves nor the greedy nor drunkards nor slanderers nor swindlers will inherit the kingdom of God.* **1 Cor. 6:9-10**

What is the world coming to? My heart is broken, a part of me will always mourn the loss of the natural order of things. Planet Earth is putting its own self under a curse. We seem to be getting further and further away from God. The Jesus inside of me is weeping aloud. I'm sure many of you who are real Christian can relate.

But God is still on the throne, he will be the one to judge what is right and what is dead wrong. Nevertheless, I say to all humans, hurry find your way back home!

Candid Snapshot

In loving pursuit of the unfaithful! Though God will discipline his people for disobedience, in this room he is paralleling Israel unfaithfulness to God, and I am doing the same here, paralleling our world today to the same unfaithfulness Israel had, nothing's changed. We are still hardheaded as ever. But just like back then, God is patient and his compassion for us never ceases, but still, come on, we can't keep acting as though we're not responsible for our behavior, just because we have a savior. That's a worldly man made lie. We are responsible and we will be held accountable too. In fact, Jesus, uses the "Apostle Paul" to warns everybody, "tell the world this": For the wages of sin is death; but the gift of God is eternal life through Jesus Christ our Lord. **Rom. 6:23** So you see, "The Wages of Sin is *"STILL"* Death!" Open your ears, are you deaf? God is not to be mocked or taken for granted, God wishes no one to perish, but we will if we do not get back to the natural order of things which includes, accepting his son Jesus Christ, "The Almighty King"!

Key Verse

The Lord said to me, go show your love to your wife again though she is loved by another and is an adulteress. Love her as the Lord loves the Israelites, though they turned to other gods and loved the sacred raisin cakes. **3:1**

Key Action

Cheaters stop cheating!
Go home to your spouse,
Rebuild your life in Christ,
Make it a 'Christian' house!

Key Prayer

Lord help me to forgive and love again.

Amen

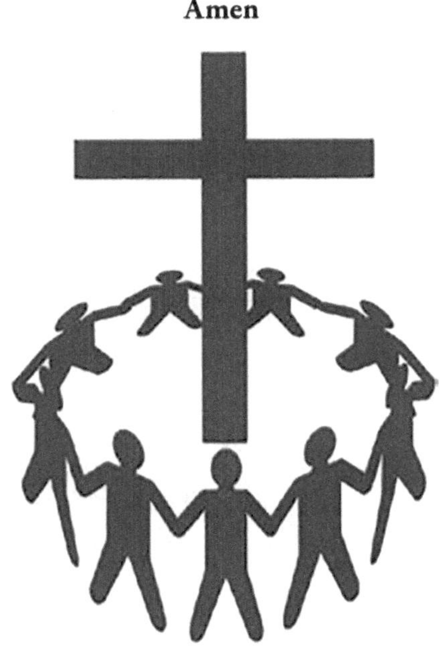

Joel

Room Twenty-nine (Old Testament)

Hello come in, come meet Joel, another prophet, Joel is out calling for repentance, with pretty much the same message and warnings, as all the others. He also sees the outcome of sinful living, "me too". Like I already said, we just can't do what we want to do! Joel joins the crew, he warns the people and the nation that if they don't 'Repent' they will suffer greatly, and food will disappear right before their eyes. And too, if they don't listen to his warnings, when destruction comes, (don't act surprised) they're going down. However, if they do straighten up and fly right, straighten up and be right, then God will bring restoration to his people, there will be blessing all around. (I jazzed the words here up a bit, but that was the core message, that was it.)

Same holds true for today, *"Turn Around"*, *"Repent" Get with Christ! Keep Your **"Feet"** Planted on Solid Ground!*

I'll say this again, if I can change, you can change, everybody can change! I was not always living right, I had my issues too, but I've changed, now every day I make it a priority to live for Christ, and for me that means reading my bible on a regular bases.

I want to encourage "Everybody, Everywhere" that wants a new life in Christ to: **G**et the Bible, **O**pen the Bible, **D**o the Bible! **God** is with **YOU!** Be the change the world needs to see, walk with thee...

Candid Snapshot

A change of heart is calling out to you and me, a beautiful life with Christ the devil doesn't want us to see. Instead it says, me, me, me, come on there's no such thing as A Jesus Christ, that's just "make believe!" But Jesus already told us the devil is a liar, a thief. He's out to kill and destroy, plus rob you of your destiny. All I can say now, is let those who have eyes finally see! I pray repentance dies with me.

Key Verse

"Even now," declares the Lord, *"return to me with all your heart, with fasting and weeping and mourning.* **2:12**

Key Action

"Change" If I Can Change, 'You' Can Change, *"Everybody Can Change!"*

Key Prayer

Lord forgive us, for we have sin against you. In repentance, I reframe from ungodly living, I will fast for seven days, restore me.
In Jesus name ***Amen***

  Miss Asondra StarN'air

Amos

Room Thirty (Old Testament)

Welcome to the Amos room, Amos was a prophet too, as you can see God had a lot of prophets didn't he, yes he did.

All these prophets were the voice of God, crying out, shouting out, "Obey and Honor Me!!!" Well here is this room Amos is dealing with disobedience, (Israelites are at it again.) just like all the rest of god's prophets and apostles; and why, the bible says *"People are in Love with their Sin!"* **Jn.3:19**

Well today, nothings change, "Sin Is In, The Devil Wins!" But, only for a little while longer, Jesus is coming back again and the world as we know it *'Will End'.*

The take home message is this, because God is holy and good, he expects the same from his people. And like the Israelites, (his people), Gentiles too (anyone who is not Jewish) Must put into practice righteous and clean living, or suffer the consequences as well.

Candid Snapshot

How we live matters to God, if we say we love him, let's all prove it by the way we live and carry ourselves. The Bible does say, you will know them by their fruit, but life has taught me something else too, "Never be impressed by a nice car or a sharp suit" **Matt.7:16**

Key Verse

Israel's Guilt and Punishment
(Ours too, if we keep on sinning against God.)

Hear this word that the Lord has spoken against you, O people of Israel, against the whole family that I brought up out of the land of Egypt: "You only have I known of all the families of the earth; therefore I will punish you for all your iniquities. (Sinful Lifestyles, Wicked Hearts.) **3:2**

Key Action

Stay devoted to God, don't let the enemy take what God is trying to give you, fight to stay alive in Christ! Even if that means you have to tell some "Good-Bye!"

Key Prayer

Dear God, please help open my eyes, this book is beginning to make me think, something is happening to me, I'm feeling conviction in my heart, I've been sinning, not living right, can you save me from myself too? I am in dire need of a savior, I am a believer, but I have not acted or lived like one, I want to come clean, I have behave badly, my home life is a mess because of how

I'm living, but I'm getting tired. Health wise, I don't feel as good as I should. Perhaps because I haven't been doing good. Well that's all about to change, today I'm asking for guidance and help in Jesus name.

Lord, please come in and be Lord over my entire life, because the way I am living, I can see it's not right, this is all wrong, give me wisdom, make me strong!

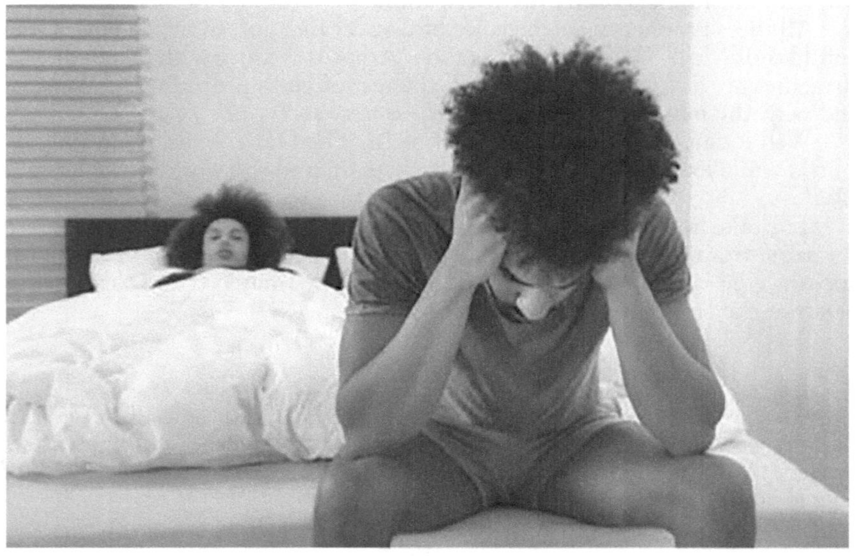

Sex outside of marriage is **WRONG!** If I'm going to do this, this person needs to be my wife. So I'll pass, **"Not Tonight!"**

In Jesus name, "help me to live right."
Amen

Break Time

So far, we have been in Old Testament rooms, which are my favorite books of the entire Bible by the way. I don't really know why except to say there's just something about traditional foundations, and the fact that God is running things, we have not yet met Jesus or have we? In these old testament rooms, we have learned that God is the one who lays down the law, not man. But often he uses a person to be his voice "his massager" and oracle if you will. I really believe he's using me right now and I hope he's using you too. Oh, and I do hope that everyone who is with us are having a great time on this tour and that you are learning a lot too. And it would be so awesome and amazing too, if some got saved along the way. I don't know how you feel, but it's a wonderful day!

Your host, Miss Asondra StarN'air

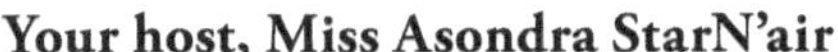

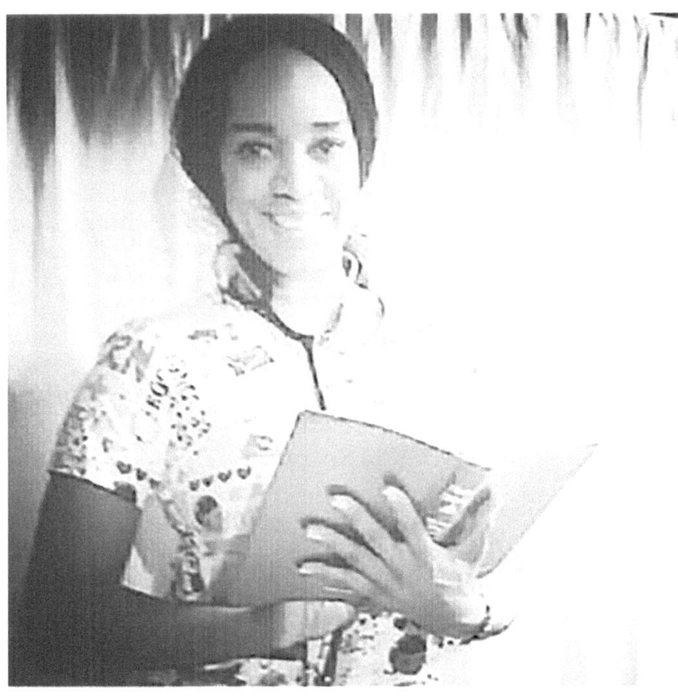

Use the bathroom, get yourself some more refreshments and meet me back here in thirty minutes, our next room on the tour is **Obadiah**, see you in there!

Obadiah

Room Thirty-one (Old Testament)

Welcome back, theme here, prides goes before destruction.

Obadiah was a prophet! Here he waste no time beating around the bush, 'You proud and deceitful nation you're going straight to hell' because you refuse to listen or obey God. Your treachery and pride is going to cost you. Obadiah was referring to the destruction of 'Edom'. (an ancient kingdom in Transjordan)

Obadiah unlike some others prophets we met on our tour, did not give hope or words of encouragement to these people, no, not at all, he made it crystal clear that the proud is going to be dealt with severely; no ifs, and, or buts about it.

Exactly what is pride, some may asked, put simply, a person who thinks they don't need God. For example, someone who believes that their hard work/education /inheritance or whatever the case may be, got them where they are at, they made it happen, not God. God is not a part of the equation, nor is he exalted. And to add salt to injury, Proud people do what they want, when they want, and to whomever they want! Let's call that kind of existence and behavior exactly what it is, "Supremacy" and that has *'PRIDE'* written all over it! Now we've all heard of 'White Supremacy' right, forget that, times are changing. Today I see Supremacy and Pride everywhere. The fact of the matter is this, supremacy or pride has no color anymore, I wonder if it ever did. Remember, blacks were kings and queens, we ran things. Today, some well to do blacks are just as bad and prejudice whites, it all boils down to that heart. For the bible says A heart full of pride, God, hates and He will not continue to tolerate. Everyone will be humbled one day. In fact, God says pride goes before destruction. **Prov.16:5** In this room Obadiah is dealing with a nation, but I'm dealing with the human heart. "Change" is the order for both, the nation and the heart. And again, Jesus is the perfect place to start!

Candid Snapshot

"Pride' God hates Pride, Enough is Enough!
"Change" Enough is Enough, that's enough!

Key Verse

The pride of your heart have deceived you, you live in the clefts of rocks and make your home on the heights, you who say to yourself, who can bring me down to the ground?
Though you soar like the eagle and make your nest among stars
From there I will bring you down, declares the Lord. **1:3-4**

Key Action

Gimme the Mic, pardon me Miss Ross, stop in the name of God, before you break his heart, think I over, hasn't God been good to you, think it over, hasn't God been true to you, then Stop in the name of God, before you break his heart. Besides, 'Pride' is an awful way to leave your mark; *'Think it Over'!*

Key Prayer

Father God, give me the courage to stop living for myself and the world, provide for me a way of escape, "Pride" I know you despise and hate.

Amen

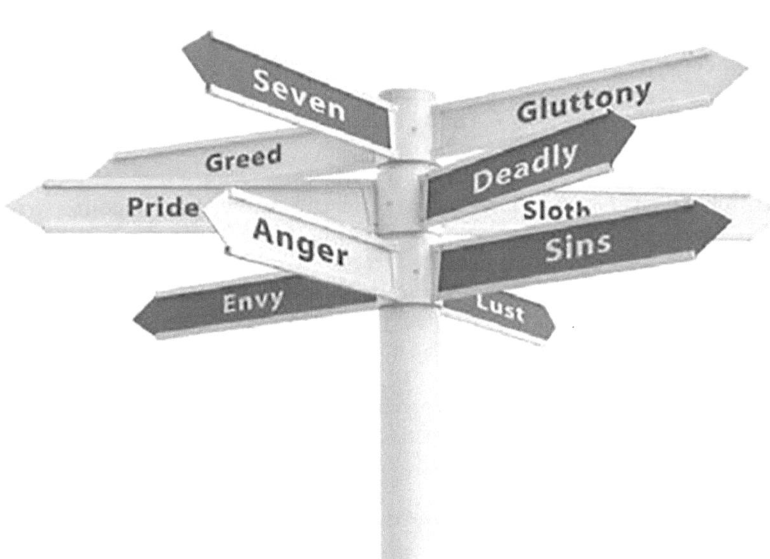

Where there is strife, there is pride, but wisdom is found in those who take advice. **Proverbs 13:10**

Jonah

Room Thirty-Two (Old Testament)

Come on in, how would you like to spend time in the belly of a whale for three days and nights? Well, then you'd better not do what Jonah did, What did he do? He ignored God's call, very interesting story, later on go back and read all about it. Why you're at it, might want to make some popcorn! The bible is full of adventure too, you are about to go inside the belly of a fish! "Have fun" bring me back some!

The moral of the story is this, if God calls us to do something, don't ignore or resist. We'd better not say 'later, I got other commitments; me and my homies getting ready to bounce up in the clubs, we bout to get our groove on. Or say something ridiculous like this: "I ain't doing nothin, I'm chillin!" Johan is lucky he make it out alive, so don't be jive! Get serious, learn from his mistake so you won't get ate. Please, please read your bibles, that's what it's for don't be passive, ***"Land On Shore!"***

Candid Snapshot

"Just Do It!" Listen up everybody, me too, when God calls us to do something, ***"Just Do It!"*** Everything else can wait, sports, your personal life, your goals and dream, school, everything. **God Must Be Top Priority!** I was in nursing school when God called me, *"Stop"*, *"write my book and call it A Caregivers Bible To Excellence"* and don't think I didn't try to run, to my favorite karaoke spot, or give him plenty of reason why I could not, I did, but God came after me too, now the rest is history!

Hey when I'm done here, does anyone know where I can get a large fish sandwich, fresh cut fries and homemade coleslaw, I'm famished; all that talk about "the belly of a whale" has made me hungry!

Key Verse

The Lord came to Jonah son of Amitta; "Go to the great city of Nineveh
and preach against it, because its wickedness has come up before me"
but Jonah ran away from the Lord and headed for Tarshish.
He went down to Joppa where he found a ship bound for that port.
After paying the fare, he went aboard and sailed
for Tarshish to flee from the lord. **1:1-3**

Key Action

You can run, but you won't get far, God will even come and
snatch you out of a bar! "Key Action" is simply this *"Don't Resist!"*

Father God, I can hear you now. Tell me what you want and which way to go. This time I will obey your wishes and not tell you no.

Amen

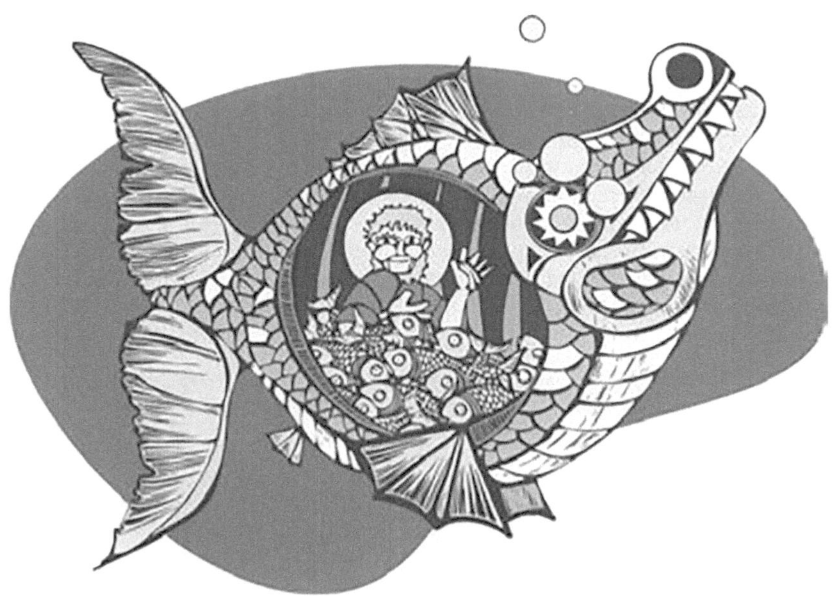

**Hello, I'm Still alive, but I've learned my lesson.
Send me, I will go....**

Micah

Here in this room we get to meet Micah he was a prophet also, he predicted the coming of Christ and the place of his birth. He also preached against oppression, pride, greed, corruption, religious hypocrisy and holy living and how God would hold them responsible for their action.

I ask you, does any of this sound familiar? What makes us think that God is going to overlook our behavior and the way we live, He's not. Many of you believe that Jesus dying on the cross for us get us off the hook, but it doesn't. Jesus dying on the cross, while true saved us, but it also defeated the world for us too, which means we can live a life holy and true if we really want to. And If we say we love God and his son then we ought to. Christ has left up with the power to do just that. "Live upright!" So you see, we are NOT to go on sinning, Jesus die for righteousness! He cares how we live our lives; Christ die so he could be our guide! All one has to do, is reject this world, get into his word, "come inside"!

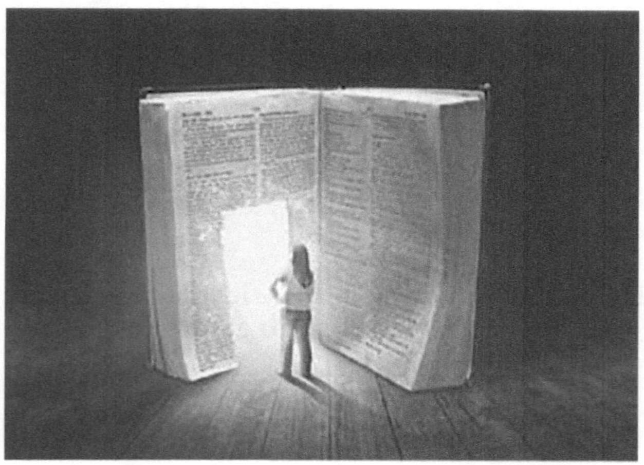

Throughout the entire bible repentance is God's cry out to us. ***Honor Me, Stop Disrespecting Me", Live Righteously!*** Everybody's been warned! This book the one you're reading right now, has my father's approval all on it. Like Malachi, me and so many others, we don't want God's wrath upon you. It's out of love that we reach out to you, the bible say in **Proverbs 21:2** *There is a path before each person that seems right, but it ends in death.* A repeat: ***Honor Me, Stop Disrespecting Me, Live Righteously!***

- Pre-marital sex and sexual mortality is unacceptable to God, we are asking for trouble, if we continue to carry on this way. **Exodus 22:16,! Corinthians 7:2, Genesis 2:24**

- Same sex marriages are an abomination to the lord. **Leviticus 18:22**
- We cannot sever this world and God too. **Matthew 6:24**
- The wages of sin is death **Romans 6:23**
- We are to tithe a tenth of our wages/first fruits to God, not doing so robs God. **Malachi 3:8**
- Be Holy, like Our Father in heaven. **1 Peter 1:16**

Let's All Get It Together!

Live For Christ, "Live Righteously."

Candid Snapshot

Using many voices over thousands of years, God sprinkle promises of the coming messiah. We are told, he will come, he will leave, and he will return. True believers awaits his return, but for the sake of this tour, let's get back to Micah, his prophecy points not only at judgment, but hope too. That hope was the birth of the messiah, "Jesus Christ", the savior of the world. The Star of Bethlehem, Imagine with me that "bright and starry night!" Soon the messiah will reappear.

Key Verse

"My people, what have I done to you?
How have I burdened you? Answer me. **6:3**

Key Action

What's your answer people?

Players, ballers, murders, drunken fools and thieves, prostitutes,
schemers, liars, cheats, haters, evil doing, idol worshipers,
pride arrogance and greed. God is asking us a question,
"What have I done to you? How have I burden the world?"

God is the one who created the entire universe and everything in it,
then he took his breath and breathe life into us He's the one who started it all,
He gave man and woman life. How can we forget about all that?
And turn our backs on God, and think all is going to go well for us,
it's not, not by a long shot! "Stop disrespecting our creator".

Key Prayer

Lord have mercy on us all!

Amen

Nahum

Room Thirty-Four (Old Testament)

The room of Nahum wants the world to know *'Evil'* will not last forever.

Nahum was another one of god's prophets. Nahum tells the people, and we should take heed too, that destructions is about to fall upon those who are out of compliance with God's will and that evil doers will have their day of reckoning.

This is why we mustn't worry about haters or troublemakers, they will soon be cut off, dealt with "gone" yes these individuals will reap what they've sown.

So let's not put any energy in these kind of people, forgive them of course and pray for them too, but move on.

In this room we learn that it is not going to go well for us if we keep pissing God off, the way we live matters to him. God's mind has not changed he is still against sinful living, always has been and always will be.

If we continue sinning against God, there will be consequences and for some, it may be severe, it may even cost some their life. Don't get it twisted, the wages of sin is still death you know, I just sayin', God's not playin'!!!!

Candid Snapshot

Evil will be dealt with, it's just a matter of time!
Get your house in order while you still have a chance.
God's patience is coming to an end.

Key Verse

Woe to the city of blood, full of lies, full of plunder, never without victims.

Key Prayer

Lord I need to come clean, all I asked is another chance to
make things right. I have recked my life and I'm ready to come clean,
I've been awful, I've been mean, I've done so really bad things.

Lord give me a chance to make things right, I've been in the dark for so long,
I know how I've been living is disrespectful and wrong.
Right now, Father God, I need a savior, "Jesus" for he's the guiding light,
come into my life and make me over tonight! I want to come back home.

Amen

Habakkuk

Room Thirty-five (Old Testament)

We are at room number thirty six of our tour, here we meet Habakkuk, a prophet as well, he poses honest questions about injustice, and why God allows evil to exist?

Attitude abounds here! People we must trust God no matter what our circumstances are. God is in control He already knows the situation, what we need, how we feel, and all that we're going through. He even knows what we're thinking before we think it. Our attitudes ought to be, no matter what, God will never leave me.

This room use to be a place I would I find myself in quite often. Every day I found myself having to fight to keep a roof over my head. At the time, I never understood why because I loved and helped everybody. But today, now I know, one will be hated if they don't belong to this world. **John 15:19**

Overall, Habakkuk message and mine also it this, We must trust God through it all, the good, the bad and the ugly side of life. Those who stay righteous always lands on top! So I say, keep doing good, keep doing God and never, ever Stop!

Attitude is everything yawl, we must rely on God to work things out in our favor. No matter what is happening to us, we mustn't fight the way the world fight; oh no, instead we hold on tightly to the word of God and allow the scriptures to do what they are designed to do, which is to protect us, comfort us, and deliver us too.

I tell you the truth, when I was being bullied, persecuted, lied on and hated back then, let me tell you, if it had not for the lord on my side, you wouldn't be reading this book today. He took what was meant for evil and used it for good; all because I trusted him like we should. Listen, "Everybody", we do not know the future, but God does. For example, who knew Christ had a book called *'A Caregivers Bible To Excellence'* with my name on it? Not me.

Trust God People!

For he knows the plans he has for each and every one of those who love him. *"Trust God!"*

Candid Snapshot

Life can be so perplexing and complicated. Many times no answers can be found. Yet we are left with only one question **"Why?"** However, it's at that time we **"MUST"** trust God and lean not on our own understanding. Furthermore, the bible says this: *"I realized that no one can discover everything God is doing under the sun, Not even the wisest people discover everything, no matter what they claim.* **Ecc. 8:17** Again, "Trust God!"

Key Verse

The Sovereign LORD is my strength; he makes my feet like the feet of a deer, he enables me to tread on the heights. For the director of music. On my stringed instruments. **3:19**

Key Prayer

O' my Lord, I am yours for the taking, you complete me, I am lost without you, the music of my soul longs to be with you. Take me my Lord and use me for thy service.

Amen

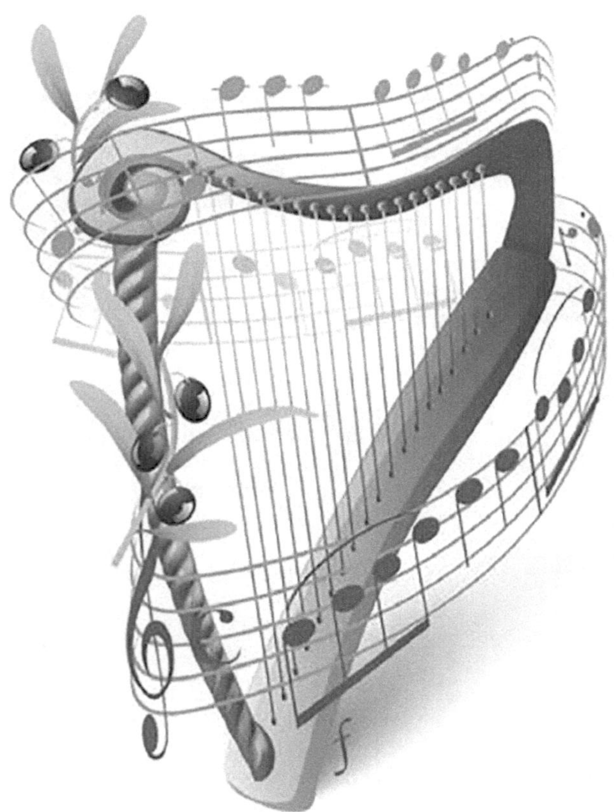

Zephaniah

Room Thirty-Six (Old Testament)

Zephaniah was another one of God's prophets. Here he speaks to us about **Irresponsibility** and **Complacency** both leading to our downfall. This is an interesting room, for Christians in particular, because we should know better than to straddle the fence. There are those who live double lives, one foot in the church, and one foot in the world doing all kinds of things. fornication, porn, lying, cheating, drunkenness, drugs, gambling, greed, hating one another, you name it. And another thing, Christan's have gotten quite comfortable watching all kind of filth and violence on television. The bible is clear that we are to guard our eyes and ears. Zephaniah's message to the people and it still holds true today is this: ***When God judges sin, those who know the most suffers the most.*** Yet there's another message too: If we change our ways, **(Repent)** God will not punish us, on the contrary, he'll help his people thrive! My advice, "Stay Alive!"

Candid Snapshot

Get right with God, Stop the facade! Those who know the most, suffers the most! We cannot live for God and this world too, "No", that just won't do.

Key Verse

Dead flies will cause even a bottle of perfume to stink! Yes, a small mistake can outweigh much wisdom and honor. A wise man heart leads him to do right, and a fool hearts leads him to do evil. You can identify a fool just by the way he walks down the street! **10:1-3**

Key Action

In order to defeat sinful living, one must stay in the word as if your life depends on it, and let me tell you, it does! Read and breathe the bible it's the only way to keep alive. Jesus is the only way and his way is through bible reading.

Key Prayer

Lord today I pray for my child, he/she's lost, I have tried everything I know to Get him/her to turn their life around, but my child won't listen, I cannot get through to them, please if I have so kindly earned any favor from you, grant me this my lord, that my child will be safe and protected out there, spared too. Don't let any harm come to them. Please God, find him/her, send one of your angels to minister the word to them, bring my child home.

Amen

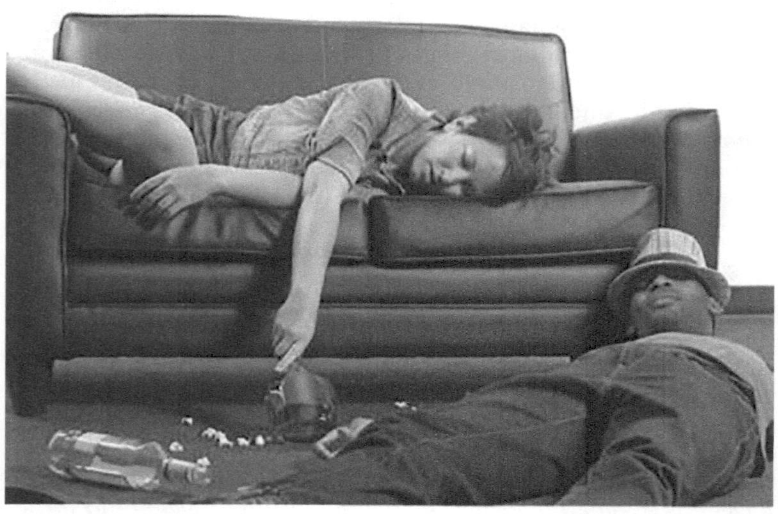

   MISS ASONDRA STARN'AIR

Haggai

Room Thirty-seven (Old Testament)

This room is about making God the first priority in our lives. God wants us to start taking him more seriously by being obedient and following through on whatever he tells us to do. Let's use an everyday life situation for our example, if he tells you to break off a relationship that he knows is going to stagnate you, then break it off!

And of course, if infidelity/fornication is involved, then you most certainly MUST break it off. That's a no, no to begin with, when we're in relationships like this, all in all we're sinning against God, not to mention too, hurting ourselves in the process. Nothing good is coming out of that one. (Tip for the ladies, If a man will lay with you outside of marriage, he will lay with others too, when he's not with you, this is what worldly men do, never trust a man like that.)

Wait on God, let's not let our fleshly desires destroy all the plans God has for us. My message to both single men and single women "wait it out", trust God to send you your soul mate. Meanwhile, let's all stay focus on excellence and righteous living.

Haggai, was sent by god to go and preach to the restored Israelite community, it seem they have forgotten about God's work, his temple/church. God wanted one built, but instead they were building their own lifestyles and God wasn't having that. So Haggai and his style of preaching got it done. Hope my style of writing is getting God's work done too. ***Rebuild The Christan Home!"***

What about "YOU", what are you working on?

Candid Snapshot

The Call to rebuild the temple!
Calling out to God's people, get back to work on the rebuilding my temple,
don't put your affairs or homes before my place of worship.
My house must be a place of worship for the good of the nation,
therefore get back to work!

Key Verse

Why is everyone saying it is not the right time for rebuilding of my Temple?" asked the Lord. his reply to them is this: is it then the right time for you to live in luxurious homes, when the Temple lies ruins? Look at the result: you plant much but harvest little. You have sacredly enough to eat and drink, and not enough clothes to keep you warm, your income disappears as though you were putting it into pockets filled with holes. Think it over says the Lord Almighty. Considered how you have acted and what has happen as a result! **1:2-7**

Key Action

"Build Something" in Jesus name! Get into a good bible teaching church. Do missionary work, help out, serve, join a ministry or create one of your own. If you can preach, "preach", if you can teach, "teach", "do outreach" whatever! "Help build", "serve", lets help get people saved and into heaven! So whatever God put on your heart, don't hesitate or wait, *"START!"*

Key Prayer

Lord, reveal to me, my calling?
Give me tools and everything I'll need to succeed.

Amen

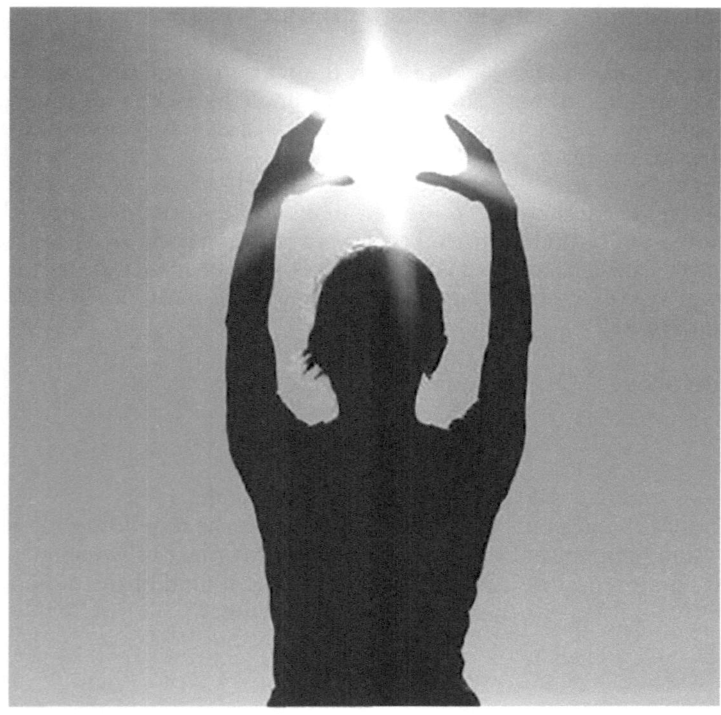

   MISS ASONDRA STARN'AIR

Zechariah

Zechariah was sent by God to help restore the community, to encourage people to live for God, That's exactly what I am doing here.

Encouraging all of you to flee from sinful living, read your bible daily and make Jesus lord over your life in everything you do, that's the core message throughout this entire book. A Caregivers Bible To Excellence is all about living for Christ, the excellent way.

Zechariah had special gifts, he could see things, he had lots of visions of things to come including the arrival of the messiah.

Preparation was the order of the day, judgment vs blessings were coming their way. However, in our microwave world today, very few people pray. many gone astray.

Jesus has come and gone, yet folks are having a party, carrying on, doing everything under the sun. Even after thousands of years and pages of instructions, people won't stop sinning. So many people are in bondage to this world's way of thinking, they have been brain washed, many loss and confused. They think that Jesus dying on the cross gives them the right to live however they want to, it doesn't, "there's a cost!"

All through the bible, there are thousands and thousands of warning against sinful living, and hundreds of *'Oracles'* in the form of Apostles, Prophets, Priest, Disciples, and somewhere in this circle, there's **"ME"**. Yes we all are speaking for **GOD**. We're saying in so many ways, the same exact thing:
'Stop Sinning Against God or Else'

But unfortunately, thousands of years later, even today, all those warning have landed on death ear. "People Are Following Their Peers." So, sad!

Candid Snapshot

I feel like singing, gimme the Mic  People get ready, there's a train a-coming, don't need no baggage, just get on board. All you need is faith, to hear the diesels humming, don't need no ticket, just thank the Lord.

"People" stay away from sinful liven, we're told all this, right from the beginning, all you need is a change of heart, Jesus is that new place to start... so people get ready, their a train a-coming........

Key Verse

The Lord Almighty was very anger with your father. But he will turn again and favor you if only you return to him. don't be like your father's were! The earlier prophets pled in vain with them to turn from all their evil ways. "Come return to me" the Lord God said But, they wouldn't listen; they paid no attention at all. **1:1-4**

Key Action

Pay attention, The Lord is calling you!

Key Prayer

Lord, come into my life, create in me a clean heart, give me a fresh start. Holy spirit, take away all that is not pleasing to you. Set me on a righteous path. "Free me from me" in Jesus name let it be.

Amen

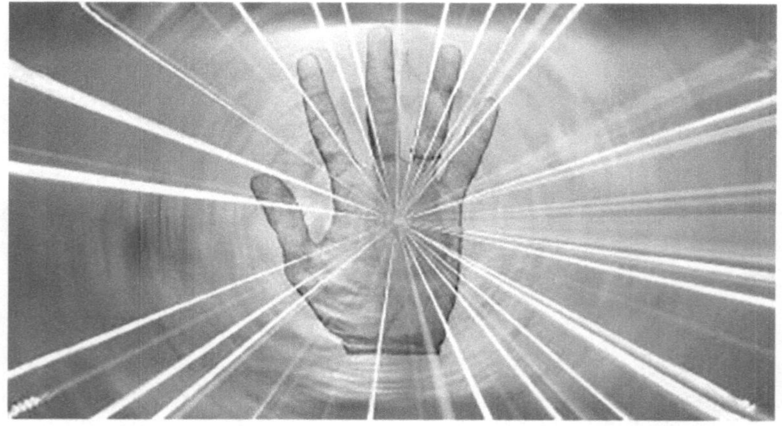

"Jesus" Lay Your Hand On Me!

 Miss Asondra StarN'air

Malachi

Room Thirty-Nine (Old Testament)

Malachi was sent as a prophet too to help bring restoration to a community that had lost its zeal. They were depressed, and weary with no hope in sight, Malachi had to do something to help bring these people out of this dark place. The basic problem that Malachi was dealing with in that community was corruption of priest, neglect of God's temple and personal sins at home.

All too often, we put our trust in the wrong people. These folks claim to be sent by God to preach or lead us in some way; yet they turn out to be frauds, schemers, and seekers of prestige and power. This is another room in my Father's house that is quite disturbing. I'm sure many of you have come across leaders that were not who they claimed to be; be it in the workplace or the church, "Counterfeits" are everywhere!

This is why we need to read the bibles for ourselves, no one should have to keep telling you about God, or what he expects from us and how we should behave down here, if you have a bible, open it up and read it for yourself.

So many of God's true leaders, such as myself we have to deal with so much, but enough is enough! Some of you out there just have to learn life the hard way, disrespecting God and his word is never okay. Look if you don't get right with God and repent, sooner or later you'll pay. The wage of sin means your life as you know it will end.

Malachi, had his hands full, so do I, with all that's going on in this room divorce, corrupt activities, the constant sinning, selfishness and insincerity, low morale, the people were down, and Malachi blamed the religious leaders, me too. The leaders are supposed to be leaders of "The Faith and Righteousness." Malachi felt the same way, the leaders of all people should have known what god required. More or less this is probably why the bible tells us not to put out trust in man.

Nevertheless, "Rest" Malachi found hope in the promise (me too) that an answer would come, and that answer is the messiah, Christ returns. Read your bibles, "Learn!"

Candid Snapshot

Never too late to change our ways, until it is too late!

Key Verse

The oracle of the word of the LORD to Israel through Malachi.

I have loved you," says the LORD. But you say, "How have You loved us?" "Was not Esau Jacob's brother?" declares the LORD. "Yet I have loved Jacob; but I have hated Esau, and I have made his mountains a desolation and appointed his inheritance for the jackals of the wilderness." Though Edom says, "We have been beaten down, but we will return and build up the ruins"; thus says the LORD of hosts, "They may build, but I will tear down; and men will call them the wicked territory, and the people toward whom the LORD is indignant forever." Your eyes will see this and you will say, "The LORD be magnified beyond the border of Israel!" "'A son honors his father, and a servant his master. Then if I am a father, where is My honor? And if I am a master, where is My respect?' says the LORD of hosts to you, O priests who despise My name. But you say, 'How have we despised Your name?' "You are presenting defiled food upon My altar. But you say, 'How have we defiled You?' In that you say, 'The table of the LORD is to be despised.' "But when you present the blind for sacrifice, is it not evil? And when you present the lame and sick, is it not evil? Why not offer it to your governor? Would he be pleased with you? Or would he receive you kindly?" says the LORD of hosts. "But now will you not entreat God's favor, that He may be gracious to us? With such an offering on your part, will He receive any of you kindly?" says the LORD of hosts. "Oh that there were one among you who would shut the gates, that you might not uselessly kindle fire on My altar! I am not pleased with you," says the LORD of hosts, "nor will I accept an offering from you. "For from the rising of the sun even to its setting, My name will be great among the nations, and in every place incense is going to be offered to My name, and a grain offering that is pure; for My name will be great among the nations," says the LORD of hosts. "But you are profaning it, in that you say, 'The table of the Lord is defiled, and as for its fruit, its food is to be despised.' "You also say, 'My, how tiresome it is!' And you disdainfully sniff at it," says the LORD of hosts, "and you bring what was taken by robbery and what is lame or sick; so you bring the offering! Should I receive that from your hand?" says the LORD. "But cursed be the swindler who has a male in his flock and vows it, but sacrifices a blemished animal to the Lord, for I am a great King," says the LORD of hosts, "and My name is feared among the nations." **1:1-14**

Key Prayer

Lord, I am defied, I have offered you substitutes, the money I put in church is not holy money, it's sin living money, money left over from the night before, that's right, but it's wrong, not even ten percent, shopping, alcohol and partying is where it all went. I realized a lot of leaders don't care where the money come from, just put it in there. But father God you know, and you reject it, nothings good coming out of funny money, money given at the last minute.

I am ashamed of my behavior, I have so much cleaning up to do, in my heart I owe you, it's long overdo, today I'm ready to commit my life to you. Take me back, help me get on track, I'm like a filthy dirty rat, I don't want to go out like that!

Amen

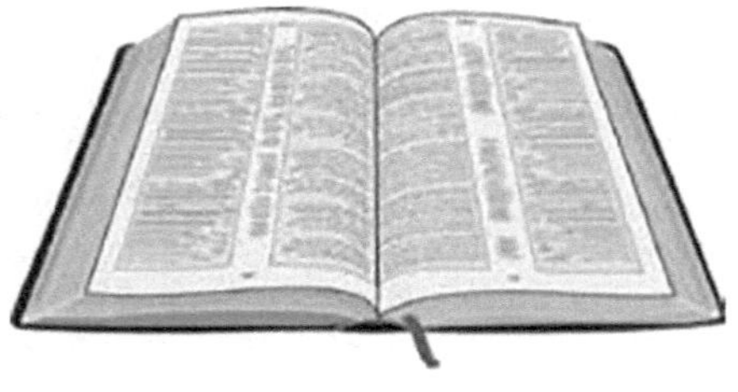

　　　　　MISS ASONDRA STARN'AIR

Let's take another break shall we.

When we come back we will continue our tour. The next four rooms are known as the Gospel of Jesus Christ. these rooms are Matthew, Mark, Luke and John, these men walked with Jesus, became his disciples. Me too!

So take a break, get you something to eat and drink, get refreshed and meet me back in 30 minutes.

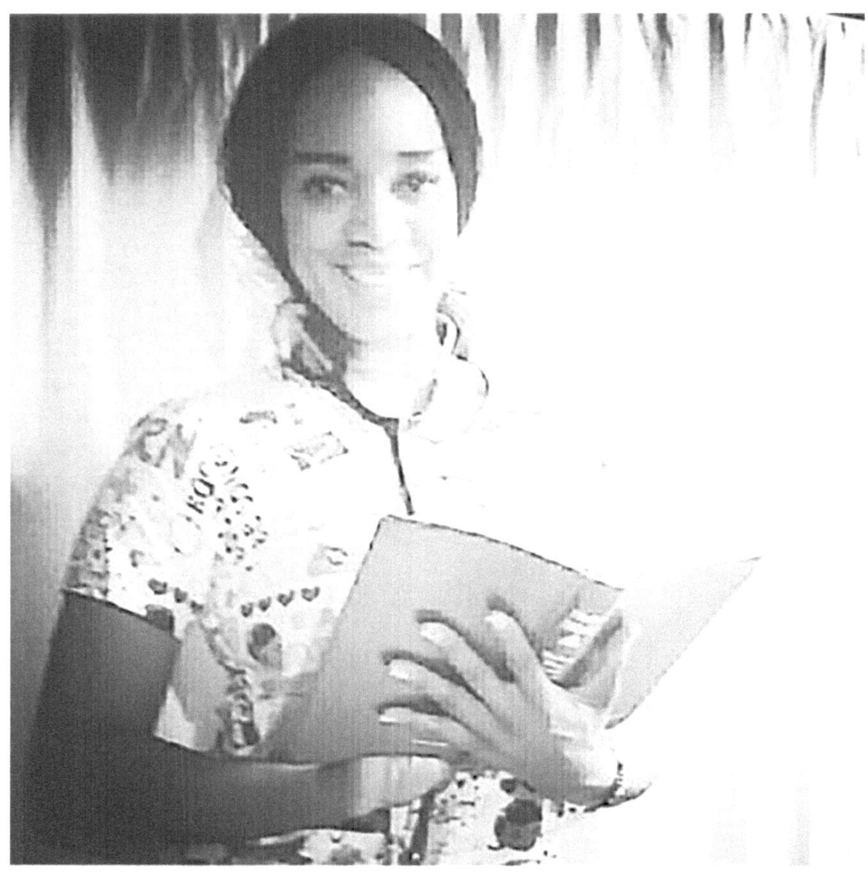

The New Testament

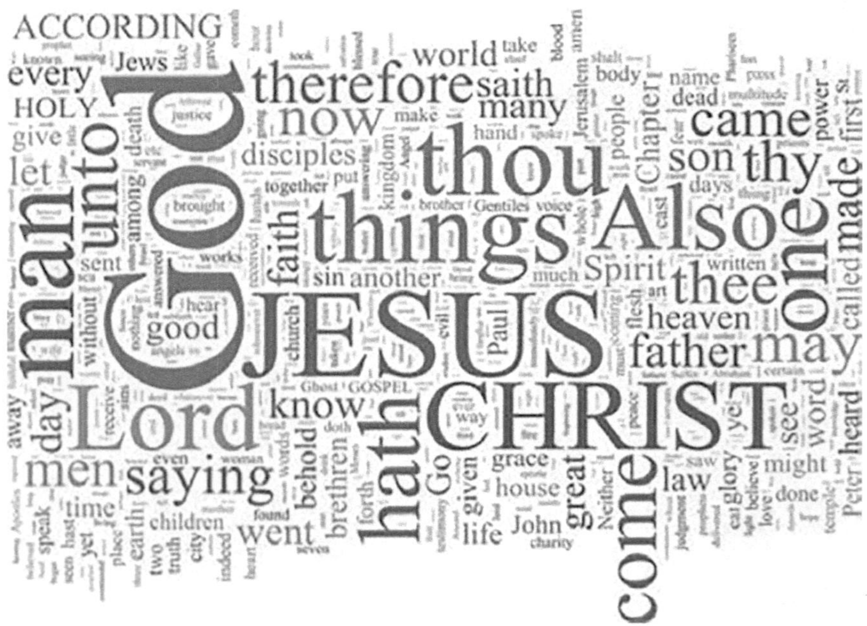

Matthew

Room Forty (New Testament)

Finally, you get a chance to meet Jesus up close and personal, his birth, his ministry and his miracles. Plus you'll get a chance to meet his disciples, Matthew, Mark, Luke and John.

First we will start with Matthew; Matthew was a tax collector, and one day Jesus saw him sitting at the tax collectors booth, Jesus approached him, and said *"Follow Me"* (leave that life behind) and he did.

Soon Mathew would discover after being with Jesus, hearing his teaching, watching him heal people and perform miracles after miracles, that Jesus was the son of God, the messiah the Jews had waited for since the old testament.

Matthew is one of the four Gospels, because he is one of the four followers, that the holy spirit decided to use to inform the world the messiah has finally come.

This room in my father's house, is all about Jesus, not about you. So when you come in here, take your shoes off, worship and adore him, for he is **LORD!** Mathew's about to tell you all about Jesus and what is expected of us, if we are to follow him. I have already made my decision, as for me and my house we shall serve the Lord.

Candid Snapshot

Jesus heals, cast out demons, walks on water, multiplies food, calms storms, and guess what, he knew who **"YOU"** before you were born.

Key Verse

How terrible it will be for anyone who causes others to sin. Temptation is inevitable but how terrible it will be for the person who does the tempting. **18:7**

Key Action

Following Christ is the order of the day, equally as important is reading his word. By doing this we become one with Christ, where he goes, we go. And don't be surprised if you feel his spirit or see one of his disciples in a bar. Take action, help win souls for Chrsit. Jesus did not come here for the saved, or church folks, no on the contrary, he came here for the sinner. The male and female prostitutes, fornicators, haters, drug dealers, nonbelievers, and the loss, not the found. take action, "see you around"!

Key Prayer

Lord, create in me a clean heart, give me a fresh start.

Mark

Room Forty- One (New Testament)

Here we meet another one of Jesus's disciples—Mark. In this room, Mark depicts Jesus as the servant of God who came to accomplish God's plan. Matthew also, but Mark Gospel is an eye witness account of events of Jesus life and his followers, unlike Mathew's and the other two, Luke and John. In here, Mark focuses more on Jesus actions than his word. So in here, you'll get a chance to see his public ministry up close and personal.

And let me tell you, when you do, you will not be the same, you'll want to change, I did.

Matthew did, now Marks on board for the Lord. *'We all Changed'!* I personally wanted to see the other side of me, the Jesus side, the one God said existed in all those desiring change. I wanted that change.

So I asked God to tear me down, rebuild me, kind of like my favorite TV series called *The Six Million Dollar Man* and *The Bionic Woman* that was an old TV series back in the early seventies.

This man, Steve Austin (the character's name), was in a crash and about to die, or be paralyzed for life one of the two but the government had the technology to rebuild him. So they gave him cybernetic parts, which gave him superhuman strength and speed. When he finally woke up and began to heal, he was faster, wiser, stronger, and had a good heart too! Now he was ready to be used, so he was sent out on a mission to help make the world a safer and better place to live in.

Question is, Can you see yourself doing that for the Lord? Well I can, so does Mark and the rest of God's disciples. Later on go back and read all about Jesus ministry, all the miracles and transfigurations. One encounter with Jesus is all it takes!

As far as my six million dollars analogy, it's real! I'm so much better than before, I'm **FASTER** at forgiving, I'm **WISER**, not having sex outside of marriage anymore, **STRONGER** too, hatred and persecution didn't stop me from getting this book to you.

Candid Snapshot

Welcome **"CHANGE"**! My testimony, I was headed in the wrong direction, Jesus called me, transformed everything about me, and now I am his forevermore. I have no problem washing feet or sweeping floors!

Let me say this, those back in biblical times are not the only ones to witness Jesus miracles and transformations on the contrary, look what God has done with me, once a black aide/slave, now free!

Key Verse

Who is The Greatest? *They came to Capernaum. When he was in the house, he asked them, "What were you arguing about on the road?" But they kept quiet because on the way they had argued about who was the greatest. Sitting down, Jesus called the Twelve and said, "Anyone who wants to be first must be the very last, and the servant of all."* **9:33-35**

Key Action

Get off you, and onto others, Jesus came here to serve, not to be served!

Key Prayer

Dear God, Fill my heart with love and compassion for others. Help me to love my sisters and brothers.

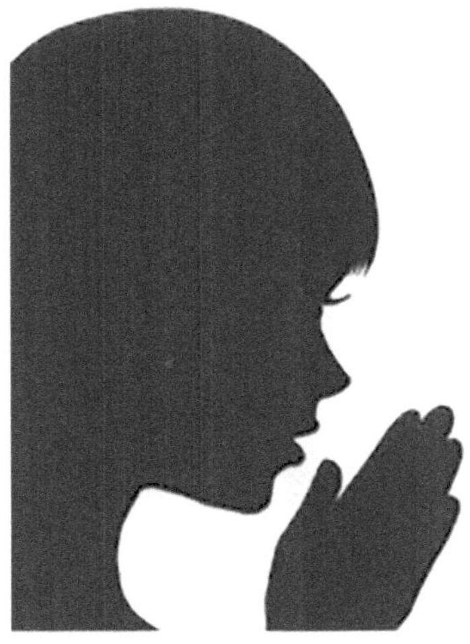

Luke

Room Forty-Two (New Testament)

We are still in the gospels, time to meet Luke another one of Jesus disciples. Luke was a physician, hey "Caregivers, we're working with a real live doctor here," a fine one at that, he cared about what Jesus cared about, getting people well. Luke's contribution to the Gospel was to show the human nature of Jesus and his place in history.

Luke was a very intellectual person and was careful to examine all the evidence and give precise dates and events.

Once you're in this room you'll notice each of these four Gospels all are pretty much saying the same thing, 'Jesus reign supreme' Jesus is the Son Of God, the Savior of the world.

In these Gospels, Mathew showed Jesus to be the Jewish Messiah and Mark showed him as being a servant of God, here Luke depicts Jesus as being one with God but also human.

And here's something else you ought to know, Mark and Luke traveled a lot with Apostle Paul, a lot of their insights on the life of Jesus came from Paul.

And a lot of my insight came from spending intimate time in his word. Today Jesus is still very much alive in the hearts, mind and soul of those who really, really love him and wants to do his will. My hope is that you want to, my prayer is that you do. God bless you, enjoy the Gospels.

Candid Snapshot

Luke was a doctor, but a Christian first! What about you?

Key Verse

One of those days Jesus went out to a mountainside to pray, and spent the night praying to God. When morning came, he called his disciples to him and chose twelve of them, whom he also designated apostles: **6:12-13**

Key Actions

If you want to fish, become fisher of men if
Christ caught you, you must catch others!

Key Prayer

Lord, I want to fish to win, show me where to cast my net? forget
"Vegas" your lottery's where it's at!

John

Room Forty-Three (New Testament)

Come, come, let's meet John, another one of Jesus's disciples! This room is filled with recorded miracles of Jesus work as well as his teachings in the upper room before his crucifixion. John describes Jesus as light, love, truth, the Good Shepherd, the door, living water, bread of life, and more.

I describe him as **"The Greatest Love of All,"** and so did the late great Whitney Huston, that song she sang, in essence was all about Christ. And she was right, The Greatest Love of All 'is' inside, that's where Jesus resides.

Here in this room, John really wants us to get it, that Jesus is really God in the flesh. And that, it's true, there is no other way to God except by this truth. Jesus is the only way to everlasting life.

John was also an apostle too! (To be an apostle in biblical days, meant one followed "Jesus"! And many of them became primary teachers of the gospel message of Jesus as well.

John was one of those apostles and of course Apostle Paul was. Paul wrote thirteen books of the bible, however modern scholars say eight, who cares they're all "Great"!

But wait, there's more!!!! Check out *"Jesus Resume"* He's done more than required, above being hired, He's "The Messiah, He's The Desired!" Go on, just look at what *He's* done, "have fun!"

Jesus Resume

- Calming the storm – Matthew 8:23-27; Mark 4:37-41; Luke 8:22-25
- Feeding 5,000 – Matthew 14:14-21; Mark 6:30-44; Luke 9:10-17;
- John 6:1-14
- Walking on water – Matthew 14:22-32; Mark 6:47-52; John 6:16-21
- Feeding 4,000 – Matthew 15:32-39; Mark 8:1-9
- Fish with coin – Matthew 17:24-27
- Fig tree withers – Matthew 21:18-22; Mark 11:12-14, 20-25
- Huge catch of fish – Luke 5:4-11; John 21:1-11
- Water into wine – John 2:1-11

Healing of Individuals

- Man with leprosy – Matthew 8:1-4; Mark 1:40-44; Luke 5:12-14
- Roman centurion's servant – Matthew 8:5-13; Luke 7:1-10
- Peter's mother-in-law – Matthew 8:14-15; Mark 1:30-31; Luke 4:38-39
- Two men possessed with devils – Matthew 8:28-34; Mark 5:1-15; Luke 8:27-39
- Man with palsy – Matthew 9:2-7; Mark 2:3-12; Luke 5:18-26
- Woman with bleeding – Matthew 9:20-22; Mark 5:25-34; Luke 8:43-48

- Two blind men – Matthew 9:27-31
- Dumb, devil-possessed man – Matthew 9:32-33
- Canaanite woman's daughter – Matthew 15:21-28; Mark 7:24-30
- Boy with devil - Matthew 17:14-21; Mark 9:17-29; Luke 9:38-43
- Two blind men – including Bartimaeus - Matthew 20:29-34; Mark 10:46-52; Luke 18:35-43
- Demon-possessed man in synagogue – Mark 1:21-28; Luke 4:31-37
- Blind man at Bethsaida – Mark 8:22-26
- Crippled woman – Luke 13:10-17
- Man with dropsy – Luke 14:1-4
- Ten men with leprosy – Luke 17:11-19
- The high priest's servant – Luke 22:50-51
- Nobleman's son at Capernaum – John 4:46-54
- Sick man at the pool of Bethsaida – John 5:1-15
- Man born blind – John 9:1-41

Raising The Dead

- Jairus' daughter – Matthew 9:18-26; Mark 5:21-43; Luke 8:40-56
- Widow's son at Nain – Luke 7:11-17
- Lazarus – John 11:1-44

Nobody But

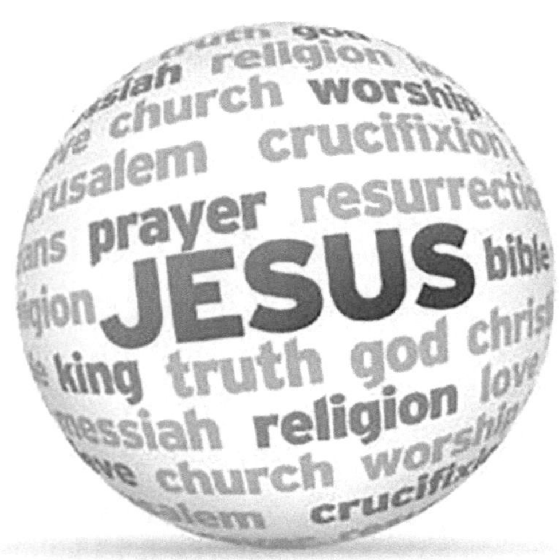

Can Do All That!

Candid Snapshot

Choose this day whom you will serve.

Key Verse

"I am the true vine, and my Father is the gardener. He cuts off every branch in me that bears no fruit, while every branch that does bear fruit he prunes so that it will be even more fruitful. You are already clean because of the word I have spoken to you. Remain in me, as I also remain in you. No branch can bear fruit by itself; it must remain in the vine. Neither can you bear fruit unless you remain in me. "I am the vine; you are the branches. If you remain in me and I in you, you will bear much fruit; apart from me you can do nothing. If you do not remain in me, you are like a branch that is thrown away and withers; such branches are picked up, thrown into the fire and burned. If you remain in me and my words remain in you, ask whatever you wish, and it will be done for you. This is to my Father's glory, that you bear much fruit, showing yourselves to be my disciples. **15:1-8**

Key Action

Look before you leap, don't go chasing waterfalls, please stick to the rivers and lakes that God has for you.

Key Prayer

Lord, I want out of this world, come take me a different route, I want to find out what your world's all about!

Amen

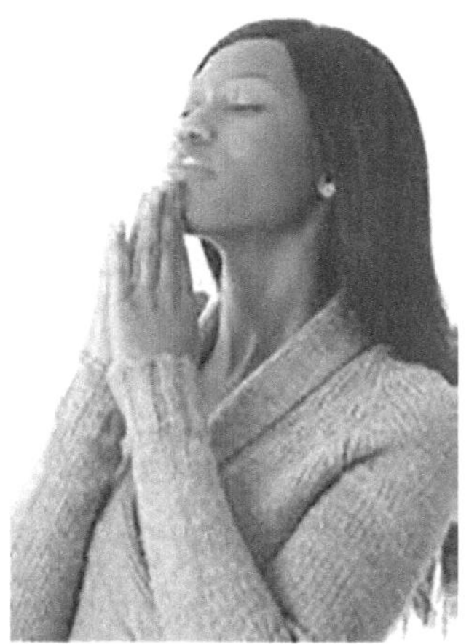

Acts

Room Forty-Four (New Testament)

Next we have Acts it is a sequel to Luke's Gospel, a continuation showing that what Jesus started here on earth will continue throughout the church.

Acts is like a history book, because it tells the story of how Christianity began and spread. You should find this room quite enlightening.

What I want to remind Christians of is this, we must not forget about the holy spirit, that's our guide to righteous living. Make Jesus Lord over your life in every way; always love and keep on forgiving.

Candid Snapshot

Jesus belongs to all people, black and white,
all are loved and equal in God's sight! So don't hate or fight!

Key Verse

'The Fellowship of Believers'

All believers were together and had everything in common **2:44**

Key Action

Get to know someone you don't already know,
invite that person to an outing or to church with you.

Key Prayer

Lord, remove behaviors of racism, hatred, jealousy, Unforgiveness and superiority far away from me, create in me a clean and loving heart.

Amen

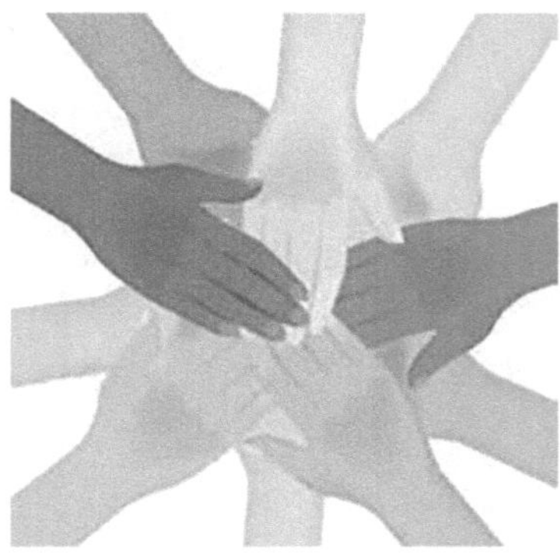

 Miss Asondra StarN'air

Romans

Room Forty-Five (New Testament)

Meet Apostle Paul, he's our guest in this room for the day, and he wanted to tell you about himself directly, Hello my name is **Apostle Paul**:

Jesus Christ's slave, chosen by God to be an apostle and sent out to preach his Good News. This Good News was promised long ago by God through the prophets in the holy Scriptures. it is the Good News about his son Jesus, who came as a man, born into king David's royal family line. And Jesus Christ our Lord was shown to be the son of God when God powerfully raised him from the dead by means of the holy spirit. **1:1-4**

okay, I'll take over from here now, what some of you may not know, because you haven't read the bible yet, Apostle Paul got converted. He was not always a servant of God before Paul he was known as Saul of Tarsus. Saul hated Christians, like some people still do today, except Saul didn't hide is hatred, everyone knew how he felt.

But one day God called out to him and said, "Saul why do your persecute me?" **9:4**

Listen, of course, I am not god, but I'm asking the same thing, **"disbelieves"** why do you persecute me and my fellow Christians? Speak up people, speak up bullies, speak up liars, "pants on fire!" Why? "Hum" why? That's okay, I know the answer, right now some of you are just loss, blind and can't see. yet, you're only destroying yourselves, and nobody else. **"Repent"** For bible teaches "we reap what we sow". Like Paul, me and others, **"Get with God and Grow!"**

Candid Snapshot

If persecutors like Saul can change, and fornicators like I can change,
then **"YOU"** can change too, so why don't you!

Key Verse

For in the gospels a righteousness from God is revealed, a righteousness that is by faith from first to last, just as it is written: The righteous will live by faith. **1:17**

Key Action

Read your bible daily, it will help strengthen your walk with God,
no more facades!

Key Prayer

The righteous will live by faith, The righteous will live by faith,
The righteous will live by faith, The righteous will live by faith!

Amen

1st Corinthians

Room Forty-Six (New Testament)

The theme of this room is **'Christian Conduct'** in a sinful world. 1st Corinthians known as: The First Epistles (letters) to the Corinthians, here, Apostle Paul had to write a serious letter to the church concerning them and the "Corinthian Community" because word got back to the apostle that so called believers weren't living the faith. (I suppose they were doing what we are doing, living like the world. I'll stop right there.) So he had to put them in their place. sometimes we can't beat around the bush, we have to tell it like it is, and here the Apostle Paul does.

What I want to say to the people of my day, if we say we are Christians, we ought to live that way! We go to church; yet outside of church, we live and act like the world "Hypocrites!" When Christians act like that, It makes us all look bad, now nobody wants to take a real Christian serious, shame on you, if this shoe fits **"YOU."** and If it doesn't, God bless you! Keep doing what you do!!!!! Today's churches as I see it, still have some of the same problems Apostle Paul spoke about in his letters—division, arguing, suing one another, immoral living, and misusing worship. I'll add a few more to this list—infidelity, babies out of wedlock, men lovers of themselves and homosexuality, misuse of God's tithes and offerings, men and women appointing themselves to be pastors and leaders but are not called by God, but using their brilliance, degrees and intellect to charm their way into the pulpit.

Seems to me too, that things have gotten worse since Apostle Paul's time in ministry. Christians have blended in with the world a lot of the congregation, and it's members do not read or own their own bibles let alone know how to really love or serve Christ; nor do they want to; they want to live for Christ and the world and they are doing it too, meanwhile, the church looks the other way.. just bring in those tithes today!

These counterfeit Christians are just as lost and miserable as the rest of the world and haven't a clue why they can't seem to get ahead or why they are so unhappy. They want to blame God too, but they're the ones trying to serve two masters, straddling the fence. And when they get caught, it's somebody else's fault.

Again, it all boils down to faithfulness to God! Apostle Paul back in his time, dealt with it all. But, today, people are still disobedient they're "off the wall" and because of it, one by one, "they fall." Unfortunately as I alluded to, not too much has changed, in fact, things keep getting worse and worse. I say this, and I do believe Apostle Paul if he were alive today would agree, that those who don't live for God, remains under a curse. Bottom line here in this room, is this: Start being obedient to our creator, by reading his word; live **_"Only"_** for him. **"Keep God First!"**

      MISS ASONDRA STARN'AIR

Candid Snapshot

Apostle Paul was a wise and skilled master builder. He help lay the foundation for what was to come, "Jesus' the messiah! And he did an excellent job, he fought the good fight and finished his race, I do believe he will see God again, face to face!

Key Verse

For the message of the cross is foolishness to those who are perishing, but to us who are being saved it is the power of God. **1:18**

Key Action

Read Your Bibles Every day!
Fall out of love with sin and let God in!

Key Prayer

Dear Lord, I am so grateful for what you are about to do in my life and for what you have already done. I am so excited about my new journey with you, can't wait to start anew. God I love you!

Amen

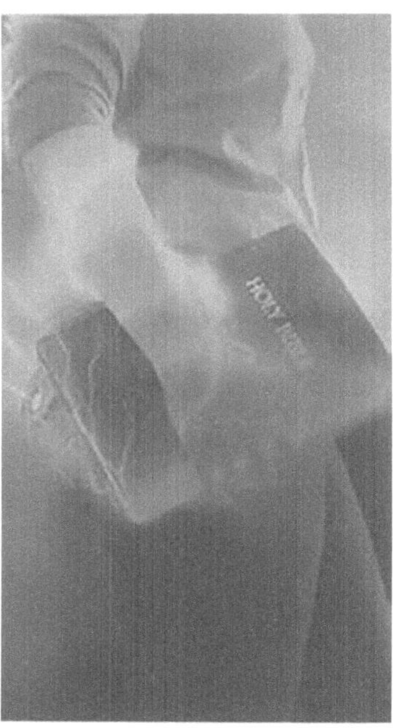

2 Corinthians

Room Forty-Seven (New Testament)

Welcome back! We're still hanging out with the Apostle Paul, now there seems to be some questions about his authority in this room, not me, I don't have any issues with the Apostle.

For I am grateful for his teaching. And I admire his commitment and loyalty to God and his son Jesus Christ, *"All"* have changed my life.

However, people love strife, yes that was going on back then and it continues today, well anyway, some leaders/people are questioning his authorities, saying things like, does he really speak for God? (I say yes, the proof is in the pudding) Seems to me, a lot of them are trying hold on to his past, and some are being schemish and wicked too, they're out spreading rumors and lies about him.

It's true, Saul, "now Paul" use to have a horrible reputation, I already touched on that, he use to hate Christians, But he got converted, God Changed his life completely and deeply. But as we all know there is always going to be people out there reminding you of your past. Some people just will not accept the change, no matter what good you do, in the world there will aways be haters and folk trying to tear or keep you down. This is probably what's being said about me as we speak, "She used to wear very provocative clothing" (that was me, I did) "Now she's a Christian?" Yep, that's right, go on,

(today I'm sing a new song! DJ, gimme the mic 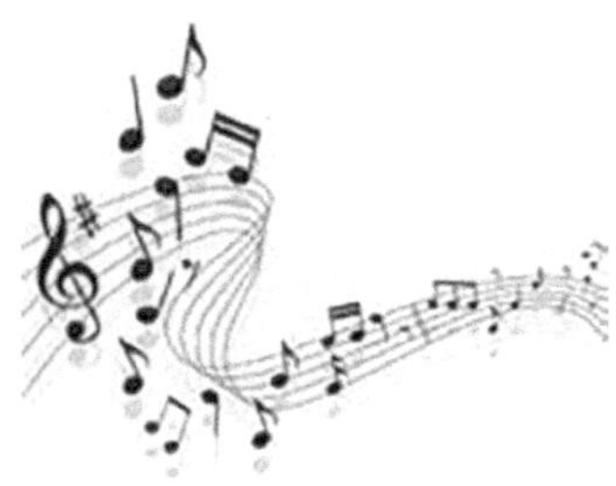 can you hear me now? Can't we all just love one another and get a long? Is that all you got? Because you know this book is hottt! With a triple t, God's been doing a lot with me. Check this out, rumors and lies, no longer affect me, I'm rollin with thee, I'm free, with two sets of double e's!

So, step back please, Apostle Paul and I, got work to do, but first, we want to relax in paradise with Jesus, **"Chill"** and feel the cool breeze! Non -believers, I'll pray for ya, but don't *'Step to Me!'*

Bottom line, Paul and I have changed, both given brand new names, but agenda's the same, *'Win Souls for Christ'*, What's your agenda, 'tender'? if it's not of God, "Return to the Sender"! That's a rap! Peace out, but remember, Jesus said pray, that God doesn't make his move in freezing cold months like, 'December!' **Mark 13:18**

Candid Snapshot

Once you start reading the bible, your eye will be open, there will be no turning back. At some point, you'll have to choose, do I live for this world or do I live to serve God?

And another thing, just because some preach powerfully, does not mean they've been sent by God. Today a lot of that comes from intellect, degrees and professional training, not Therefore, we *MUST* use discernment, and weed them out, look past all those plaques and degrees on the wall because I assure you, those not sent by God *"shall fall."* **Our Sins Shall Find us All Out!** Fact: Apostle Paul wrote many books in the bible, what about his accusers? **NONE!** The proof is in the pudding, **"I'm done!"**

Key Verse

Paul's Hardships

We put no stumbling block in anyone's path, so that our ministry will not be discredited. Rather, as servants of God we commend ourselves in every way: in great endurance; in troubles, hardships and distresses; in beatings, imprisonments and riots; in hard work, sleepless nights and hunger; in purity, understanding, patience and kindness; in the Holy Spirit and in sincere love; in truthful speech and in the power of God; with weapons of righteousness in the right hand and in the left; through glory and dishonor, bad report and good report; genuine, yet regarded as impostors; known, yet regarded as unknown; dying, and yet we live on; beaten, and yet not killed; sorrowful, yet always rejoicing; poor, yet making many rich; having nothing, and yet possessing everything.

We have spoken freely to you, Corinthians, and opened wide our hearts to you. **6:3-11**

Key Action

If anyone has experience hardship from leaders or have stumble because of them, don't worry, god will most certainly deal with them one by one, but in the meantime we must forgive them, pray for them too. Please listen, Satan does not care who he corrupts, he is no respecter of persons; he is known as an "angel of light", which Paul says simply means, sometimes Satin himself masquerades as an angel of light. In other words, sometimes people makes it look like they actually stands for good instead of evil, but truth be told, they are after something, your money or your soul, not in really saving souls. Start reading the bible for yourself, listen and do what you're told.

Key Prayer

Lord, I will bless you at all time, your praise shall continually be in my mouth! Keep me in your perfect care, let me know when a snake is there.

Amen

Time to take our last and final break,
see you back in 30 minutes!

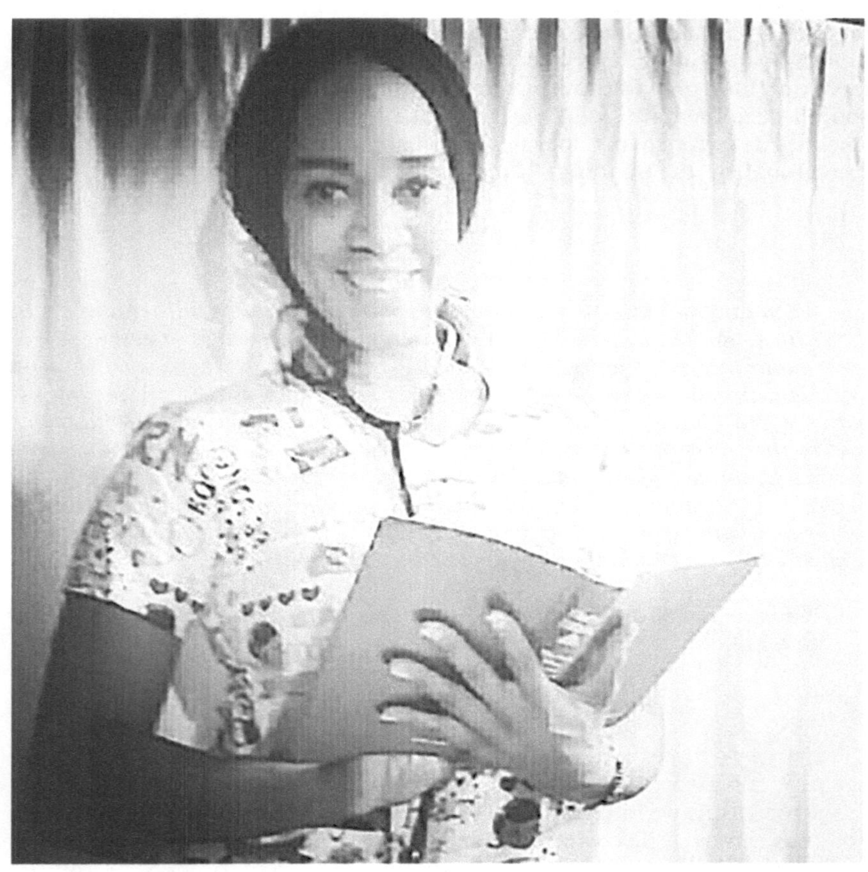

   Miss Asondra StarN'air

Galatians

Room Forty-Eight (New Testament)

Before we go on any further, it's important that you know **Apostle Paul** is the author of the Epistles, also known as *letters*. Although thirteen of the books of the New Testament are traditionally ascribed to Paul, modern scholars think that he only wrote eight of them: **Romans, 1 Corinthians, 2 Corinthians, Galatians, Colossians, Philippians, Philemon, and Thessalonians.** These ancient letter were written by Paul to an individual or groups. Many of them were *Didactic* which means, they were intended to teach, particularly in having moral instruction as an ulterior motive.

Well I guess one could say, *"Me Too"* because I also have and ulterior motive, and it's the same as Apostle Paul and so many others, I want people saved and I want them to *"Stay Saved."*

Okay, now let's go in and check this room out and let me point this out too, the **"Epistles"** rooms are smaller than the others but just as powerful. So here we have prejudiced behavior and hatred going on in this room. The Jews were tripping shall we say, (they exhibited entitlement like behavior, e.g. superiority, prejudice, whites enslaving blacks "you get the picture!") they hate *'Gentiles'* which means any person who is "Not" Jewish—you and me, black or white. Well in this room there's some bickering going on, the issue was whether we non-Jews can be part of the promise.

What's the promise? In one word, *'Heaven!'* along with the thousands and thousands of promises in the bible, like prosperity, freedom, peace, success, safety, favor, togetherness, unity; no hatred or strife, "Live Forever", receive "Eternal life"!

So, Apostle Paul responds by sending back a letter, an epistle, letting them know that God belongs to Everybody, Everywhere, that will serve and do what he ask. (I am paraphrasing) But that was the bottom line.

Anybody who wants to become a Christian and be part of that promise can be *'BUT'* mind you, you must be born again, we cannot live for this world and God too, that's not going to do, Jew or non-Jew!

Candid Snapshot

If you want God,
Signed, Sealed, delivered
He's Yours!

But He comes with a manual, *'The Holy Bible'* read it daily, it's our:

Basic Instructions Before Leaving Earth! "Book"

Before the coming of this faith, we were held in custody under the law, locked up until the faith that was to come would be revealed. So the law was our guardian until Christ came that we might be justified by faith. Now that this faith has come, we are no longer under a guardian.

So in Christ Jesus you are all children of God through faith, for all of you who were baptized into Christ have clothed yourselves with Christ. There is neither Jew nor Gentile, neither slave nor free, nor is there male and female, for you are all one in Christ Jesus. If you belong to Christ, then you are Abraham's seed, and heirs according to the promise. **3:23-29**

Key Actions

Become a servant of God, not of man!

Key Prayer

Lord, come into my heart, take over my life,
I'll make you my Lord and savior. **Amen**

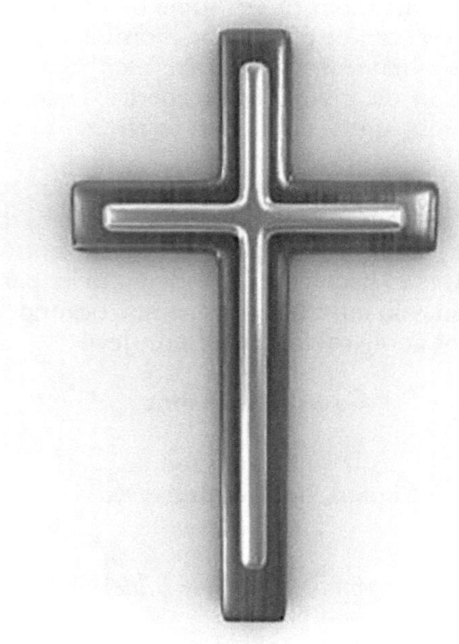

Ephesians

Room Forty-Nine (New Testament)

Welcome to the room of encouragement! Hello come on in, relax for a while, if you need some encouragement well you've come to the right place. You are not alone in your suffering, Christian all over the world have suffered and been persecuted, many have died. But you are still alive, dry your eyes!

Ephesians reminds us that God's eternal plans is in full effect, through his son Jesus Christ and his body 'the church'. If you are a believer, you are safe, you're saved, you got it made! No need to be disappointed or grieve our God is with us and he's given the believer everything he or she will even need. It's up to the believer to believe.

Some of you are weak in this area, mainly because you won't read. Reading God's Word, is a must, in fact, *his* word is the only thing we can trust!

Before we leave out of this room let me say this also, to me, this room represent stability. In here you will get the motivation and direction you need to help you to stay focus on your walk with Christ. This room may be small, but once you come out of it you'll be standing strong and tall!

Candid Snapshot

Stay with God, and God will stay with you. He has provision for all those who remain true. If we say we are God's people, then we should know that we are not allowed to do whatever we want to do for example, fornicate and lay with whomever we choose, (had to throw that one in there) no, no, no, you'll lose! Real Christians, we don't roll like that! If you want God's provisions, "Tip' ***Make Smarter Decisions"!***

Key Verse

As a prisoner for the Lord, then, I urge you to live a life worthy of the calling you have received. Be completely humble and gentle; be patient, bearing with one another in love. Make every effort to keep the unity of the Spirit through the bond of peace. There is one body and one Spirit, just as you were called to one hope when you were called; one Lord, one faith, one baptism; one God and Father of all, who is over all and through all and in all. **4:1-6**

Key Action

Live and love like Christians, encourage each other. No need for jealousy or competition. Take action, stay true to 'The Mission'. "Spread the Gospel of Jesus Christ' Win Souls, Go Fishing!

Key Prayer

Lord, remove anything that is not pleasing to you out of my heart and out of my lifestyle. Lord help me to be a better person, help me to love the "Christian Life" I pray for change. *"Teach Me Your Ways".*

Amen

Philippians

Room Fifty (New Testament)

This is the happy room, "NO More Tears!" For it is written, we are going to suffer, experience trials and tribulations of various kinds down here, but we shall overcome it all.

Apostle Paul can attest to this, it seems he spent most of his ministry behind bars. And while in there he wrote lots of letters too, (also known as epistles) well now he's writing to Philippians, another community of believers I supposed.

In his letters, he's encouraging everyone to rejoice in the good and bad times. His overall mindset was this, if we living for Christ, we are alive *"Celebrate," 'Don't Worry, Be Happy'!* God is with us! He sent his son to die for us and too, provide for us, give us everything we need. But like Paul said, if we die, we can rejoice because we will be with Christ forever!

So get it together, stop all the worry and despair, you are never alone, God is there. This is a happy room therefore, no more gloom. Dry your eyes, 'No More Tears and No More Fears, The Messiah's Near!

This room will help you deal with some of those fears, make you strong, give you peace of mind too, and remind you of how much god loves you. So, *'No More Tears', Only Happy Lives Here!!!!!!*

Candid Snapshot

From: Apostle Paul,
"Finally, brothers and sisters, whatever is true, whatever is noble, whatever is right, whatever is pure, whatever is lovely, whatever is admirable —if anything is excellent or praiseworthy, think about such things." **4:8**

"Ahoy" Tears Of Joy!

Key Verse

Rejoice in the Lord always. I will say it again: Rejoice! Let your gentleness be evident to all. The Lord is near. Do not be anxious about anything, but in every situation, by prayer and petition, with thanksgiving, present your requests to God. And the peace of God, which transcends all understanding, will guard your hearts and your minds in Christ Jesus. **4:4**

Key Action

Keep your head up! Fight the good fight of faith! Let the world know, your walk with Christ will never be a mistake!

Key Prayer

Lord I praise your 'Holy' name, I praise you, I praise you,
I praise your 'Holy' name! For you are God Almighty, Lord of lords,
King of kings. Tell me what you want, I'll do anything!

 MISS ASONDRA STARN'AIR

Colossians

Room Fifty-One(New Testament)

Come in and have a seat. There are some very disturbing things going on in this room. It seems there are some strange theories creeping in the world about Jesus authenticity. Making Jesus out to be some sort of angel, and not the son of man. And still today, we have some who don't believe he ever existed; and if he did, many question whether he did all that the Bible says he did.

Well as for me and my house this bears repeating, we will serve the LORD! So many today have gone astray by mixing the gospel message with worthless beliefs. Apostle Paul reminds us here that the way we live is important, and that we ought to keep our focus on Christ, that's the only way "Home"!

Listen everybody, it is very important that each of us read the bible for ourselves, I can't stress this enough. Don't be afraid anymore to do that, don't let others and their negative comments keep you from finding out the truth for yourself. And don't worry about all the big words etc. And if you want to know the truth about it, check this out, I don't go around quoting scriptures after scriptures, but I know my way around my father's house; (The Bible) the holy spirit brings the scripture to mind automatically for me when I need it. And here's another thing too, I still can't pronounce many of the names, or follow all that's happening in the bible myself, the holy spirit breaks most of it down for me, so that even a child can understand. I love it! Each and every time I read my bible, I get new insight, and I began to understand and see more light! All this can happen to each one of you if you let it, so"let it!" And please don't feel intimidated by this incredible life awakening huge book, no on the contrary, do what I did, *"Get Hooked!"*

That's right, get yourself saved by any means necessary; okay, so I've had my say on the matter, now it's up to **"YOU"** to reject the latter, for the world can't save you; nor can I, but I'm trying.

We've all heard it said, *"you can lead a horse to the water but, you can't make it drink!"* Ah, but my job as an oracle of the Lord, is to at least make people "think" is there really a place call hell? Yes, so I implore you,"hurry" get to know the bible well!

Candid Snapshot

People are going to challenge your beliefs. Don't let anyone stray you from the truth, be ready to defend the gospel at all times. Just as important, be forgiving, loving and kind. Stay on the righteous path, walk the thin line.

Key Verse

I want you to know how hard I am contending for you and for those at Laodicea, and for all who have not met me personally. My goal is that they may be encouraged in heart and united in love, so that they may have the full riches of complete understanding, in order that they may know the mystery of God, namely, Christ, in whom are hidden all the treasures of wisdom and knowledge. I tell you this so that no one may deceive you by fine-sounding arguments. For though I am absent from you in body, I am present with you in spirit and delight to see how disciplined you are and how firm your faith in Christ is. **2:1-2**

Key Action

"Stay Discipline In Christ!"
Keep reading and doing his word, every day and every night! *"Live right!"*

Key Prayer

Lord please give me the words to say when I don't know how to express myself, I am not eloquent in speech like others, sometimes I stumble. I need help in expressing myself. Please give me all that I need, when I need it!

Amen

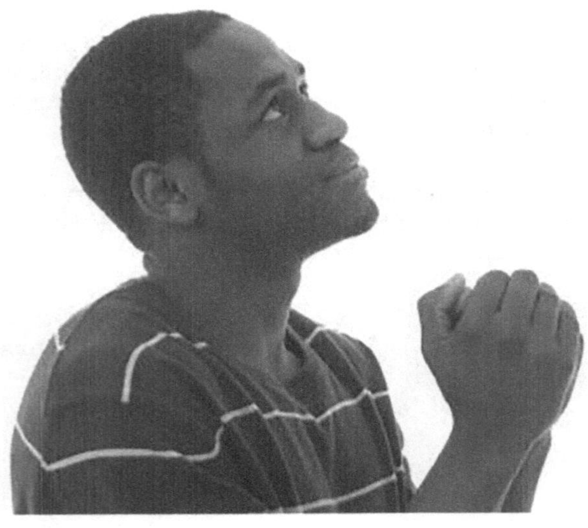

 MISS ASONDRA STARN'AIR

1 Thessalonians

Hello and welcome, meet the Thessalonian's, The *Thessalonian's* were a community of believers who pretty much were babes in Christ, newbies, shall we say, they had only been Christians for a short period of time, no more than a few months. We may have some "Me too's" out there! So because these newbies were new believers in Christ, Apostle Paul kept close watch on them. He sent letters back and forth to Timothy to address some of the newbies concerns, for example, would believers who died miss out on the resurrection? There were also reminders from Paul that Christians must stay with their faith in spite of persecutions.

Today if you are a believer, take heed to those words also, when I was being persecuted, lied on and falsely accused, bullied, whatever, I did what Apostle Paul suggested, I held on to my faith, I stayed focus on the task, I did not hate nor retaliate. We as Christian must remain a *"light"* in a dark world.

This is a good room to chill out in, especially if you're a newbie too, "just got born again." And I must say, there are a lot of do's and don'ts inside this room but, there's also lots of inspiring conversations too, you'll enjoy this room, hope to see you back soon.

Candid Snapshot

Stay with your faith in spite of your suffering. God is with his people!

Key Verse

Be joyful always; pray continually; give thanks in all circumstances, for this is God's will for you in Jesus Christ. **5:16**

Key Action

Pray continually, spend time with God daily, meditate on his word.

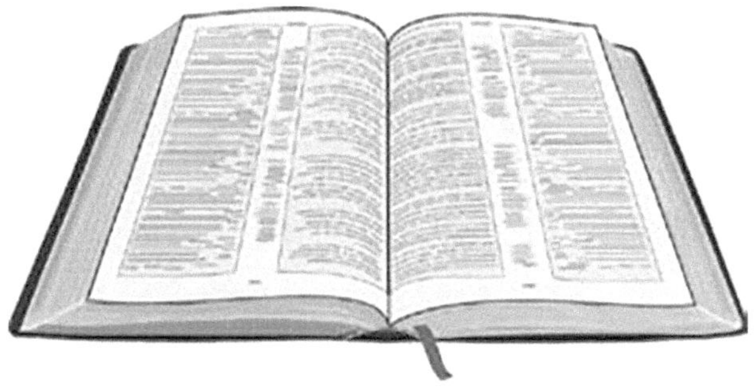

Key Prayer

Lord may my lips speak only righteousness, help remove all gossip and slander from my mouth, make me worthy to be your servant.

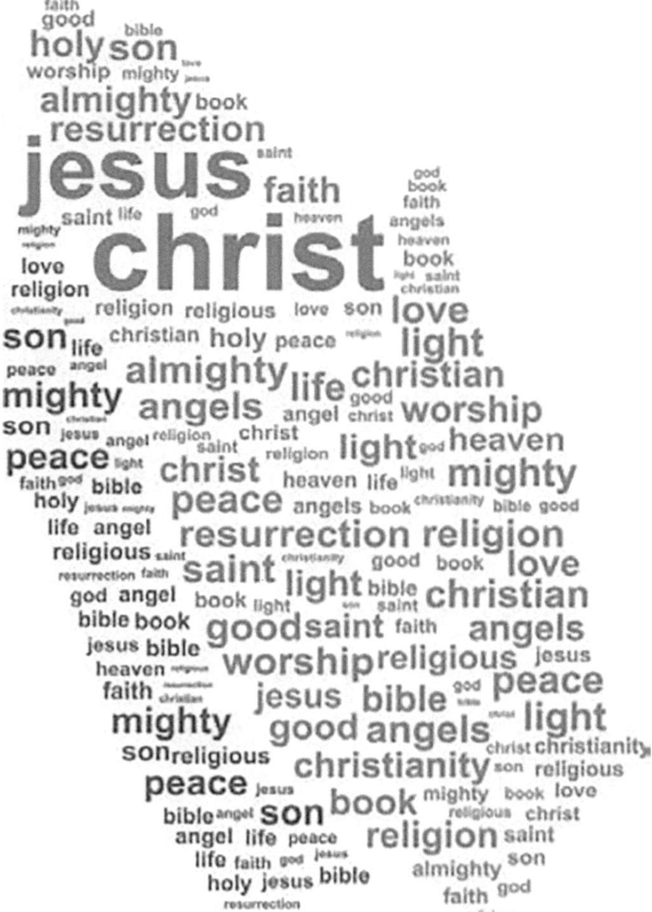

Amen

2 Thessalonians

Room Fifty-Three (New Testament)

Here in this room, we have an issue of concern—whether or not God's people, (*'Christians'*) should continue to try to build their lives down here in this wicked, evil and corrupt world, or should we just be still and wait on Christ return?

The Thessalonian's wanted to know the answer to that and how about you? Do you want to know? If you do stay in this room and read what's saith the Lord. Today this is still an issue, I have heard it said, why should we build anything here on earth when this is not our home? Why strive to do anything in this wicked old world? He's coming back soon.

Well, I'll tell you why, in my own words. *'Let Your Light Shine'* to me, means doing excellent work in Jesus's name so that others can see the difference between Christians and the world. People should be able to clearly see that you are different and do not belong to this world. One of the ways we do

this is through our everyday life, which includes our careers and dreams. We never stop working, especially if we want to eat.

Furthermore, we are expected to not only go on and build/work, we are expected to do it with excellence, no matter what, because our Creator is Excellent. We are not the children of a lesser God, the world is.

I know it's tough living here on earth, like Christ, many of us have some of the scars to prove it. But here's the thing, we are not alone in our sufferings; Apostle Paul suffered too, and also true, God is with his people, we're in this thing together, we got the kind of love that last forever. Therefore, we must carry on, we must keep building. If you have a dream, live it out, keep learning, keep growing, go back to school if you desire to, keep reaching for the stars, but wait, not the stars of this world, the star of Bethlehem, the *Star N air* that died for you and me, the only star I want to see.

In this room you'll get a chance to read Apostle Paul's letter encouraging faithful Christians to hang in there, to keep working, and continue living righteous lives, Hey did I mention, there was a time, Jesus opened blind eyes? And he still does, Listen, I was once blind, I wouldn't read the bible, I thought it was a waste of time, "I was blind". However, once I began to read it, "I could see", now the rest is history! I'm saved, I'm free, the devil has to flee! Now before I end this conversation, here's something you ought to know too, the bible tells us in **Matt. 24:36** that no man or even the angels know when Jesus will return. So with that being said, its becomes quite obvious that we should keep on keeping on. We should continue to work and strive to living the best life possible while here on earth. So, go ahead "Everybody", "Build, Build, Build" and if you have special talents, "go for it" reach for the stars, I hope you catch *'Jesus!'*

And let all of God's people say
Amen!

Candid Snapshot

Get Back to Work, "Build" Remember, You Don't Work, You Don't Eat!

Key Verse

Concerning the coming of our Lord Jesus Christ and our being gathered to him, we ask you, brothers not to come easily unsettled or alarmed by some prophecy, reports or letters supposed to have come from us, saying that the day of the Lord has come. **2:1-2**

Key Action

Don't Ever Stop Building!

Key Prayer

Father God, give me the strength and everything else I need to carry on. Give me insight, *"Grant Me Wisdom"*, *"Holy Spirit"* Please "Turn the Light On!"

Amen

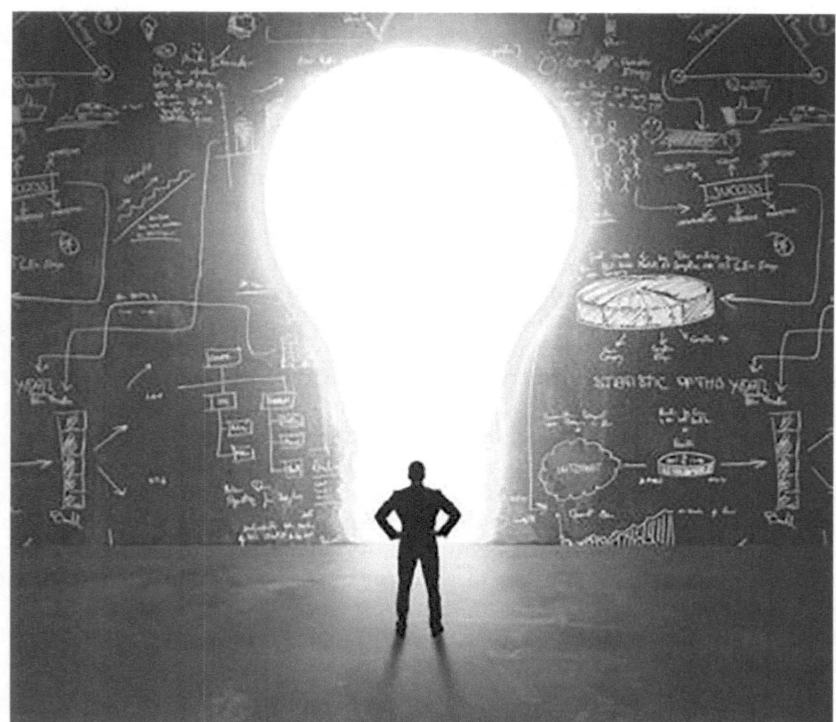

1 Timothy

Room Fifty-Four (New Testament)

Come in here, meet "Timothy," what a mighty, mighty good man! I'd love to marry someone like him, he was All- In for Christ! He set out to serve the one and only true God, to me, he had some of the characteristics as Abraham; like I said, he was a "mighty, mighty good man!" Timothy also was a faithful and true friend of Apostle Paul. They worked very closely together, Paul would send Timothy to continue on with his work in the churches, delevering messages that needed to be addressed. Timothy was someone who was strong and active in his faith and a willing participant in the cause of wining souls for Christ. But he struggled "me too" it wasn't easy for him either; he became weary in his Christian life. Apostle Paul's advice to young Timothy was, instead of giving up and thinking, *What's the use?* (like I have thought several times and I'm sure some of you have too) instead, live wholeheartedly with God's bigger picture in mind.

And let me tell you, there is a bigger picture. For example, I never thought I would be called by God to write *A Caregiver's Bible to Excellence.*

God has a plan for each and every one of us, so we mustn't give up!

When you feel like giving up, *"don't"!* Just grab your bibles and come right back in here and reread Paul's letter to young Timothy, and just pretend Paul's talking to you, I do. Stay strong, listen: *"Let us not become weary in doing good, for at the proper time we will reap a harvest if we do not give up."* **Gal.6:9**

Candid Snapshot

Sometimes I know that life can be so very overwhelming at times but still, this is *'Not'* the time to give up. Not at all, perhaps all that's needed is a little rest, nevertheless, we mustn't quit. Christian brothers like Timothy had Apostle Paul, but who do **"YOU"** have to encourage you or catch you when you fall? Well Jesus told me to tell you *"He's there"*, if you need him *"Just Call."*

Key Verse

*Fight the good fight of faith; take hold of the eternal life
to which you were called, and you made the good confession
in the presence of many witnesses.* **6:12**

Key Action

Keep Fighting The Good Fight Of Faith, Don't Quit!
No Matter What, You Got What It Takes!

Lord, keep me a soldier in your army, rejuvenate me, send me back out to be a light, in a dark world.

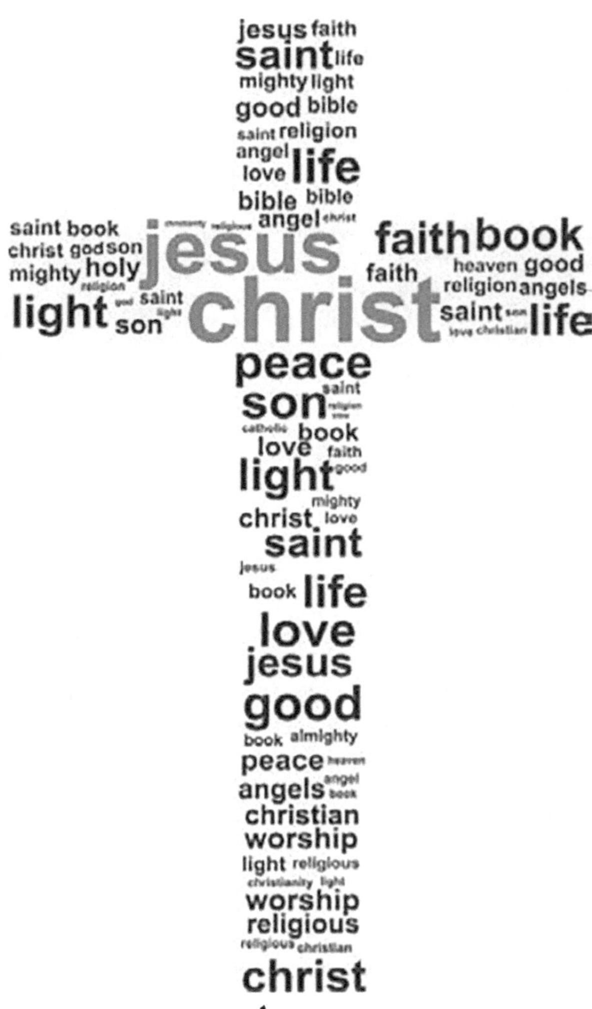

2 Timothy

Room Fifty-Five (New Testament)

Come in, welcome back, It is with great, great sorrow that I inform all of you in this room that this would be the last letter to young Timothy that Apostle Paul wrote before he died. It's a personal letter, expressing Paul's deepest feeling. He also wanted to assure Timothy that, although his earthly life was coming to an end, he would be with God—that he had been given the promise of eternal life and had fought the good fight. He also wanted Timothy to press on, to stay focused and firm in facing the persecution headed his way.

It seems to me that Paul was a warrior all the way to the end. Whatever the cost, he was willing to pay it. I have never met anyone like him and don't believe I ever will. I am inspired by him. It's as if I'm a young female Timothy in some way he talking to. I have been persecuted so much that I have become invincible, unmoved, and even more determined to serve God, also until the end. If you too are on the same path to eternal life—as you can see, it will not be easy—you are going to have adversaries trying to stop you, and unfortunately, it will be the ones whom you least expect. People in high places and "Fake Smiling Faces" (FSF) is the best humanistic way I can describe it.

I don't want my comment here to confuse you, so let me elaborate a little here. It is true, according to the Bible (Eph. 6:12), that we are not fighting against flesh and blood but against the ruler (Satan), against the authorities, against the powers of this dark world, and against the spiritual forces of evil in the heavenly realms.

But these forces need people to do their dirty work. Yes, these unseen demons, like Satan or fallen angels if you will, all need "flesh" individuals, humans, unbelievers, haters, liars and deceivers to allow these principalities to enter their minds and take over their souls and do their destructive work against God. So, no, we are Not fighting against flesh and blood, we are to pray for the souls that have been captured by these dark forces, plus forgive them too especially if someone has hurt you. Every day, all of God's people must wear the full armor of God because the bible says,: *God's light has come into the world, but people loved the darkness more than the light, for their actions were evil.* **John3:19** Therefore we must protect our minds, body and soul. Here's a sad fact, unbelievers are all under the influence of the evil ones. The farther away we are from our God, the closer we are to Satan. I don't know how else to put it!

My Caregivers' cry is that no one be left behind yet it looks like I'll be weeping for quite some time.

Nevertheless, like young Timothy, loss souls, is what we *Must* help find.

Candid Snapshot

Apostle Paul is gone, yet his spirit lives on, he did what he came to do now the Apostle's torch has been pass over to Timothy and **YOU**, "Me Too". If you say you love Christ, then we all have a unique job to do. The motto: **Each One, Reach One, Teach One!** "It's My Turn Now" 'A Caregiver's Bible To Excellence', has stepped up to the plate, Denounce Unforgiveness, Jealousy and Hate". Apostle Paul is Dead, it's **YOUR** turn now, like Timothy, serve "Don't Hesitate!"

Key Verse

Paul, an apostle of Christ Jesus by the will of God, in keeping with the promise of life that is in Christ Jesus,
To Timothy, my dear son:
Grace, mercy and peace from God the Father and Christ Jesus our Lord.
I thank God, whom I serve, as my ancestors did, with a clear conscience, as night and day I constantly remember you in my prayers. Recalling your tears, I long to see you, so that I may be filled with joy. I am reminded of your sincere faith, which first lived in your grandmother Lois and in your mother Eunice and, I am persuaded, now lives in you also. For this reason I remind you to fan into flame the gift of God, which is in you through the laying on of my hands. For the Spirit God gave us does not make us timid, but gives us power, love and self-discipline. So do not be ashamed of the testimony about our Lord or of me his prisoner. Rather, join with me in suffering for the gospel, by the power of God. He has saved us and called us to a holy life—not because of anything we have done but because of his own purpose and grace. This grace was given us in Christ Jesus before the beginning of time, but it has now been revealed through the appearing of our Savior, Christ Jesus, who has destroyed death and has brought life and immortality to light through the gospel. And of this gospel I was appointed a herald and an apostle and a teacher. That is why I am suffering as I am. Yet this is no cause for shame, because I know whom I have believed, and am convinced that he is able to guard what I have entrusted to him until that day. What you heard from me, keep as the pattern of sound teaching, with faith and love in Christ Jesus. Guard the good deposit that was entrusted to you—guard it with the help of the Holy Spirit who lives in us. **1:8-13**

Key Action

Join Timothy and I as we continue to fight the good fight of faith. Wear The Armor of God.

Key Prayer

God be with us as we continue on where others have left off.
Lord keep your people safe and strong!

Amen

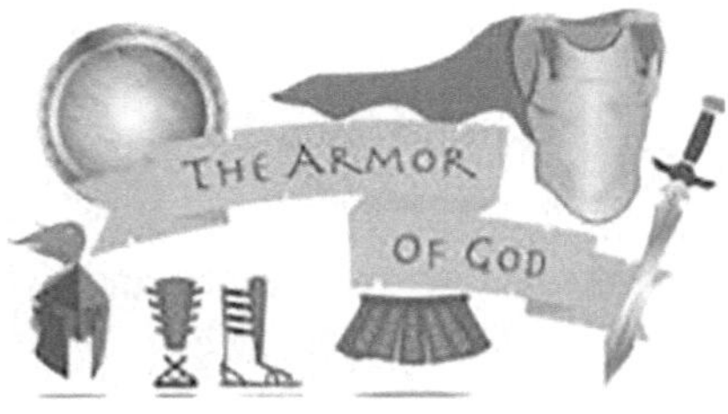

 Miss Asondra StarN'air

Titus

Room Fifty-Six (New Testament)

Here in this room, we get a chance to meet Titus, another one of Apostle Paul's associates. Titus's task was to help select leaders of the church and present the qualifications given by Paul to ensure leaders were in compliance with those qualifications. Titus was also to help instruct the believers in basic Christian teachings.

This world is still evil and will be until Christ return, so all of us today had better learn how to conduct ourselves down here. In a nut shell, *The Way We Live down Here Matters To God!*

Candid Snapshot

Those who walk upright has a responsible to help others walk upright! You do not have to be a leader of a church, you are the church, older woman are to teach younger woman, if their clothes or behavior is inappropriate, say something, but do it the Godly way of course, but do it. In the same way, older men are to do the same with younger men; help teach that young man respect and honor. Encourage marriage, godly homes, don't just let them run wild or roam. "Mentor Them", if you see something, say something!

Key Verse

Remind the people to be subject to rulers and authorities, "to be obedient, to be ready to do whatever is good" to slander no one, to be peaceable and considerate and to show true humility to all men. **3:1-2**

Key Action

Get Involved, Help others find their way!

Key Prayer

God use me in the service!
Send me, I will go....

Amen

Philemon

Room Fifty-Seven (New Testament)

Hello, and welcome to the room of *'Brotherly Love.'* Here, in this room, we celebrate freedom. Yes, we are no longer slaves. In God's eyes, if you are a Christian, both the slave and the master have now become one.

What this means is everyone no matter what your status in life is whether you're a caregiver, doctor, lawyer, butcher, baker, candle stick maker —each matters. And your nationality doesn't matter either—be it Jew or, like me, Gentile—it doesn't matter. And color ain't nothin' but a thang! Anyone who puts their trust in Christ, he or she will become God's people. Yes, a new creature in Christ, if you will. Therefore, let us all, come together as one body of Christ, and respect and love one another.

In this room you will learn about Philemon he was a slave owner. One of his slave just took off and ran away. His name was Onesimus, but during his escape, he ended up in Rome where Apostle Paul was. And one day he got a chance to hear one of Apostle Paul's Christian messages. After that, he was forever changed! Yes Onesimus became a true believer, almost kind of like what happened to me except I wasn't running from a person, I was running from the world. So, apparently, Apostle Paul got a chance to know this slave and became convinced that he was not the same person, he had changed, and ready to be a good and loyal servant of both Philemon and God. So Apostle Paul sent back a letter asking Philemon to receive him back, and he did.

But something amazing happened too, whereas before, their relationship was slave and master, "Now" it's *"Brotherly Love"*—they became equals, no slave or master mentality. Both developed the kind of love and respect that only comes from above *"Agape Love"*!

Let's Get us Some!

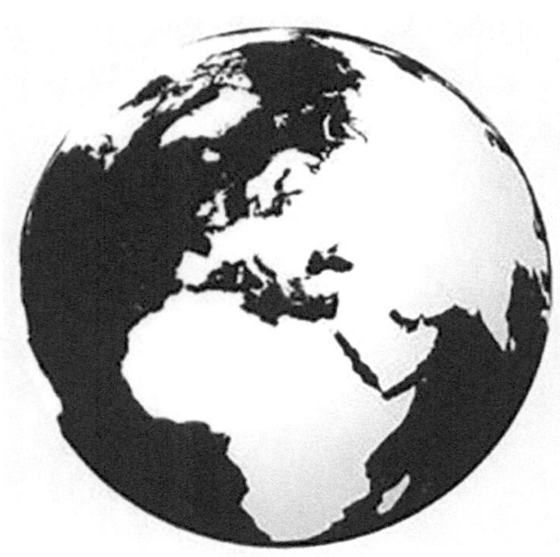

 MISS ASONDRA STARN'AIR

Candid Snapshot

Without Jesus in the mix, there can be no real Brotherly/Sisterly Love.
Jesus is the source of it all!

Key Verse

*Perhaps the reason he was separated from you for a little while was that you
might have him back forever— no longer as a slave, but better than a slave, as
a dear brother. He is very dear to me but even dearer to you, both as a fellow
man and as a brother in the Lord.* **1-15-16**

Key Action

Get with Christ, like so many of us, become his slave, if you do, you've got
it made!

Key Prayer

Lord, place me on *"YOUR"* potter's wheel, make me over,
this time I want to live for you and serve *"YOU"* for real.

Amen

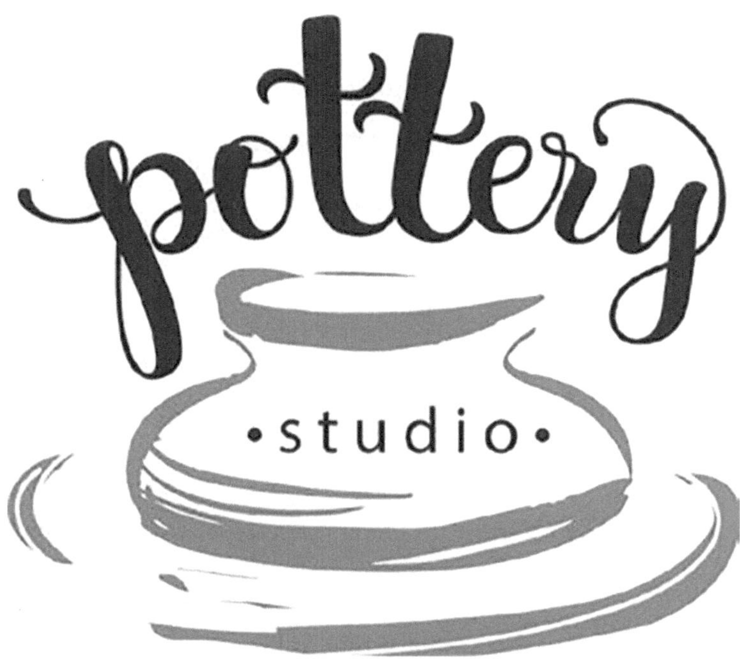

Hebrews

Room Fifty-Eight (New Testament)

In this room, we lift up our voices and sing, Hallelujah to the King!

Yes, Jesus died to restore everything—no more Old Testament or you returning to your old life. No more animal and crop sacrifices "All Done!" Today, because of Jesus's death on the cross, we now have it better than those who paved the way before us. What one does with this information, is now up to each individual. However, don't get it twisted, the wages of sin is still death. But this time **"YOU"** will decide, eternal life or death by the way you live. Not me, not Jesus, not God—you and you alone must choose this day whom you will serve.

In Hebrews, it clearly shows that, through the blood of Jesus, we have been saved. And we are no longer under the Law of Moses or the Jewish customs. ***"We Are Free!"*** *Hallelujah, Hallelujah, Hallelujah!* This is why, when I come in here, I get so excited!!!! World, I just can't hide it, (I'm not one of the pointers sisters,) but, *"help me Jesus"*, I'm about to lose control and I think I like it!

It says in Hebrews 1:1, "Long ago, God spoke many times and in many ways to our ancestors through the prophets, but now in these final days, he has spoken to us through his son" Jesus"

What that means to me is that Jesus is the one in charge—not me, not you, not the president, not my boss, whatever the cost, Jesus is the ruler over man and all things, hallelujah to the King. If you're down with that, stay on board! Say it with me:

JESUS IS LORD! JESUS IS LORD! JESUS IS LORD!

Candid Snapshot

Jesus Is The Only Way!

Key Verse

In the past God spoke to our ancestors through the prophets at many times and in various ways, but in these last days he has spoken to us by his Son, whom he appointed heir of all things, and through whom also he made the universe. **1:1**

Key Action

Read your Bibles daily, get to know Jesus, he is God's son, superior to angels, kings, billionaires, movie stars, actor's alike there is no other like him and no one will ever love and care for us the way he does. This is what I want you all to do, "Take Action!" and "No More Excuses!", Go out this week and buy yourself a nice bible and commit to one full year of reading it for yourself. If you don't do anything all year, do that! I promise you, your life will feel brand new, and remember, what God says in his word, *"He'll do!"*

Father, God, I am seeking wisdom, I have always be intimidated by the bible, I can hardly pronounce many of the words, not to mention the fact that, there's over a thousand pages. One thousand three hundred seventy-seven to be exact, and in some bibles a few pages more. That's been a little overwhelming too. But this time I'm not going to let that stop me, my prayer is this Lord, hold my hands. Ease my fears and anxieties, my mind tells me, I will not comprehend all that I am reading. So, Christ, if that does happen, help me Lord, reveal its meaning, explain the parables too, just don't let me quit, and go back on my word. Jesus, it is my hearts hope that I will fall deeply in love with you, like others have. Today, I am totally open and ready for the journey, excited too! I love you Lord and I want to get to know you better, right down to the letter! Help me do just that. Give me what I need, right now I desperately need you in my life, "I'm ready" there's no turning back!

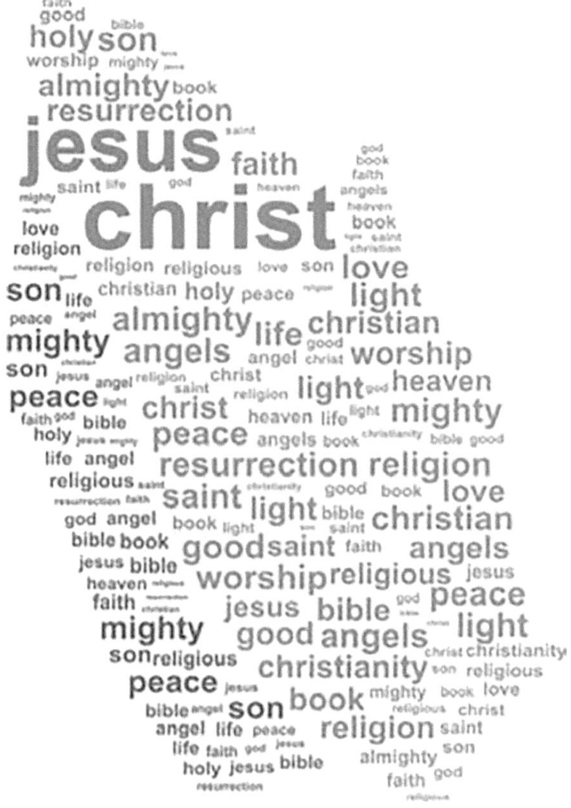

Amen

James

Room Fifty -Nine (New Testament)

Come, come, lets meet Jesus half-brother James. James also supported Jesus ministry. Here, James gives us some practical things we can use to help keep us living the Christian lifestyle. In this room James covers an array of topics and one that comes to mind that I think is of great importance is *'Faith and Deeds'* James says, and I quote" *What good is it, my brothers and sisters, if someone claims to have faith but has no deeds?* **2:14-26** "Later on, go back and read". What he is simply saying here is, faith always has something like *"Action"* to show for it! For instance, like what I'm doing writing; God called me to write this book, and I took *"Action!"* It is by faith that this book will be in the hands of millions and millions of people. And it's my hope as well, many will get saved. So because I acted, and like "Abraham", *"Believed God"*, I have something tangible to show for my faith, you're reading it now *'A Caregiver's Bible To Excellence!'* "Hence Faith and Deeds", Tell me now, how many more examples do **"YOU"** need? **Faith Without Works Is "DEAD!"** From now on, "don't just talk", do something with your mouth instead!

Candid Snapshot

Use these practical guidelines given by brother James it's there to help us in our Christian walk, and also help set us apart from the rest of the world. Just as important we must began to exercise our faith like we exercise our bodies in the gym; It's going to help take us places we've never been.

Key Verse

Is anyone in trouble? he should pray. **5:13**

Key Action

Exercise your faith daily, which means you *MUST* read your bibles.

Key Prayer

Heavenly father, send your holy spirit to help guide me, as I prepare to take action. Once called, I know you will give me everything that I need to succeed.

And by *"Faith and Deed"*, I shall proceed!

Amen, Lord be with me!

1 Peter

Room Sixty (New Testament)

Today, in this room, we meet another apostle. His name is Peter.

I like being with Apostle Peter, he is someone who through all his suffering, triumphed. He did not let his trials and tribulations get in the way of his commitment to God. Here Apostle Peter remind us that suffering will be part of the Christian's walk. That's true, hey, there's no way around it and I'm a witness to that fact, unfortunately, one cannot be a follower of Christ and not suffer—**"YOU"** will suffer.

Hopefully you've read *'A StarN'air Story'* in the book of StarN'air but, if you haven't yet, go back and read; because now I know for sure now, that all that persecution and pain I endured was really a confirmation that I didn't belong to this world. Had I belonged to this world, I wouldn't have suffered as I did. **John 15:18-19** This Apostle reminds us that when under attack, we must stand firm in our faith, do whatever it takes. And two, we *Must* continue to spread the gospel all over the place. Stay focus and strong people, run your race!

Not to change the subject, but I know that there are lots of distractions out there, we live in a world where each day has its own troubles. But that's where God comes in at, just like in biblical times we will be faced with all sorts of inconveniences and challenges, that's life. But God knows all that is occurring, and his plan for us goes beyond our present troubles.

I can't say this enough, *"TRUST HIM"* denounce sinful living, be all loving and forgiving! Be reminded also that some of the things we are faced with are there to teach us lessons, build our faith and help us mature.

Over the years this room has help build a more solid foundation in my walk with the Lord, yes it has, it gave me a more tenacious grip on how I am to conduct myself here on earth. Stay in this room long enough and it'll do the same for you —maybe more.

Nevertheless, although we suffer, Peter's letters also brings encouragement, hope and grace for believers like you and me who sometimes feel abandon by God. God has not abandoned us, he wouldn't ever abandon his people. So never think like that, instead we are to keep on fighting yet still, find a way to rejoice in our suffering too; God loves you! Furthermore, we celebrate, we rejoice because his people know Jesus is coming back soon and his people will one day rule.

I leave you with this my sister's and brother's, *Good* is more powerful than evil, *Love* is more powerful than hate and everything God promised to his people will be given to us by works, good deeds and faith.

Candid Snapshot

When life throws lemons at you, ask, is that all you got? If it is, make lemonade! When life throws stones at you, don't falter, pick them up, and build God an altar. Then, after you have done all you can do, "Stand" God will single out whose who?

Like Peter, we got a job to do, so never, ever lose focus on who you belong to! "Stand Strong in Your Faith!" Don't Retaliate or Hate.

Key Verse

Therefore prepare your minds for action; be self –controlled; set your hope fully on the grace to be given when Jesus Christ is revealed. As obedient children do not conform to the evil desires you had when you lived in ignorance. 1:13-14

Key Action

When persecution, hated or mistreated, keep doing good.

Key Prayer

Heavenly Father, *"Holy Spirit"* and all your goodness, please come to me, help me. Don't let me grow weary in doing good, keep me on the battle field, renew my strength, right now I feel all alone, wounded, left in the woods. "Come rescue me!"

Amen

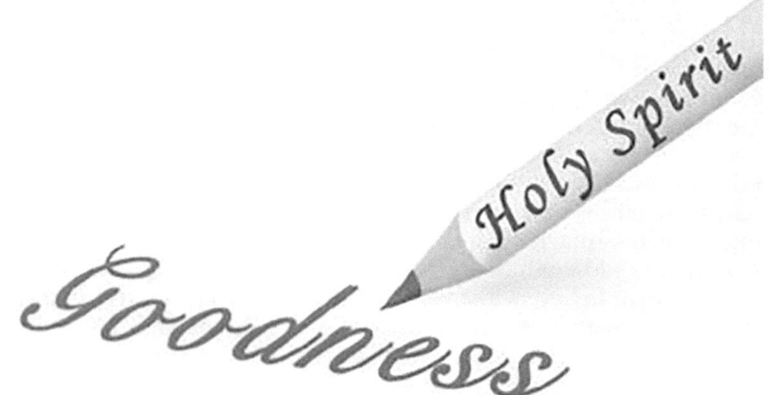

2 Peter

This is the last letter from Apostle Peter, telling Christians to beware of false teaching and those out to destroy the truth by adding their own ideas ahead of the church teaching. He also told us to stand strong in the midst of numerous pressures to conform to this world—don't. But remember, Christ is coming back and He will do away with the current world as we know it. Therefore, do not become attached to it, is his message.

He also informs us that the world is seeking to undo all that God is doing, but we, as Christians, must resist all such pressure and continue to live godly lives.

Candid Snapshot

Hold on to the truth, false teachers promoting moral compromise and doctrinal errors, is a disgrace to us all. We must stand strong in the truth, protect it to by no way of compromise.

Key Verse

But there were also false prophets among the people, just as there will be false teachers among you. They will secretly introduce destructive heresies, even denying the sovereign Lord who bought them—bringing swift destruction on themselves. **2:1**

Key Action

Be a responsible Christian, read the bible for yourself. Protect what you have with Christ, don't gamble or roll the dice!

Key Prayer

Lord, give me the gift of discernment!

Amen

1 John

Room Sixty-Two (New Testament)

In this room, John addresses those who are dear to him as little children—like the way God sees us. I love this. He gives us practical instructions for Christian living. He tells us Jesus was really God in human form. In other words, those who know Jesus also know the Father.

John's core message is the same message, as far as I'm concerned, with all the other apostles, leaders, and believers—Jesus is the only way to the Father. In fact, Christ says, *"I Am the way, the truth and the life. No one comes to the father except through me."* **John 14:6.** So there you have it, and with that being said, if there's anybody out there that wants to be saved and see God face to face one day, then come from amongst them. Who is the *"THEM"* we're referring to? What else, **"The World"** of course and all its lures, for example, let's take your lover, the one you're not married to, how about that one, or hey what about this one, your drug dealer, and the bottle of gin, you think is your friend — Lord have mercy, will the madness ever end! And let's not forget about the **"My Way"** selfish lifestyles, "oh no", wait a minute, don't touch that dial! Lastly, what about **"The Proud"**? For crying out loud, does Christ dying on the cross mean anything, Lord have mercy, let the angels sing. **"Repent"**, worship *"The KING!"* I do believe that if John were still alive today, he'd say the same thing.

Candid Snapshot

Live in God's love, Love in God's Love, Stay in Love this way!

Key Scripture

Do not love the world or anything in the world. If anyone loves the world, love for the Father is not in them.
For everything in the world—the lust of the flesh, the lust of the eyes, and the pride of life—comes not from the Father but from the world.
The world and its desires pass away, but whoever does the will of God lives forever. **2:15-17**

Key Action

Come Out of The Darkness into His Marvelous Light, "Live Up Right!"

Key Prayer

Lord I am a sinner who can't seem to stop sinning, I party just about every weekend, drugs and alcohol fornication and all; I've been at this most of my life now, every bodies doing it, living this way, it's fun, but there are side effects. I experiencing them right now, I don't feel healthy anymore. I want to

 Miss Asondra StarN'air

change, but I don't know how to change, my way has become the norm, not just for me but my friends too. Lord, if you can handle all of what I'm telling you and changed that for me, please do, I want you too. Lord I am sorry, so, so very sorry about how I have lived, I haven't honored you at all and I've been horrible to a lot of people too, Lord I need you. Please help me turn around, I want to come out of the world. I am in desperate need of a savior right about now, my life is a mess, nothing but drugs, thugs, booze and the blues. And too, I'm tired of feeling sexually used and abused. I can do better, and I can live better too. Lord this is my cry out to you: Jesus come in my life, clean me up, do what you need to do, Lord, I'll surrender to you.

Amen

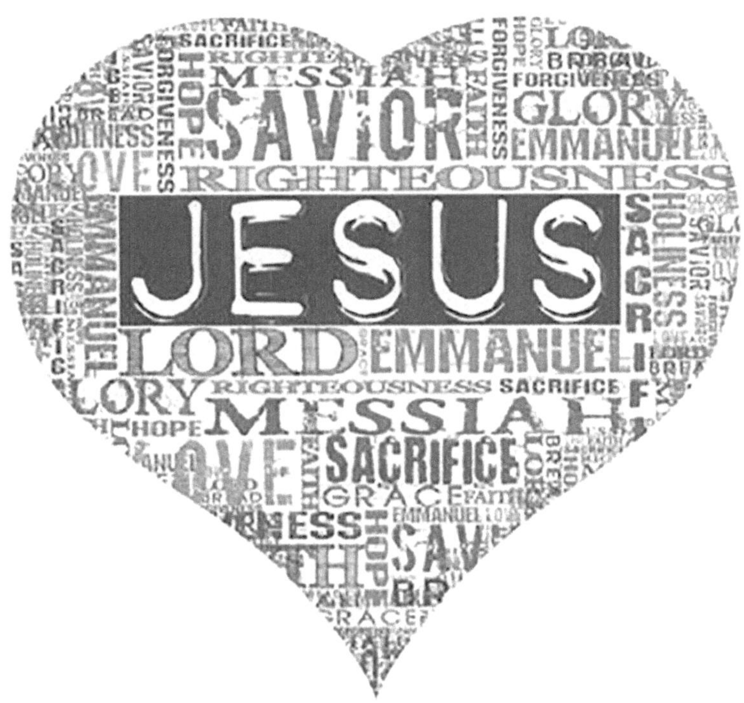

2 John

Room Sixty-Three (New Testament)

Here, John sends a second letter to a Christian woman to encourage "Christian Love!" And in that letter he also spoke about discernment, and how we are to make sure we are well-read in scriptures so that we will not be deceived by false teaching.

Furthermore, John also asked that believers do not participate in evil endeavors and to stay strong and committed to doing what is right.

I believe what he's simply asking us here is to **"Live In Truth!"**

Fast forward to **"NOW"** today's world is the devil's playground. 'Real Christian' really has to be on guard 24-7. We have got to start looking at lifestyles and behavior, not just what comes out of a person's mouth. Be wise, anyone can say I love you. And take heed too, some bible scholars, with their sophisticated devices, and large following may not be who you think they are? Don't be fooled, "Pride" and "Money" rules this world. All in all, hear this: Don't Be Impressed with Anybody! Not even me, 'JESUS" is all you need to focus on and see! Be smart, play it safe, because there are too many wolfs in sheep clothing out here, and once they hook you, there may be no escape.

Pick up a bible, it's never too late!

Read Your Bibles Every day!
Rebuke the devil and he'll stay away.

Candid Snapshot

The best way for us to keep on keeping on is to follow Johns call to obedience, truth, love and hospitality toward one another. We must ***"Read Our Bibles Daily"*** so that we will be certain of what we believe without compromise or faltering, this is the hallmark of Christianity!

Key Verse

Grace, mercy and peace from God the Father and from Jesus Christ, the Father's Son, will be with us in truth and love. 1:3

Key Action

Let no one read the bible for you, if you can read, **READ!**

Hear this, if you don't read, you don't grow, if you don't grow, you don't know nothing! People can tell you anything and they will. Ain't no such thing as purple rain!

 Miss Asondra StarN'air

Key Prayer

I am in need of change, come into my life and rebuild it in Jesus name. Teach Lord, how to live according to your word.

Amen.

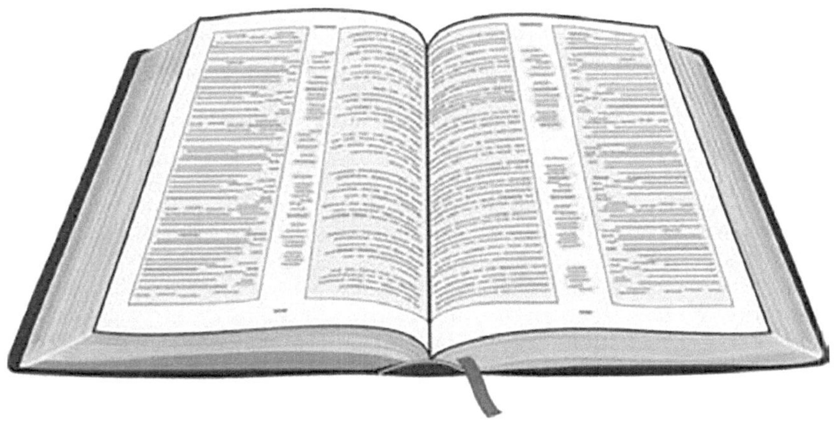

3 John

Room Sixty-Four (New Testament)

This is John's third letter, this time to a friend named Galus. John wants Galus to help support preachers who were traveling to preach the good news and to help provide food and shelter for them and anything else they might need, I would imagine.

He also wanted Christians to support one another, John said those Christians working against one another—it is the same as working against God, and they are actually doing the work of Satan.

Personally, I don't want to tell you how many times I have seen this, Christians hating on other Christians. In my opinion, these are not real Christian we do don't act or behave like that. I agree with John, that's the work of Satan, stay clear of that.

Outside the church, it gets even worse. How does one find unification in a world that plots and schemes, using Christians too as their prey? Warning, there are corrupt and evils minds out there, and many times it's the ones you least expect, not everyone is true blue if you know what I mean, so beware! The Bible says this "You Will Know Them By Their Fruit" by I say too, don't be impressed with a "Big Office" and ah "Fine Suit!"

In the meantime, let's love and care for each other. If another Christian needs help, anyone for that matter—help them.

Candid Snapshot

Today, we live in a high-tech age where we can communicate in so many ways. Emails, cell phones, face-book, chat rooms, tweets, texts and who knows what else will link in... but what about good old fashion face to face, Christian friendships?

It's missing, it's not there, it seems to be a thing of the pass. Every ones seems quite satisfied with five minute friendships, over some kind of tech device. If we want real friendships we must make time for it! And that means spending more face to face time together. Friend are not to be taken for granted, we must get back to building quality friendships, no one should be without one. Just like no one should be without Jesus, He's the best friend you will ever have.

Key Verse

Dear friend, do not imitate what is evil but what is good. Anyone who does what is good is from God. Anyone who does what is evil has not seen God. 1:11

Key Action

Find someone to build a real friendship with, start with Jesus first! He will show you what love and loyalty looks like.

Key Prayer

Dear God bless my life with the gift of friendship, for those who have chosen to be my friend, " I am so very grateful"!

Make me worthy of their friendship as well. Together let us rejoice in the name of Jesus Christ our Lord and Savior, Please Lord grant me this favor.

Amen

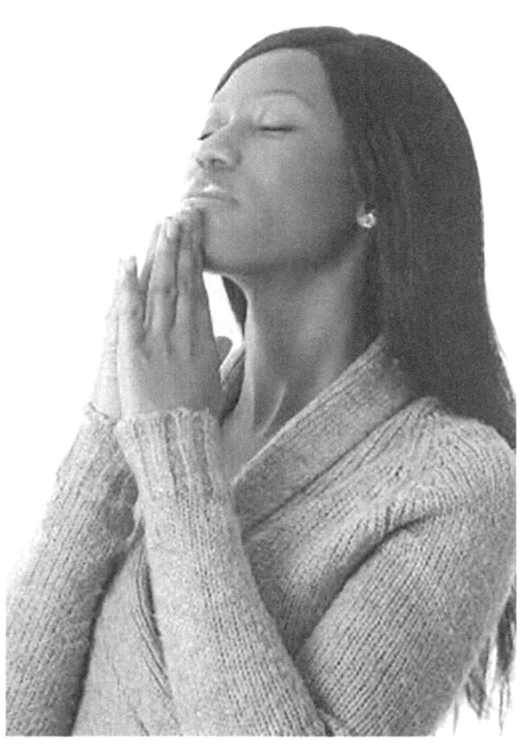

Jude

Room Sixty-Five (New Testament)

In this room, it's not what you say that matters but how one lives that determines who a person really is. Jude is urging believers to stand firm on God's Word and reject false teachers and false doctrine.

But allow me, to take it a step further, do not only reject false teachers and false doctrine but also reject entities and people who participate in glorifying sin.

Jude is sending a cautionary letter to the people, so am I now. We both agree that we must stand strong in the faith, and not be swayed by smooth talking leaders/preachers that tell us that Jesus dying on the cross over looks our continued sin, these preachers are tickling your ears, telling you what you want to hear, so that, that money keeps coming in. This world has become a casino to anyone who can figure out how to become rich!

Now hear this, our tour is about to end, so this is the last time I will say this, **READ YOUR BIBLES DAILY!**

Look ah here, If you allow someone else to tell you what's in the bible, they can tell you anything, to get those big houses, cars and diamond rings, 'I'm just sayin, God's not playin!' You must read his word for yourself, the bible is really our friend, a protector, it's wisdom never the ends, and when all else fails, *'The Holy Bible' God* and his Son *"Jesus Christ"* will all be there. Now before you leave this room, I think you ought to **"Listen"** to what the Lord has to say:, *"Beware of false prophets, who come to you in sheep clothing but inwardly are ravenous wolves.* **Matt.7:17**

So there you have it, you've been warned, okay, enough of that, it's time to celebrate, it's ***"Revelations"*** time!" The last room in my father's house awaits us, let's get this party started! I'll meet you all over there, my work is done in here, I'm out!

"The Take Away", get to know God and his Son *"Jesus Christ"* for yourself, find out what his word is all about; again, "I'm Out!"

Candid Snapshot

Get a bible
Open the bible
Do what it says
Is with you!

Key Verse

Dear friends, although I was very eager to write to you about the salvation we share, I felt compelled to write and urge you to contend for the faith that was once for all entrusted to God's holy people. For certain individuals whose condemnation was written about long ago have secretly slipped in among you. They are ungodly people, who pervert the grace of our God into a license for immorality and deny Jesus Christ our only Sovereign and Lord.

Though you already know all this, I want to remind you that the Lord at one time delivered his people out of Egypt, but later destroyed those who did not believe. **3-5**

Key Action

Give your life to Christ, live faithful and upright!

Key Prayer

Father God, mode me into the kind of person you want me to be, from now on I shall look to thee.

Amen

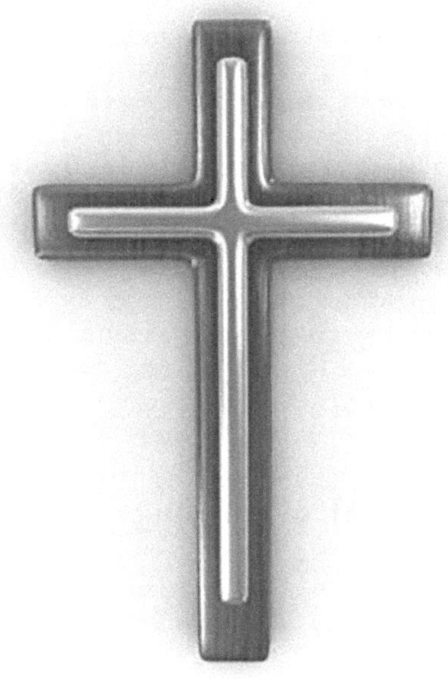

Revelation

Room Sixty- Six (New Testament)

And now the end is near and so we face the final curtain. This room will question and judge our lifestyles on that we can be certain.
Revelation is a complex book, it was written by the Apostle John. It has two major sections, the first being letters to the seven churches the second being a series of visions, awful vision too, and it remembers all those Christians who were persecuted, mistreated and murdered, according to *'Revelation'* will live again. There is so much in this room, plus the overthrow of evil and the return of the messiah. This my friend, is the most anticipated room in the house, this room is for true believers, (meat eater) babes can't handle this room. For we are the mature ones, we don't waiver or go back and forth, or need to be pacified with lies from the outside.
We already know which way to go, like I said, we are the mature ones, and the loyal and faithful ones too, how about **"YOU?"** We have fought the good fight, held on to our faith and have waited for his return The Revelation is this: ***"He's Coming Back Again!*** But if you sit in this room long enough ital feel like he's already arrived. Oh, just sit back, put your feet up, have a glass of wine, tea, or go for it a banana split and just imagine, "no more pain or suffering" it's finally over. We won't have to deal with white power, black power, no more of that crap, no more rich and poor, supremacy will not exist. nor will prostitutes, drug dealers, murderers and thieve, no more abortions, political hierarchies, illness or handicaps No more tears, no more caregiver's cry, we can kiss that all good-bye!
World, now you know why I live for Jesus and why I'm not afraid to die. I met him a long time ago, I saw his Star N air, oh how I long to be there!!!!
But until then, it's time to celebrate, Rejoice, "Revelation" do your thing, the Messiah's coming back for us, "let heaven and nature sing.

Hallelujah to the King of kings!

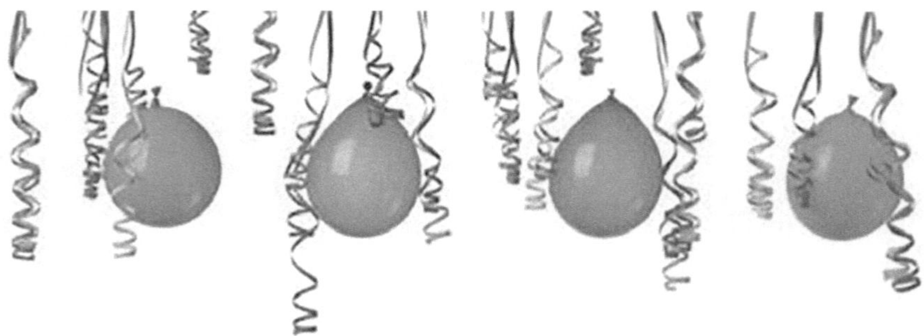

       MISS ASONDRA STARN'AIR

Candid Snapshot

Jesus will have the ***"Last Laugh"***! And so will his people.

Key Verse

"Behold, I am coming soon!
Blessed is he who keeps the word of prophecy in this book." **22:7**

Key Action

Keep doing good, keep loving your enemies, keep building,
keep striving for excellence, do it all in Jesus name!
Let the believers all say, **Amen!**

Key Prayers

"Pray then like this: *'Our Father in heaven, hallowed be your name. Your*
kingdom come, your will be done, on earth as it is in heaven. Give us this day
our daily bread, and forgive us our debts, as we also have forgiven our debtors.
And lead us not into temptation, but deliver us from evil.'"
For thine is the Kingdom, and the glory, forever and ever

Amen

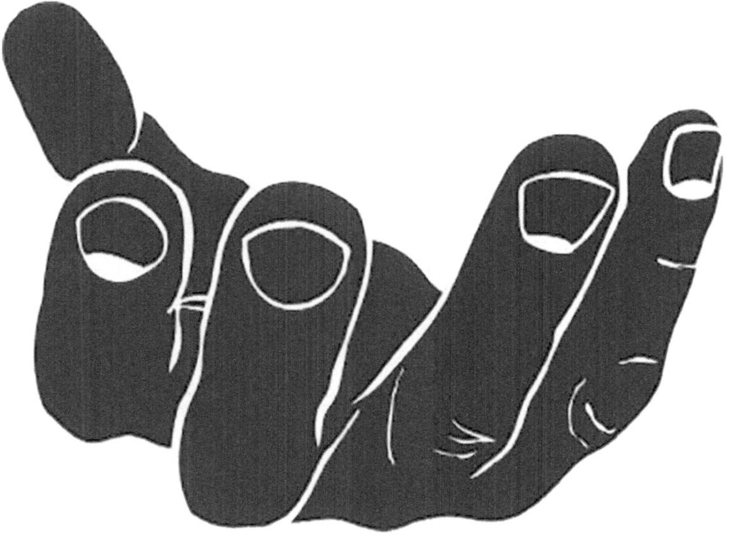

Winding down

Hope you enjoyed the tour, next time bring a friend
until we meet again *"God Speed!"*

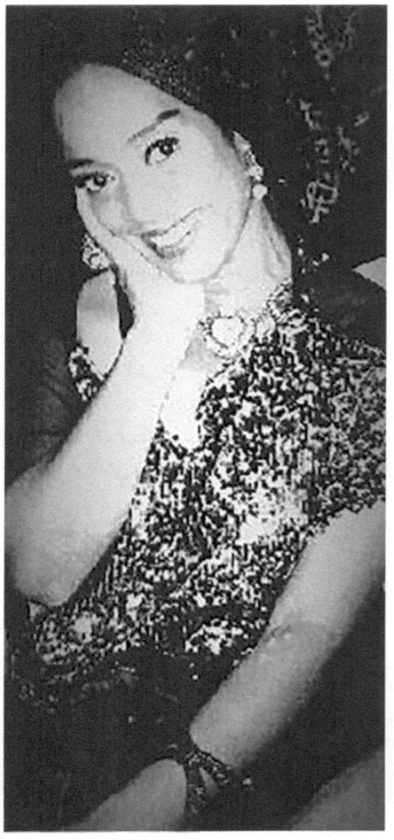

          Miss Asondra StarN'air

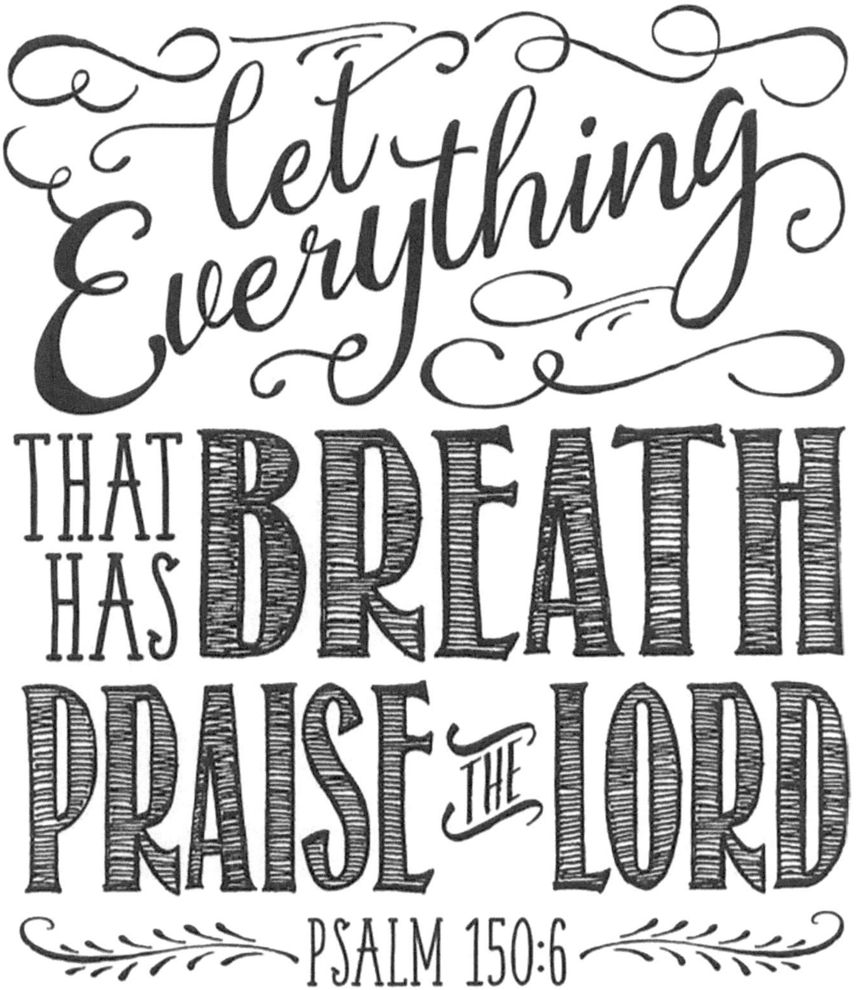
Let Everything
THAT HAS BREATH
PRAISE THE LORD
PSALM 150:6

Choose Whom You Will Serve!

Ok, now that you are almost finished with this entire book, it's time to make that change I talked about earlier in the book of StarN'air, I made that change and so can you. Making that change is easy, all you have to do is switch lives, yours for Jesus. Once you do that, the Holy Spirit takes over and does the rest. He will take all your mess, your pain, all your burdens, disappointments, debts too, and make you *"Brand New."*

Get Saved!

"Now therefore fear the Lord and serve him in sincerity and in faithfulness. Put away the gods that your fathers served beyond the River and in Egypt, and serve the Lord. And if it is evil in your eyes to serve the Lord, choose this day whom you will serve, whether the gods your fathers served in the region beyond the River, or the gods of the Amorites in whose land you dwell. But as for me and my house, we will serve the Lord." **Joshua 24:14-15**

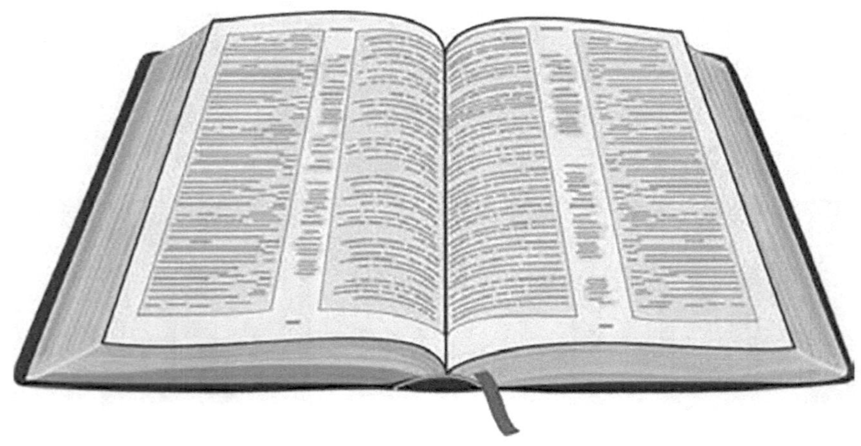

How to Study the Bible

Basic Instructions Before Leaving Earth

There are many different ways one can approach bible reading. Some like study groups, where everyone is reading the same thing and then have discussion afterward.

I think, if this is your first time reading through the bible, it should be just you and God, not a group.

Whatever is comfortable for you is the most important I suppose. But here's the thing, you want to make sure you and you alone are developing an inti- mate relationship with god in your own unique private way which means what he says to you, he may not say to others.

Groups are great after you have studied the first year with God alone. Because now you are ready to share testimonies, revelations, ask question and fellowship with other Christian and not feel lost or intimidated by "Christian Intellects", there are those who know it all, full of pride and dug into the bible for the wrong reasons.

By studying God's word the first year by yourself, just you and god, you will be able to weed out "Counterfeits" everyone in a bible study group are not necessarily there for real Christian living, some have hidden agenda.

Again, get to know God for yourself first and foremost then join study groups. Fellowshipping is very important and encouraged.

Tools You Can Use!

TURN THE TV OFF AND TURN GOD ON

- God will meet you where you are at. So find a book in the bible that speaks to your current situation.
- Or start at the beginning that's what I did. Genesis
- Find a special place in your home to begin your journey with god. Give yourself at least a year to get a solid foundation.
- Don't worry about full understanding, that will come as you continue to live for Christ.
- Ask God to penetrate your mind, body and soul to want to change and follow Christ.
- Commit to the same time and days to study your bible without any distractions.
- Let you family know on this day at this time, you will not be available.
- Pray, tell God how much you need him and how you are lost without him.

Listen for God, he will speak to you, God may want you to read from the New Testament first, then the Old Testament.

Don't get in front of God, surrender to God and allow him to slowly mold you into what he wants you to be.

About the Author

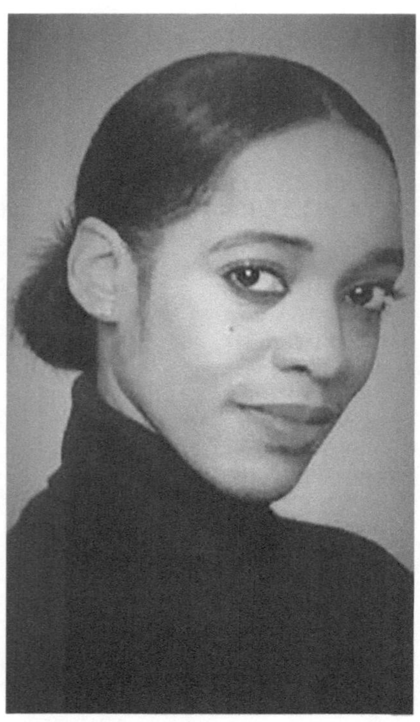

Miss Asondra StarN'air

Miss Asondra StarN'air has been in the health-care industry for more than twenty years now. She's single and hopes to remarry someday. She would also like to travel the world doing whatever God calls her to do. Whether it's, sing, write, speak, wash feet, whatever! Miss StarN'air felt the dire need to write this book and believes it was a calling from God that she did so, to help open the hearts and minds of caregivers all over the world and introduce them to Jesus as well.

Star Nair's loves the work of ministry, she's ordained and can perform marriages. By trade She's a certified nurse assistant, and too, an advocate for both seniors and caregivers nationwide. She lives in the state of Ohio and enjoys Christian living and pursues **"Peace"** at all cost. It is her heart's desire that those who are suffering, lost, bullied, or abused find salvation in our Lord Jesus Christ. She hopes this *"Caregivers Bible"* will help with all that. Miss Asondra StarN'air also known as 'Star', says, if this book can get one person saved, just one, then it was worth all the days and nights she cried, asking God to take this body of work from her. Like Moses, in her heart she felt, I'm not sharp, I am slow in speech and tongue, I'm not an RN, I'm just ah aide.

A Caregiver's Bible To Excellence pushed her beyond limits, but it also took her to a higher place. A lot of time, sweat, and tears went into this book. The pain and suffering was real, plus all the wisdom inside. Well, now she can't hide, God has spoken: *"Write my book"* and call it *'A Caregiver's Bible To Excellence!'*

So, world, here it is!!!!!!!!

This incredible, incredible book is a book of Excellence and Triumph. And a movement toward 'Change'.

Miss Asondra StarN'air is her name!

★ StarN'air ★

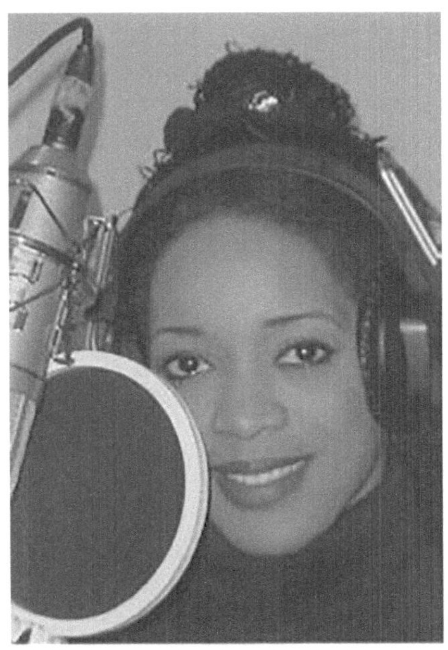

An Artist Too!

I once dreamed of becoming a global recording artist, but all that changed, when I changed and gave my life to Christ. My life shall not become a roll of the dice. When I decided to give my life to him, I didn't have to think twice. I will never choose money, music or fame over Christ! Yes indeed he's worth every sacrifice. He's the Star N air I can't wait to see, where he's at. I long to be. As you can see, I still have a lot of music in me, but now it's up to God, what shall be, shall be! My biggest mission in life is to help set others free! Stay tuned, this will not be the last you've heard from me.

Live, Peacefully!
With love, Miss Asondra StarN'air

Dedication Page

This book is also dedicated to my daughter, Jazz. You are so loved. It is my heart's desire that you also get saved and leave this world behind. God wants to introduce us to a whole new way of living. God has so much in store for those who will follow him, but everyone must come on their own. Please forgive me for any mistakes I have made. All mothers make mistakes—I'm no exception. But one mistake I did not make, and that was having you. You are my Jazzy Jazz, and I love you.

*Always remember, those not in Christ, are a playing a dangerous game with their life. Live to please God, **"Live Upright!"***

You are your mother's daughter. If you fall, get back up. You are loved—more than you will ever know.

Jazzy Jazz

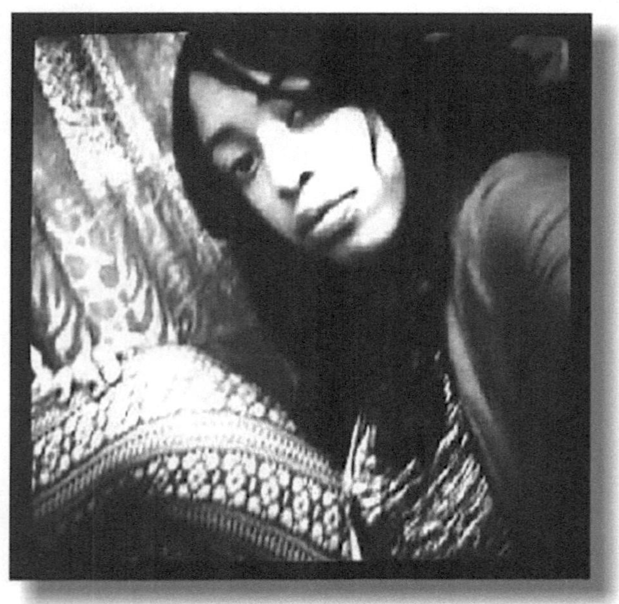

 MISS ASONDRA STARN'AIR

It's So Hard to Say Good-bye!

Well, it's that time—time to say good-bye. It seems we've been together for a long time. Writing this book was not easy, but with the holy spirits help I got through it. This was quite a journey, I must say, we covered a lot, hope you learned a lot too, I did. Lots of work and research went into this book. I am so glad I made it through, what about you? Oh, how I do hope you love your Caregivers Bible, I was called to write it just for you. And I also hope everyone follows through on being the best care- giver ever, these pages will help you get it all together. Today a new generation of caregivers are on the rise.

Never Stop Living For Christ!

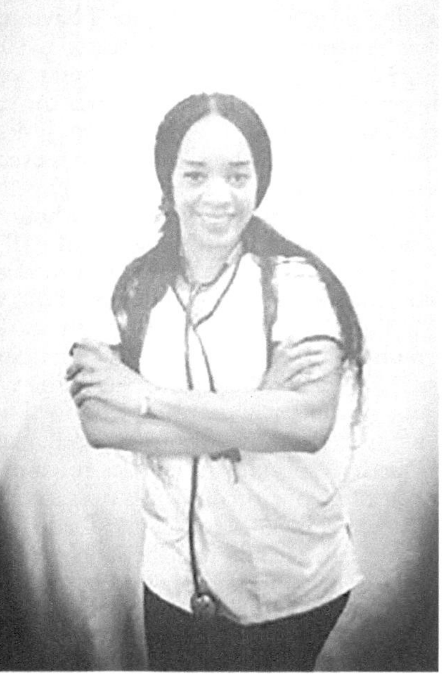

We are the 'Brightest' well trained and skilled healthcare workers of our generation. We must lift up our voices and make our request known. **"We Want Economic Equality"** and we want to be included professionally with the entire health-care team. That means professional pay and benefits for "ALL" health care workers, we mustn't leave (**HHA's**) Home Health Associates out, home care workers are a part of the entire team.

"We Are All One" I know after this book comes out, my work out in the world has just begun! It is my heart's desire to get out there and help fight for change, higher wages for all healthcare workers, home care name change, keep the initials **HHA** but remove Aide to **Associates**: Health Health Associates that's a more professional and dignified name. The word "Aides", keeps us impoverished and slaves, we are not slaves. So as you can see, from here, I still have a lot of work to do. I want **"CHANGE"** and caregivers, change takes action. **"Be Smart, do Your Part!"** As for me, finally, I want to help take 'Caregiving' in a whole new direction, with Christ leading the way! If you are with me, get ready to fight, everybody, **"Together"** says **"Okay!"**

In Jesus Name, Amen
Moving Forward, Working Towards Change,
Don't Ever Stop, Go All The Way!

The Close

Finally, it's time to release this book out into the world and hope it finds you. I made it my heart desire to take everything I have learned about caregiving and then some so that caregiver's like you all over the world would be armed with information and tools you can use. I hope I have accomplished that here.

Adding to that, I also wanted to challenged everyone to keep growing and reaching new heights to become the best caregivers ever. We are in such high demands, let's become pros. This book prepares the caregiver to excel. To be the very best, not only professionally but personally too. Jesus says in his word, be perfect like my father in heaven is, "being perfect" includes excellence I'm sure. **Matthew 5:48** It is from that premise "A Caregiver's Bible to Excellence" emerged, a new let there be revelation if you will, but of course, not without Christ, oh no, not without **'Almighty'** Jesus, **The Greatest Love/Caregiver of All!**

Jesus is the role model of excellence for all humanity, no matter what, if he's not leading the way, you're not going very far, nor will you stand out from the rest. Mediocrity today still rules on this dark planet, haterd too. But hopefully by the time you have finished reading and participating, studying, working toward change and striving for excellence in Jesus name you'll began to see, the real me too, I love all of you, no matter what you say or do. The ultimate goal for me here is twofold, I want caregivers to move toward "Excellence" and I also want caregivers to move toward "Christ", especially if they desire a more prosperous and happy life. (live right!) Yes, I want to help win your souls over to Christ, get you back home to him, where you've always belonged. Come on, "Really", you didn't think it was going to be all work and excellence and no Christ? No, on the contrary, when it all said and done, it's all about Christ! From now on, let him run your life!

Now I leave you with this **"A Caregiver Bible To Excellence"** yours for the taking, for you can lead a horse to the water but you cannot make him or her drink, but I drank, and I drank. And now I'm "sprung out" flying high on Jesus!

Taste and See that the LORD is Good!
Psalms 34:8

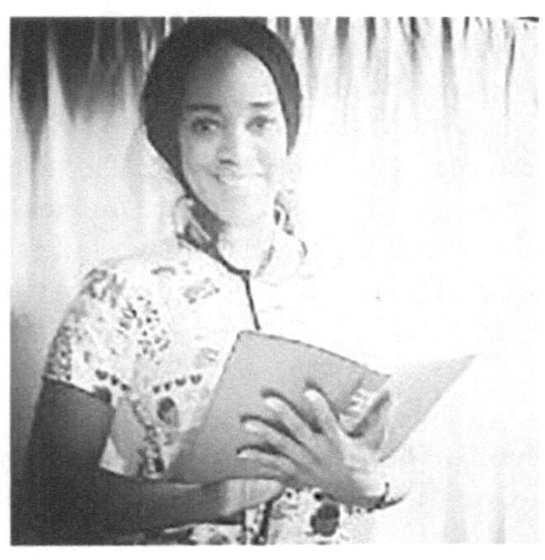

      MISS ASONDRA STARN'AIR

An Invitation To Caregiving

In today's healthy economy, if you want to work, you can work! Anyone can find a job at any age. People are living a lot longer these days, and there are lots of opportunities out there. One for sure is the "health-care industry." It's booming, and there are no signs of it stopping anytime soon—probably not ever. People will always need people to help care for them and lend a helping hand—always. That's what Jesus was all about. He was a caregiver of the Most High: ***"The Greatest Caregiver of All."***

Why not learn to become like him? Let him show you how wonderful serving others can be. Watch him turn you into the kind of caregiver the world longs to see.

But, first you must **"CARE"** and second, you must be **'A GIVER'**, "get it", **'A CARE GIVER'** but not just any kind of **CARE -GIVER**, but one who will be there, do the job, deliver! If this is you, Jesus wants you to join his team, and if you are loving, kind and great, you can ask him for anything! God has his own reward for those who love and serve him well, look at me can't you tell! Well, this invitation is for you. Black, white, brown, yellow—blue, whatever your color, God loves and wants you. **Female** or **Male**, anyone and everyone who loves and desires to be a **CARE-GIVER** *God Is Calling'* He called me, now he's calling **"YOU."**

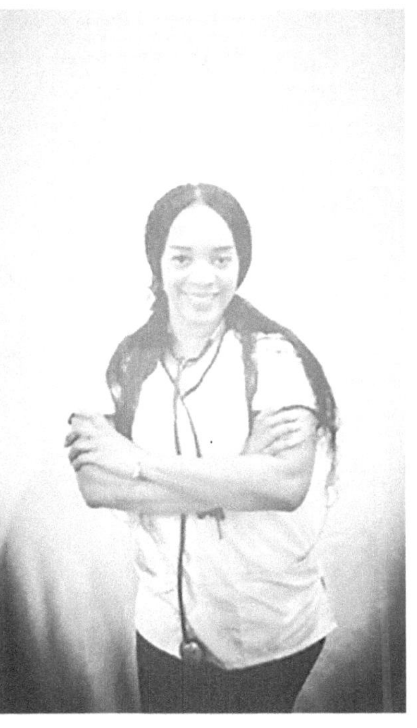

Together, let's see want *A Caregiver's Bible To Excellence* can do!

In Jesus's name, say it with me.
AMEN!

Good-bye! Love always, *Miss Asondra StarN'air*

Have "No Fear"

Caregivers, as we move forward toward change, we will be faced with opposition, but don't be afraid, let that not stop us. If we want equality, our voices heard and respectability which includes higher wages for all the hard work that we do then we must fight for it, knowing that God is with us. We must cross over to the other side, prosperity await us. Remember have no fear, God says he has not given us a spirit of fear, but power and love and of a sound mind. **Tim/2 1:7** In God We Trust, Get on the bus! Help fight for a 'Better Tomorrow!'

In Jesus's name, Amen.

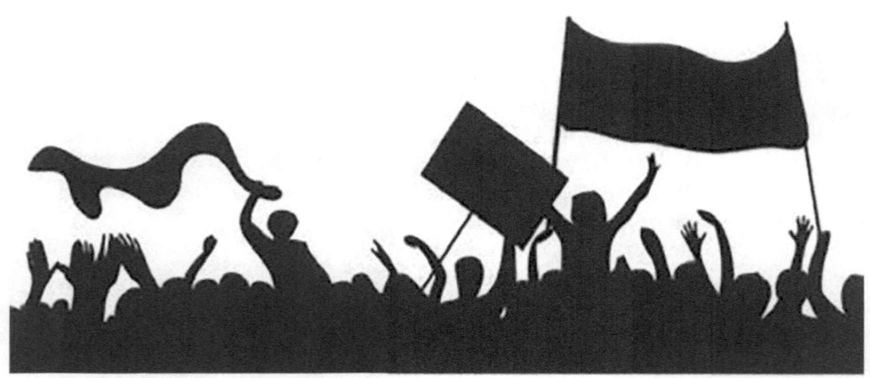

 Miss Asondra StarN'air

Love One Another!

This is an intro to a song I wrote almost twenty years ago and seem so appropriate here in this book… it goes like this
"Love One Another Like Your Sister's and Brothers"
love one another like your sister's and brother's
…you've been told this over a thousand times
…why does this kind of compassion
always leaves your mind?
and you for get to be kind
always out to find
a reason not to
love one another like your sister's and brother's
but once you do… a new world, you'll discover
God gave his son…
the only one
there's no other
who can teach us
how to love one another
like our sisters and brothers…
But you've been told this over a thousand times
Why does this kind of compassion always
leave your mind and you forget to be kind.
Always got to be reminded, in your heart, why can't you find it, good to,
love one another like your sisters and brothers!

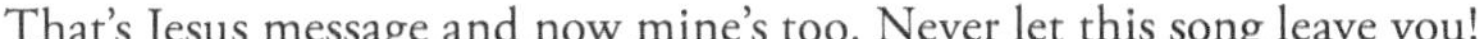

That's Jesus message and now mine's too. Never let this song leave you!

"Love One Another Like Your Sisters and Brothers"
In Jesus name **Amen!**

Seek the Kingdom of God above all else, and "caregivers," we must live righteously, and all these things will be added on to us! (Personalized)

—Matt. 6:33

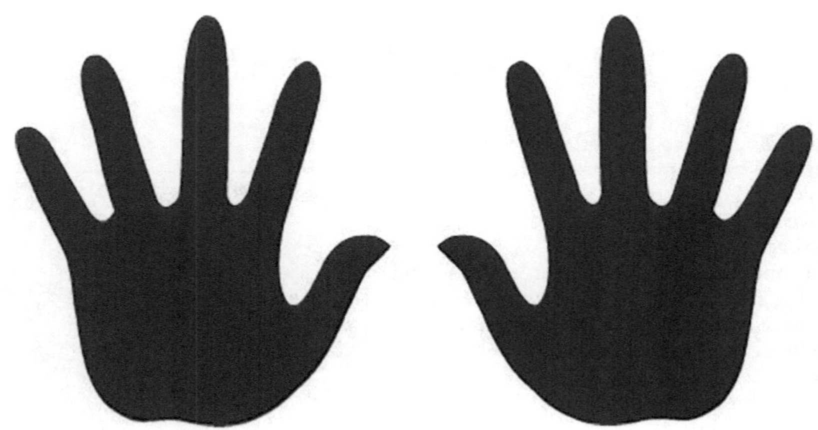

The Prayer of Protection and Blessing for Caregivers
Your hands are my hands
Go and heal the wounded and the sick

 Miss Asondra StarN'air

You have been given power like Moses—his rod, his stick
It's there for you when you need it
I'm with you, along for the ride
You have been given all you need: peace, power, protection, strength
Just let love be your guide
Remember your hands belong to me
So be gentle and kind
No harm shall come to those with God on their mind
"His holy spirit speaks"
I've made each one of you unique—one of a kind
beautiful, bountiful 'Sunflowers' together you shine
You're protected, you belong to me,
keep believing, *"Have Faith"* although you cannot see
It's caregivers like you that make this world a better place to be
May you prosper in all you do
And remember God loves and will always take good care of *"YOU!"*

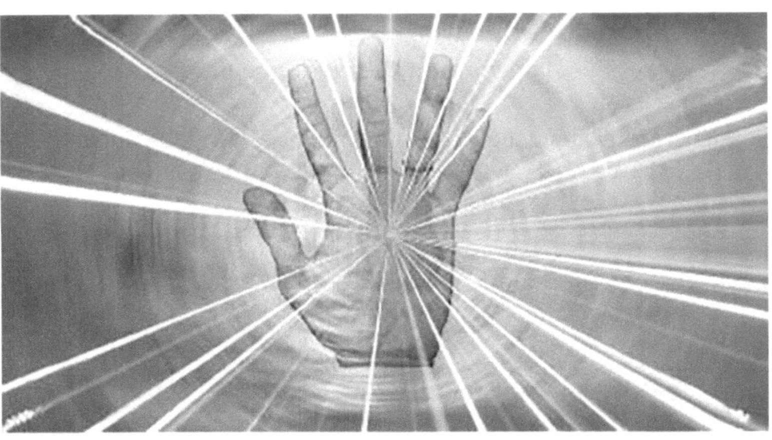

Go In Peace!!!!!

StarN'air Tears...

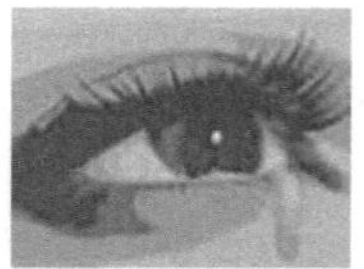

The time has come for me to say good-bye
I don't want to go, but I must… God has more
work for me to do. I love all of you.
Hopefully, somebody, one body, anybody, will read
this book and become a better person.
and fall madly in love with Jesus like I have, if that does indeed
happen, just know I also came back for that **1** person
And let me tell you, it was worth all the hell this world

tried to put me through to find **YOU.**

You are worth dying for, you are worth crying
for, you are worth saving too,

My work is done, now may Love, Peace, Power, Prosperity,
Protection and Grace be with **"YOU"** forever, in Jesus name, **"AMEN"**

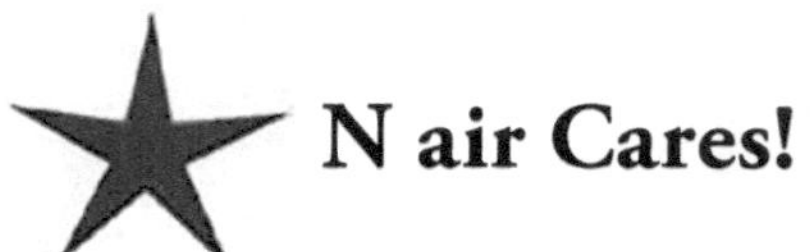

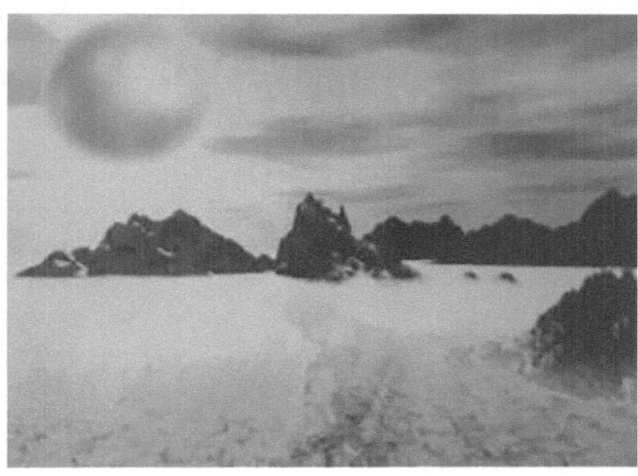

Miss Asondra StarN'air

Peace On Earth

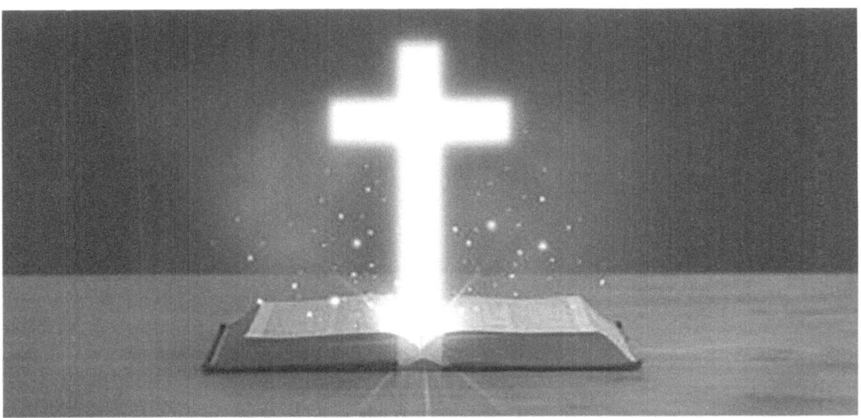

Peace I leave with you; my peace I give to you; do not let your hearts be trouble, nor let it be afraid. Let my perfect peace calm you in every circumstance and give you courage and strength for ever challenge. **John 14:27**

In Jesus name, Amen.

Count down Time!

10

Never stop working toward a better day, fight to WIN!

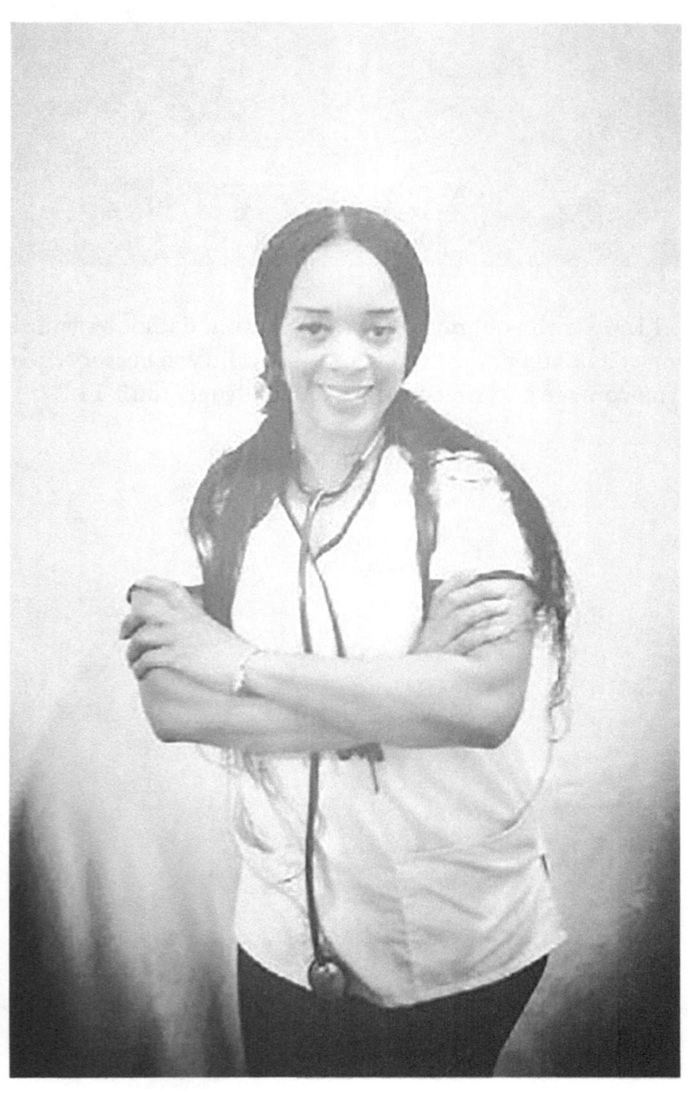

Keep Hope Alive, Read Your Bibles, "PRAY" and You'll Be Fine!

8

Love, Forgive, No Matter What, Never Hate.

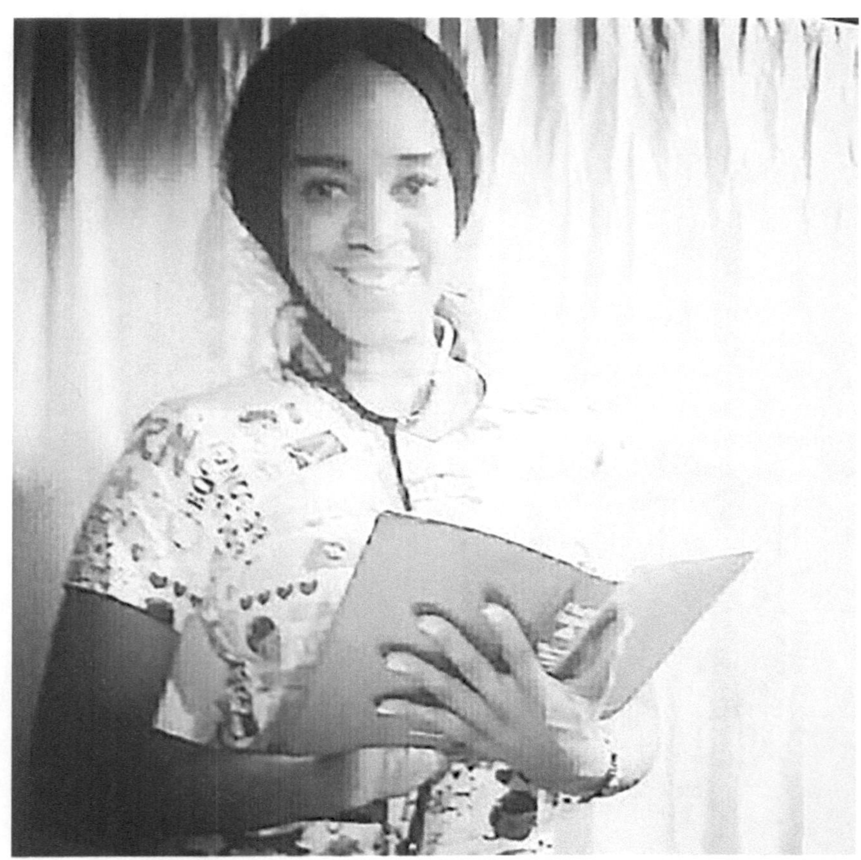

Miss Asondra StarN'air

Repent, Say No to Sin!
Be Perfect Like Our Father in Heaven

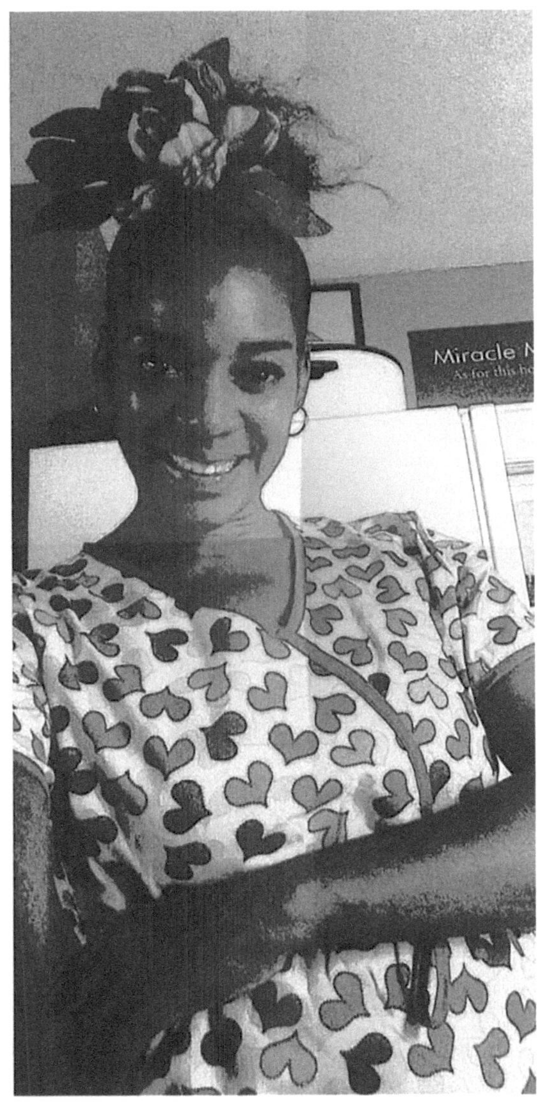

6

**Don't Straddle the Fence or Mix,
Stay True to the one and only True God.
Think you can handle this?**

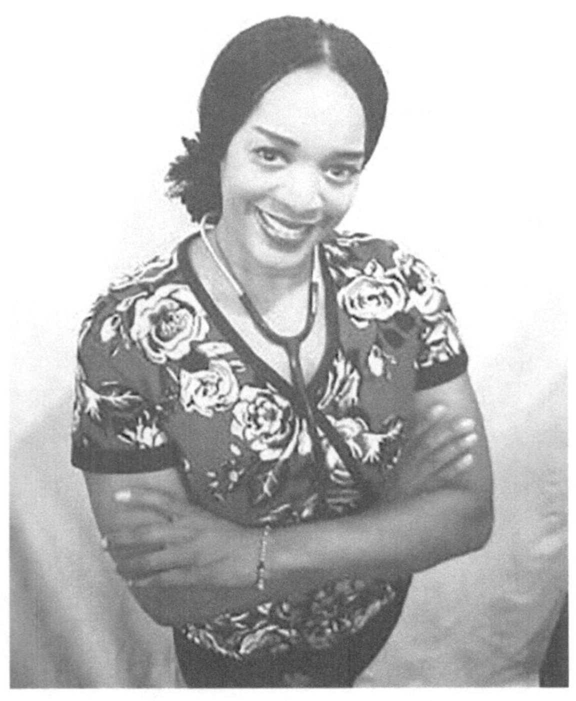

I'm Still Standing

  Miss Asondra StarN'air

You've Arrived, Keep Evolving, Growing, God IS with 'YOU'!

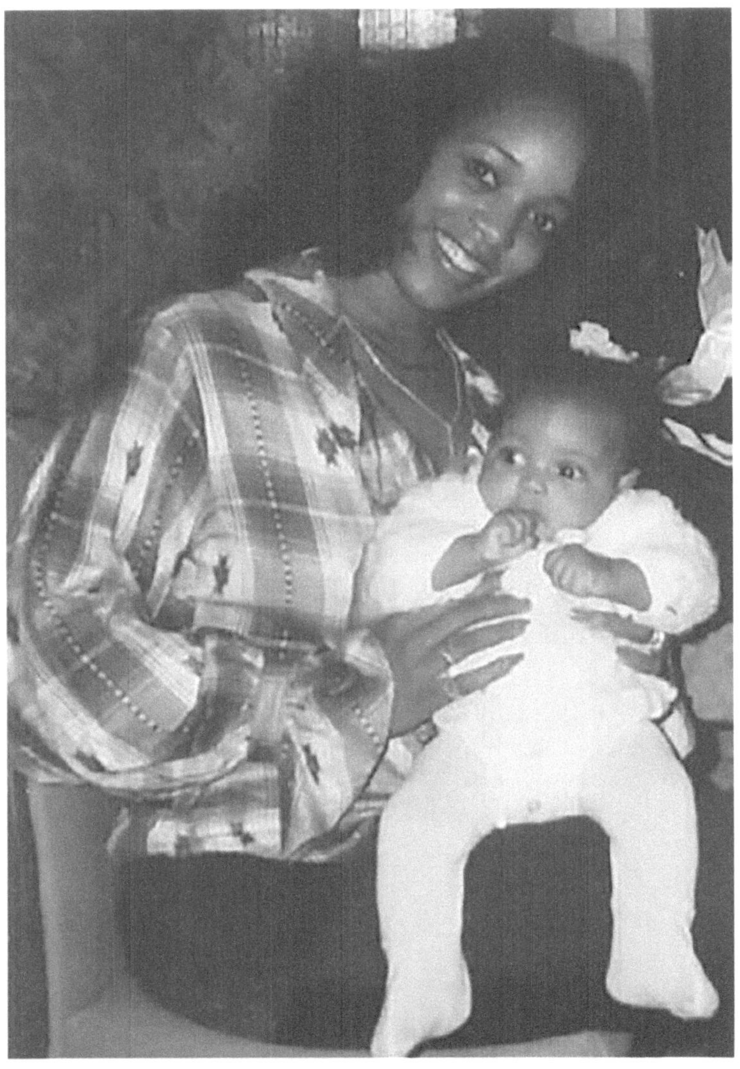

**We have to be a good example for our children.
We have so much work to do!**

Don't Be Afraid Anymore, Walk Through This 'Open door'...

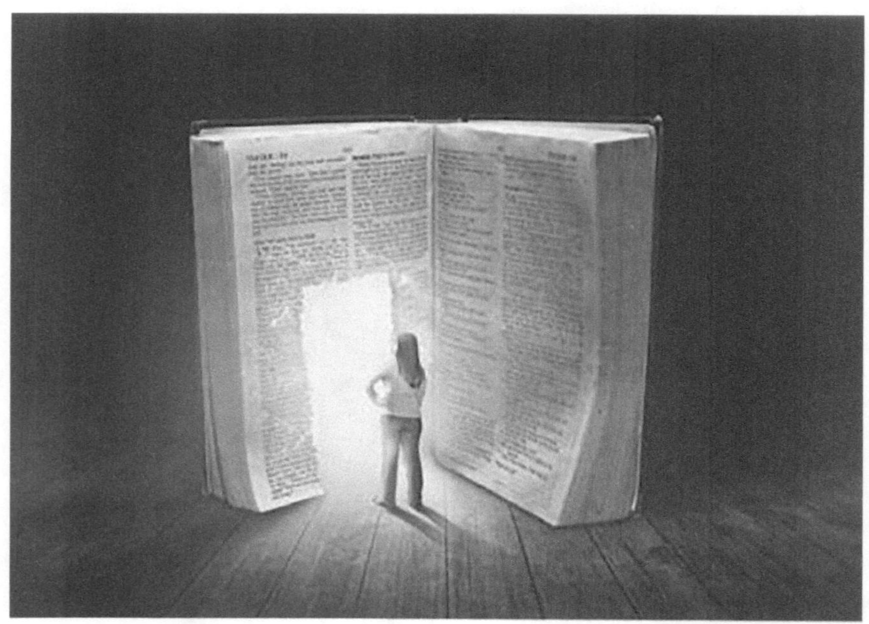

Get the book of life
Open the book of life
Do the book of life
Is with **YOU!**

3

Remember, Life is not about you or me!

It's about the one who died so we could be free!

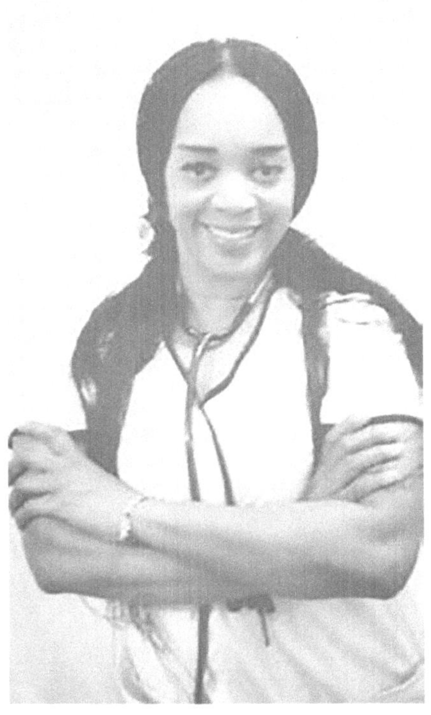

It's about Jesus, caring and giving, serving others in need.

That what makes us his Caregivers!

His 'Sun Flowers of life!

Always remember from now on we are working for Christ, not man, Christ!

2

Now I'm feeling blue,
I'm getting ready to move on, and I'm going to miss you!

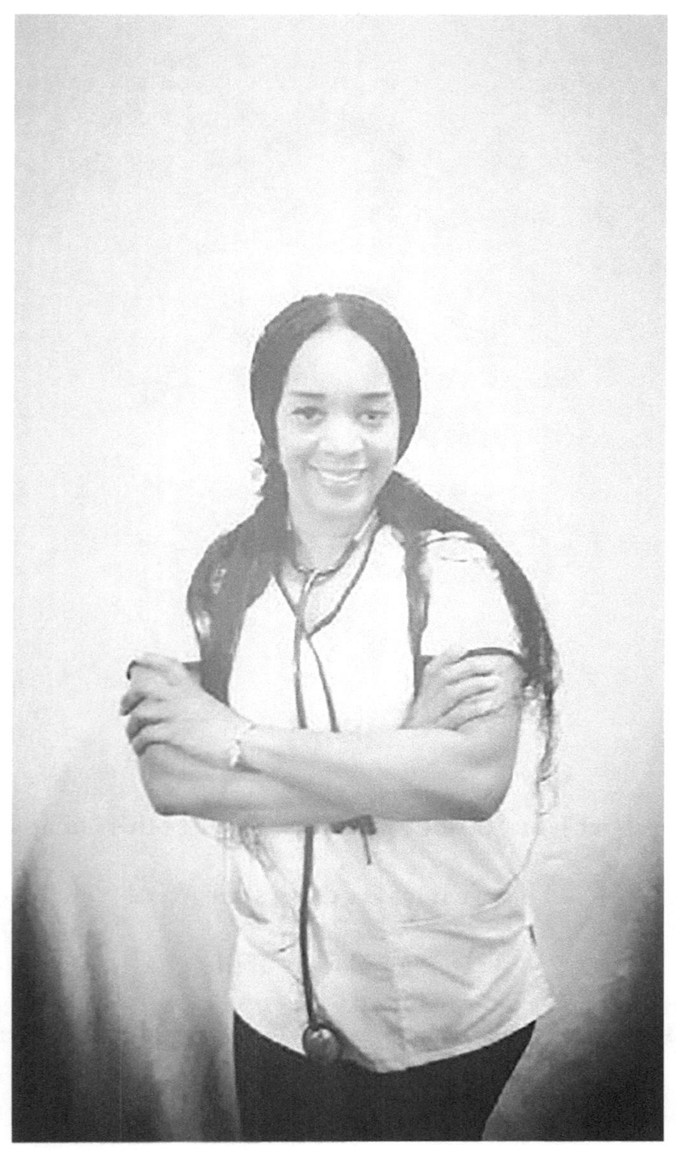

 Miss Asondra StarN'air

Time to say good bye...

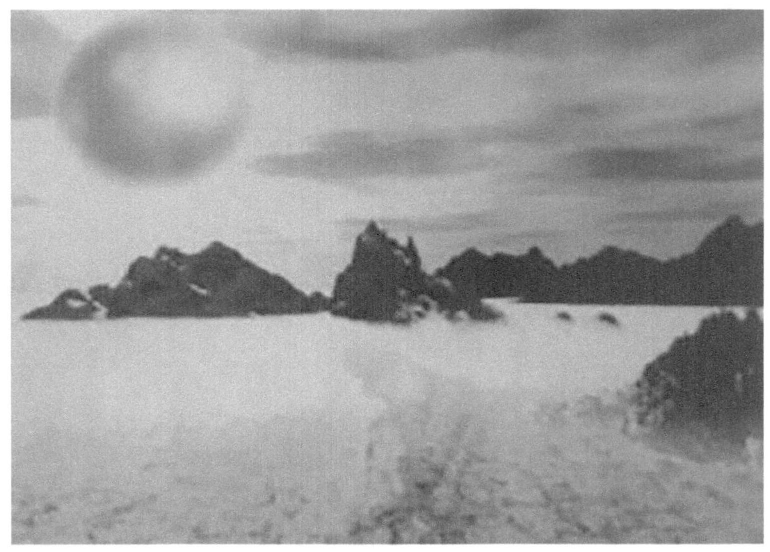

Miss Asondra StarN'air , It is finished!

Now "YOUR" Work Has Just Begun!

Well done, My Good and Faithful Servant!

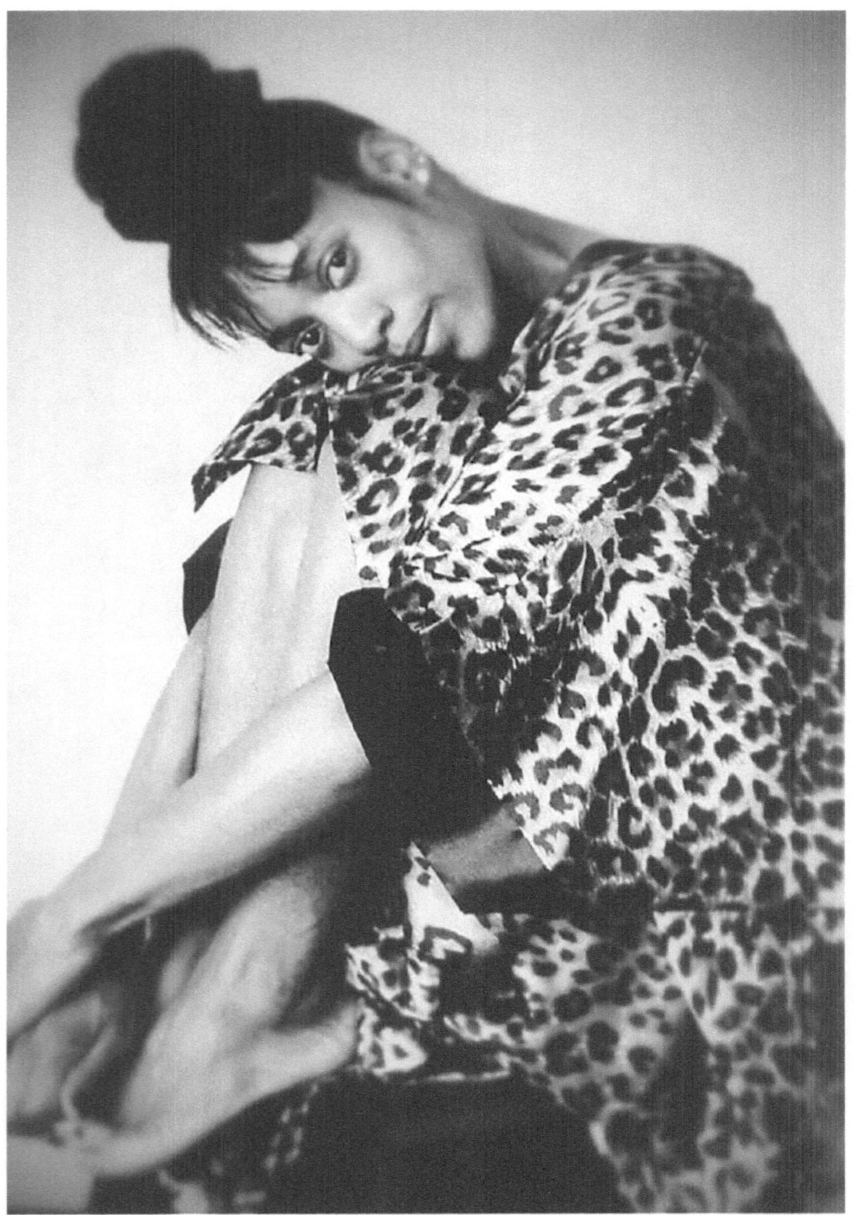

Well done!

 Miss Asondra StarN'air

Halo

It's Been Pleasure, Writing and Caring for All of You!

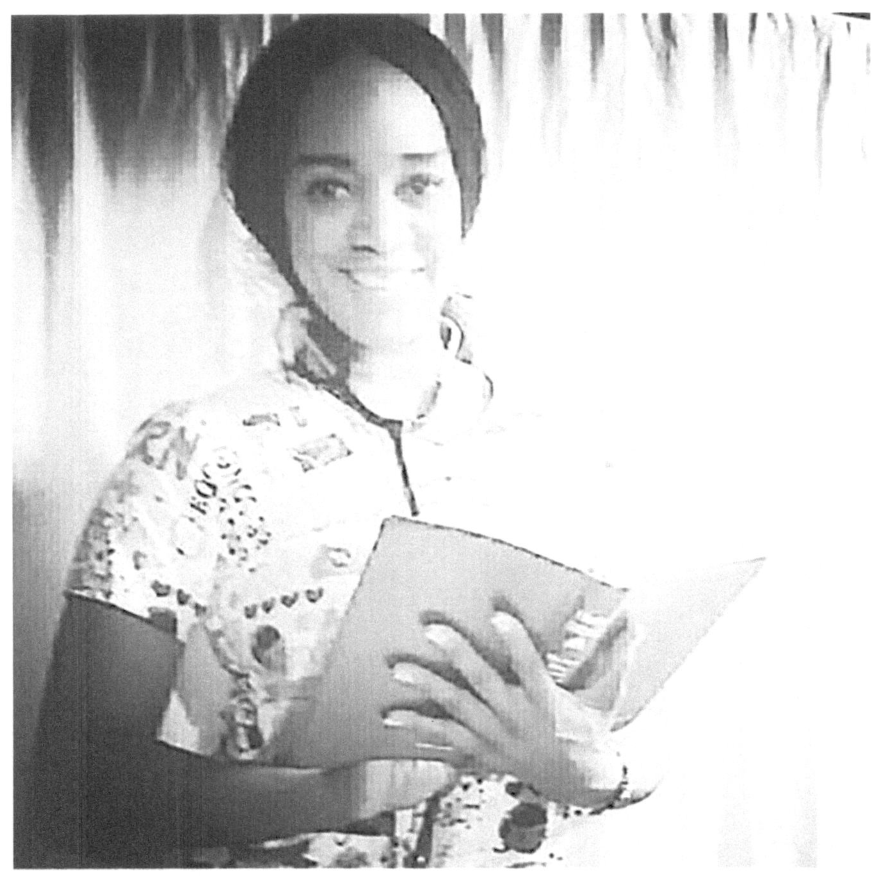

Good-Bye!

**Now may the God of Abraham, Isac and Jacob be with you all.
Love and Peace Always,**

Miss Asondra StarN'air

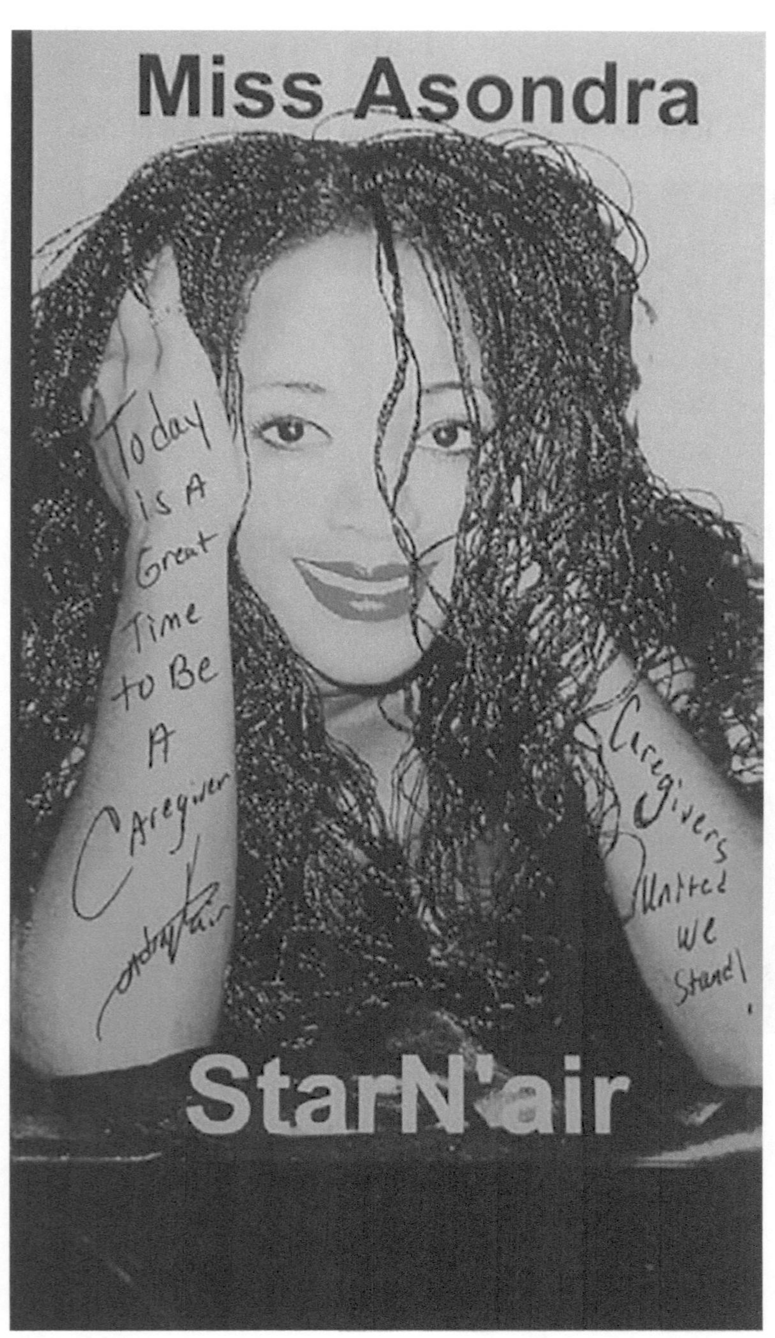

Miss Asondra
Today is A Great Time to Be A Caregiver
Caregivers United We Stand!
StarN'air

Revolutionary Book

It's finally here!

A Caregiver's Bible to Excellence is a revolutionary book—no other like it on the planet. it's so heartfelt and inspiring. Words cannot describe what God has done here with Miss Asondra. She's a genius! Everyone in the world should own this unique and incredible book.

—Janette Louis, LPN

Florence Nightingale would be proud! Many of you will not be able to put this book down, because it is more than a book. It's a new day for caregivers, yes indeed. It's a new way of life. Jesus has risen; he is leading us now.

—Tabatha Wilkins, Caregiver

Unity is what we need—a kind of coming together that is so much needed in the world today.
Will never part with this book, ever! All I can say is WOW!

—B. K. A., DD

This is a great time in history for caregivers. God is about to do something amazing. Got my Caregiver's Bible, I'm ready! "Incredible Book" It's true—nothing like it on the planet. Nothing! What a blessing she is to us all.

—Lisa Anderson /Caregiver

For we know that giving care is one of the highest expressions of love one can give to another. That's what Jesus was all about! Jesus loved and healed the oppressed and the sick; he wore his heart in his hand. In Moses's time, he was given a scroll with the Ten Commandments. Now look what he has given us . . .

A Caregiver's Bible to Excellence

StarN'air, you did it this time; talk about becomig a household name, you are amazing. We salute you for answering the call. You made your mark on the planet. You gave us something worth fighting for—a vision of excellence. May God bless you beyond your wildest dreams.
Love always.

—Ms. Chapman/ A real friend!

Miss Asondra StarN'air

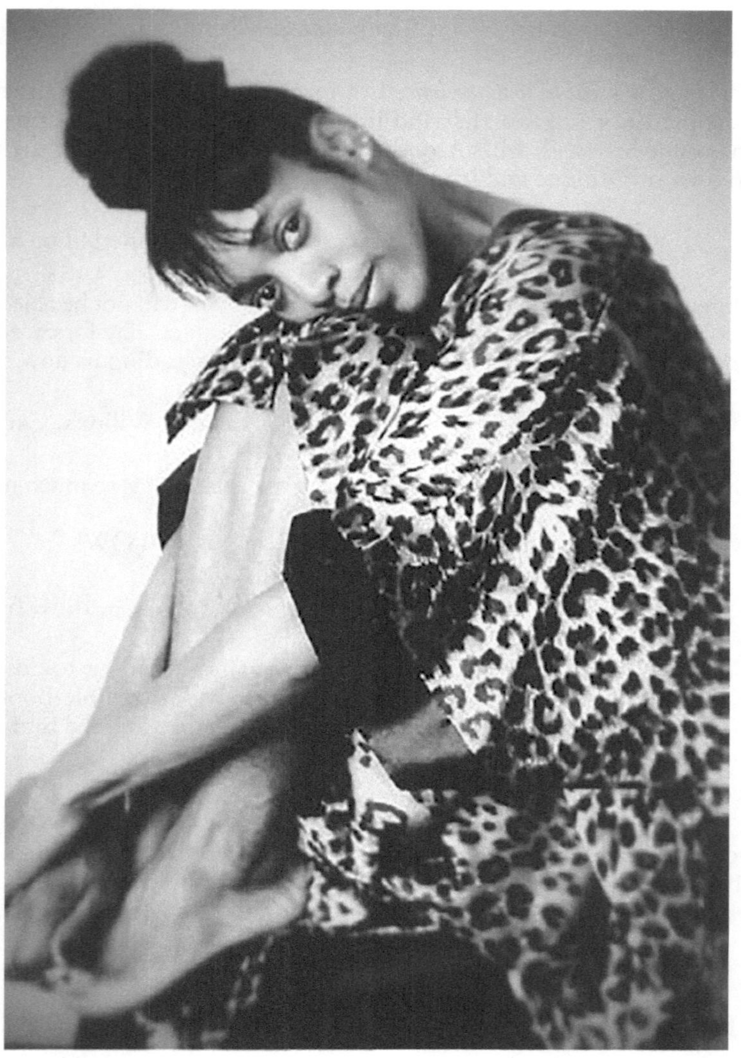

Changing the way we do caregiving—one caregiver's heart at a time.
Get this book; walk the straight and narrow line.
Remember to be loving and kind!
Good-bye!

REVOLUTIONARY BOOK, It's True!

A Caregiver's Bible to Excellence is a revolutionary book—no other like it on the planet. It is so heartfelt and inspiring, you will not want to part with this incredible book, trust me.

Florence Nightingale would be proud of Miss StarN'air. Florence believed everyone—women/men nationwide—should have basic caregiving awareness skills. Hey, you never know when someone you love will need help. This book gives you all that and more, plus it helps prepare the working caregiver for ultimate achievement and professional success.

Caregiving is one of the highest expressions of love one can give to another; that's what Jesus was all about.

Everyone Should Open Their Hearts And Help Care For Others!

But I rejoiced in the Lord greatly,
that now at the last your care of me hath flourished again;
wherein ye were also careful, but ye lacked opportunity.

—Philippians 4:10

"Bright Star"

Worldwide, this book will opens your eyes! And for caregiver especially, it's a must have.

Why do I recommend this book?
Oh my god, we need a book like this . . .
Along my journey, I have been fortunate to meet a positive, fierce, compassionate, charming person named Star. StarN'air is the reason that gives us all not only a voice, but caregivers a real respect for our craft. Star helps motivate all of us to give all we have—to go above and beyond as caregivers. God called the right person to write this incredible book. Miss Asondra StarN'air is not only a gift to the world, she truly is a **"Bright Star"**!

Truly spoken by Sharon Commings

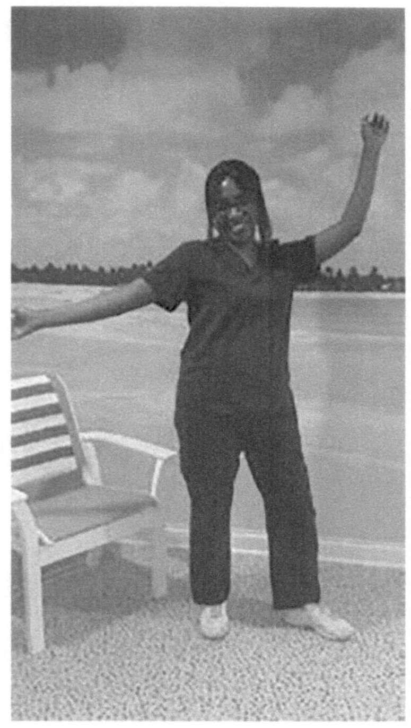

We Are New day Caregivers!

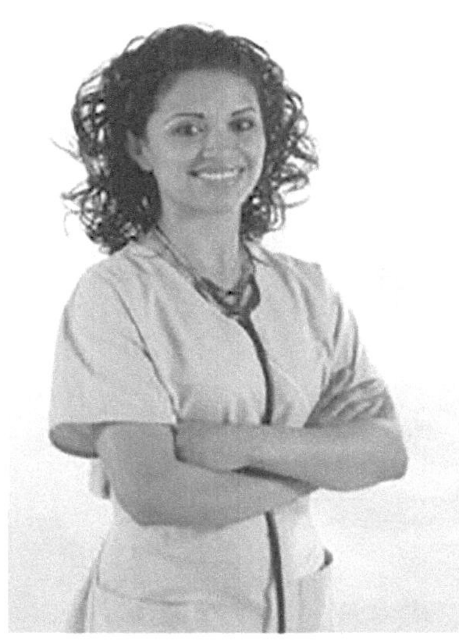

It takes a lot of guts to stand up for what is NOT right! Miss Asondra StarN'air is a true pioneer.

Never before in history has there been anyone to fight for caregivers this way, and under such constant pressure, losing one job after the other, while still fighting for equality.

Most people would have given up a long time ago, changed professions—but not Star. I agree with Asondra. Once a caregiver, always a caregiver—especially if you know it's your calling. And it certainly is hers. My advice to caregivers is to "Unite" become one body, because that's what it's going to take for real change. I love being a caregiver; it is such a rewarding career.

It offers so much flexibility and provides many opportunities for those perusing nursing degrees, like me. What an incredible book! Never seen anything like it or met anyone like Ms. Asondra StarN'air.

This is a truly a Caregiver's Bible to Excellence.

All I can say is "wow!!!!"

Maria Chapel

Joy To The World

Joy to the world! *A Caregiver's Bible to Excellence* has come. Let us give all the glory to the King. Let every caregiver rejoice and sing; all the praises go to our King! All the praises . . . goes to our King.

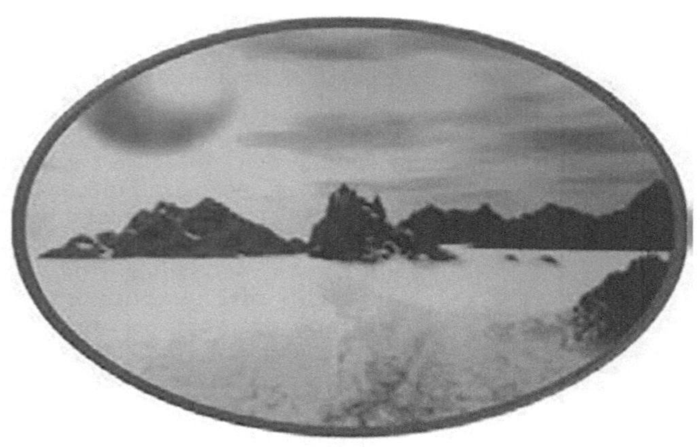

Joy to the world,
A New day has come
Let prosperity and economic growth
For caregivers ring
Let every caregiver
Receive their share,
Of the American Pie
Of the American Pie
Of . . . the . . . American . . . Pie
Joy to the world,
A "New day" has finally come
if others can make their mark, so can I!

 Miss Asondra StarN'air

TESTIMONIES

How has this book helped or inspired you?

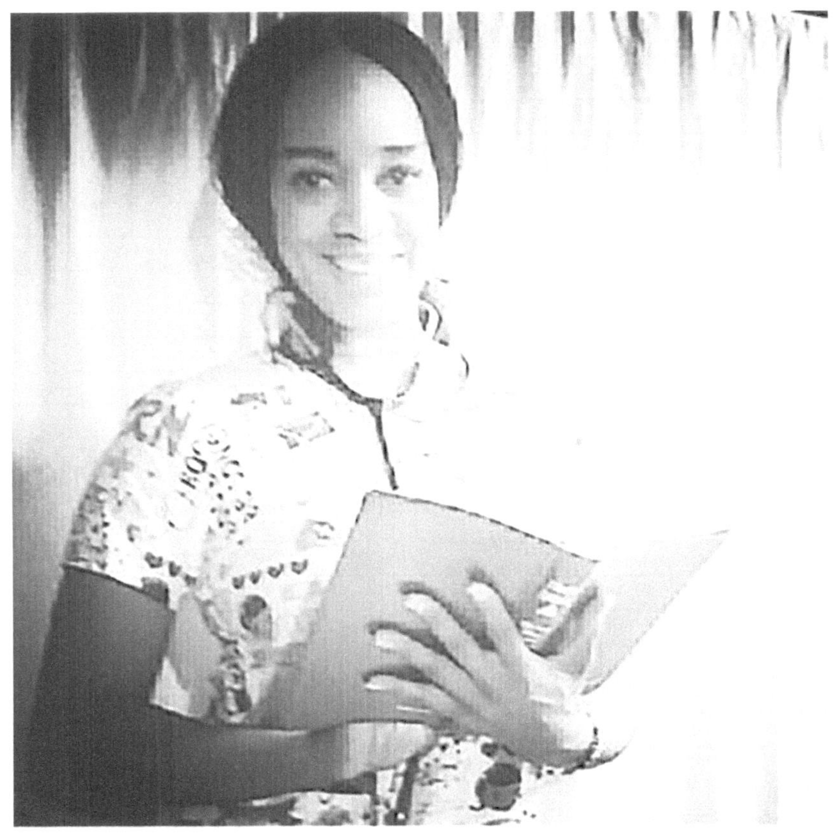

Tell us, Tell Everybody!

Signed, sealed, delivered ________________________ Jesus, I'm yours!

All About Me!

Caregiver's Introduction: Hello, my name is _______________________ | 475
____

Now tell us how long you've been a caregiver and why you decided to become
a caregiver? ____
____
____
____
____
____
____
____

What do you like the most and least about your work as a caregiver?
____
____
____
____
____
____
____
____
____

What changes would you like to see? _________________________________
____
____
____
____
____
____
____
____

What would you say to new caregivers?

____
____
____
____
____
____
____
____
____
____

What would you like to say to management?

____
____
____
____
____
____
____
____
____
____
____

Words to the author, "Star."

____
____
____
____
____
____
____
____
____
____

What state do you live in? ____
Contact information: e-mail ________________ phone ______________

I grant release of writing and photos to Miss Asondra StarN'air for future projects. Signature _________________________ Date ___________

Caregiver's Bible To Excellence "Testimony"

____

Please email back this Caregiver's Introduction sheets along with a picture for website posting etc. to: OnlyOneStarNair@Gmail.com and please include a number you can be reached at, I may want to use you and your testimony for future projects. Here's wishing you all the best, with all my heart and love, ***"God Speed!"***

 Miss Asondra StarN'air

A Caregiver's Bible To Excellence!

A Caregiver is simply someone who **"Cares"**,
Someone that wants to be there," **A Giver."**

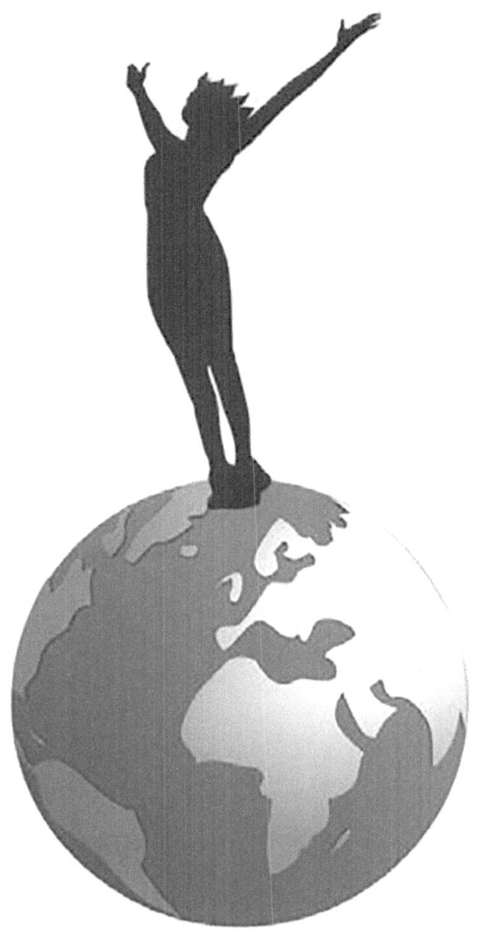

Someone Who Will Deliver!

Holy One
The Word
The Sacrifice
Firstfruits
Mediator
Son of God
Living Stone
Light of the World
Prince of Peace
Living Word
Deliverer
Beloved
King of Kings
Almighty
Lord of Lords
Lord
Emmanuel
ETERNAL ONE
Judge

JESUS CHRIST

Savior of the World

Begotten
Worthy
Living Water
Beginning and End
Master
Redeemer
Alpha and Omega
Holy Child
Advocate
Unchangeable
Great I Am
Son of Man
Prophet
Cornerstone
Annointed
Rabbi
Morning Star
Lamb of God
Great Physician
Lion of Judah
Good Shepherd
Healer
True Vine
Lord of all
Messiah
Bridegroom
Example
The Way
Bread of Life
Ancient of Days
The Truth
Living Water
The Life
Lilly of the Valley
Wonderful
Word of Life
Our Passover
King of the Jews
Chosen One

MISS ASONDRA StarN'air

A Caregiver's Bible To Excellence!

Become More and More like **'Jesus'**
Let's all live in a world where "Everyone's" **A CAREGIVER!**

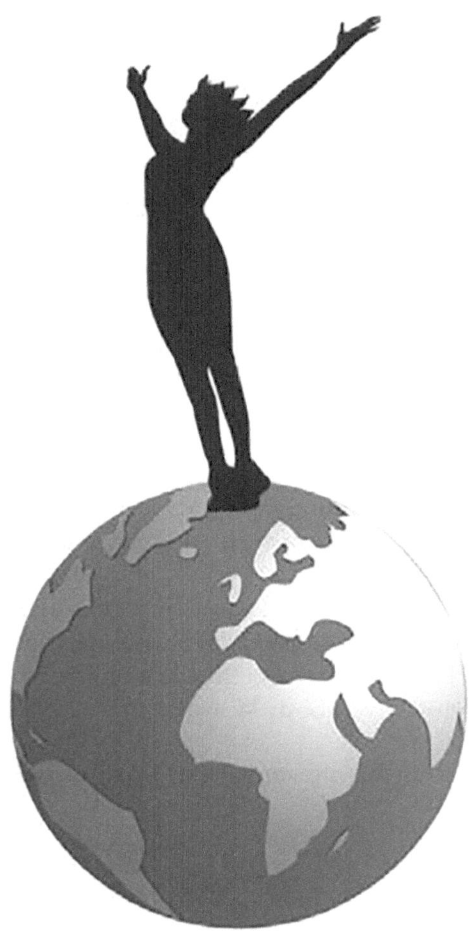

Never Stop Spinning The Globe Of Excellence!

Remember

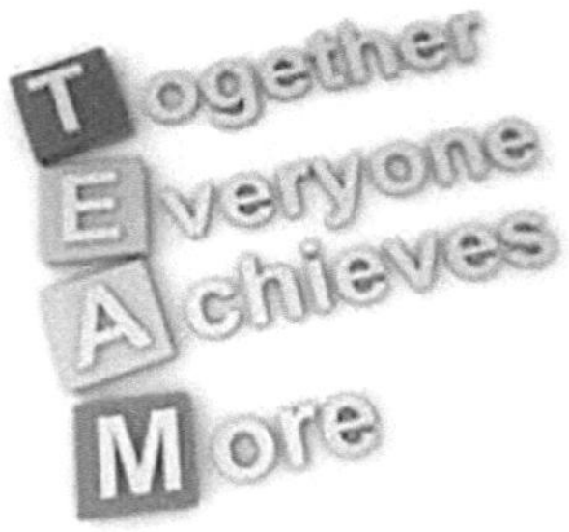

Tribute Page

This Tribute goes out to all those who are on a righteous path, those who are honest and fair in their dealing with others.

And to those businesses that are really out to make a difference, who see the vision of a color blind world and equal opportunities for everyone, **'Caregivers Matters!'**

Finally, I like to also acknowledge our Unite State Government, we have certainly come a long way, from the new deal era.

Today there are many more opportunities for us as caregivers, and we're glad, thank you.

But still, there is more work to be done, Home Health Aides must become professionalized, **'New Day Caregivers'** is a movement in the right direction and with the help of this Country and President of The United States we will keep **"America Great", "Everybody Wins!"**

So I say to you all, lets run this race together, let's not let anybody struggle of fall!

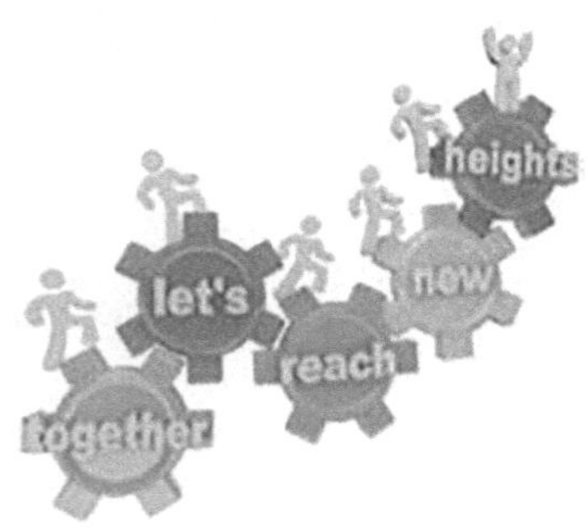

 MISS ASONDRA StarN'air

Special Thanks, Special Page!

I want to reach out and thank everyone who purchased this book. You are more than a customer to me, you are my new family. Together we can help change the world. **Special Thanks, Special Page!** If you are with Christ, and I hope you are, **"We Got It Made!"**

Love you, this is "Your" page!

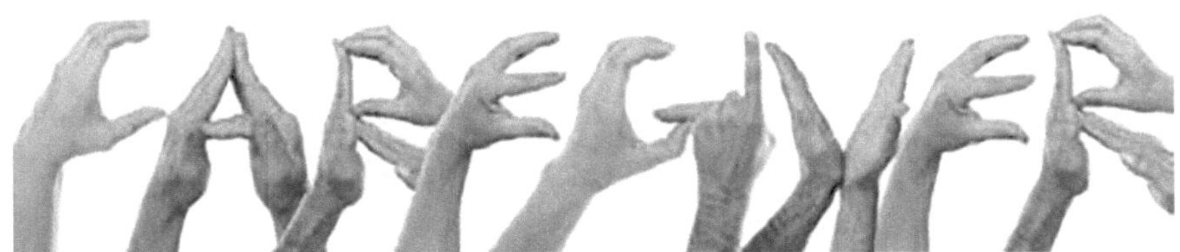

"We Deliver"!

God Bless You All!

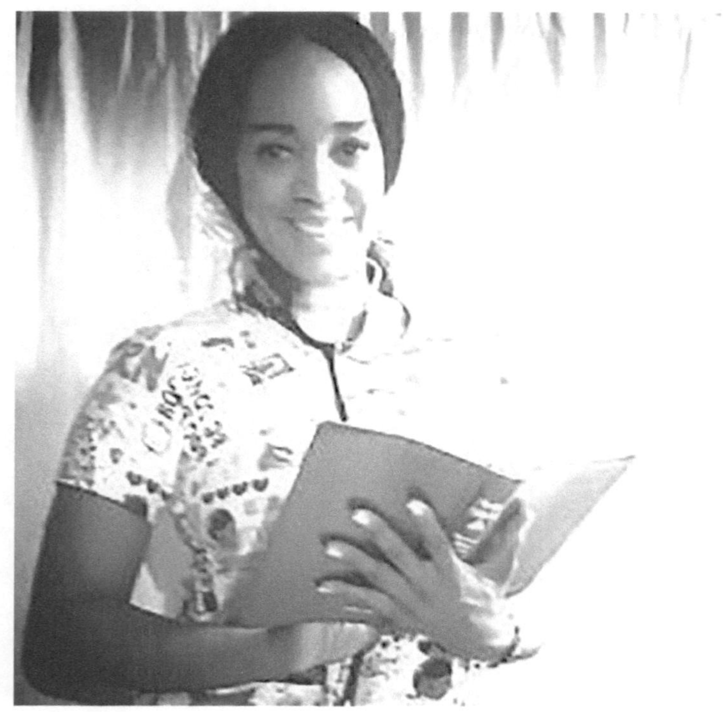

"Farewell"
Miss Asondra StarN'air

Good Bye!

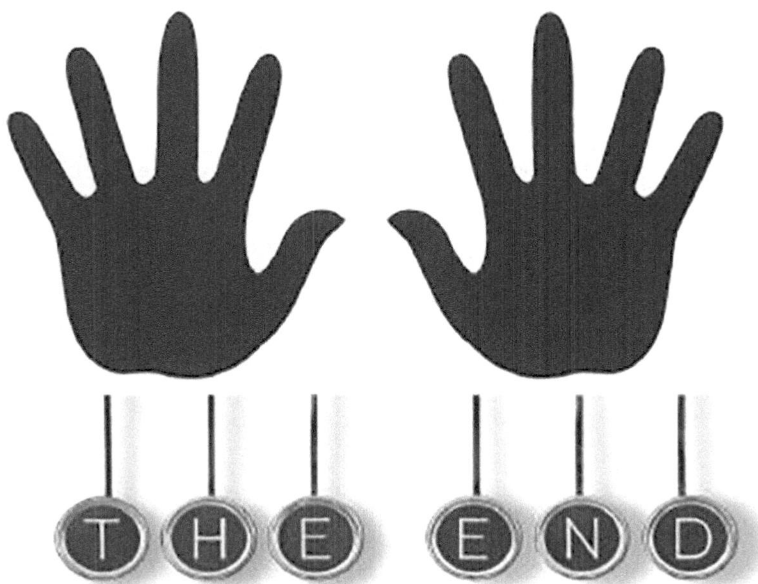

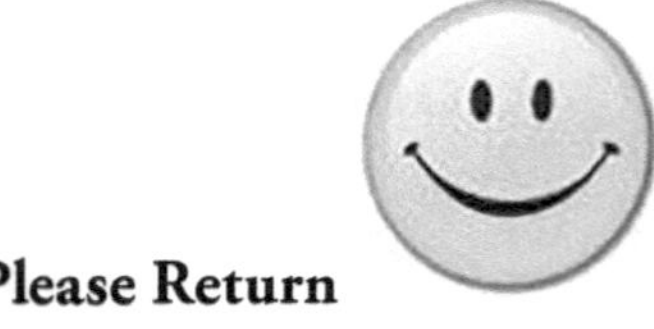

Please Return

If someone finds my book, please return it to me!

My name is ____

My address is My contact number is ______________________________

My e-mail address is ____

Thank you so much. We need thoughtful and honest individuals like you in the world.

May God bless you for what you have done. This book is very, very special to me and my family!

If this book is not lost, I leave this book behind to the ones I love: my family. I want ______________________________________ to have this book. This book is a blessing From God; may you always cherish it like I have.

Signed, sealed, and delivered—it's yours! I will never forget how much I love you. Until we meet again. Good-bye.

Signature ________________________________ Date ________________

Be Blessed!

     Miss Asondra StarN'air